"Highly recommended for the novice user to get started on the right path, as well as long-time aromatherapists. There's something for everyone in this book!"

— SYLLA SHEPPARD-HANGER, LMT, founder and director of the Atlantic Institute of Aromatherapy

"Beautifully designed and put together, you will refer to this book again and again."

— DR. STEVEN FARMER, best-selling author of *Earth Magic, Animal Spirit Guides,* and *Healing Ancestral Karma*

"I highly recommend to anyone that has an interest in aromatherapy and exploring the energetic and vibrational aspects of essential oils that they add this book to their aromatic library."

— KELLY HOLLAND AZZARO, RA, CCAP, CBFP, LMT, registered aromatherapist, aromatherapy educator and past president of the National Association for Holistic Aromatherapy

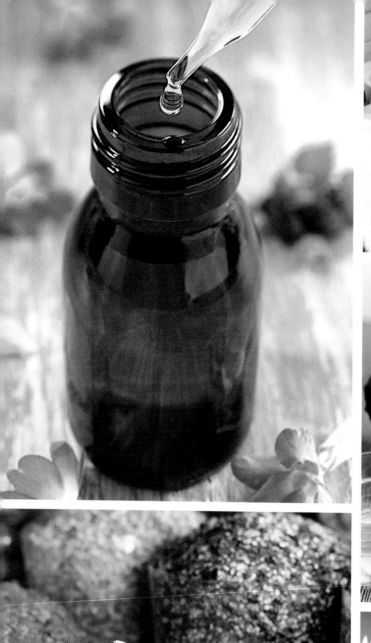
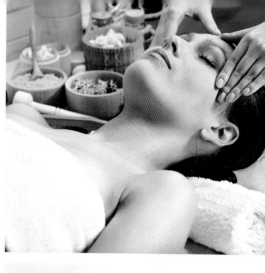
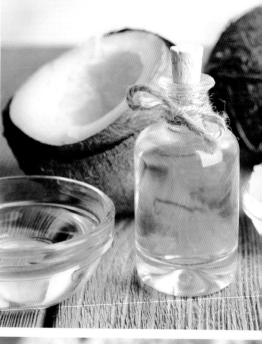
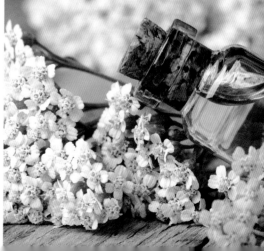
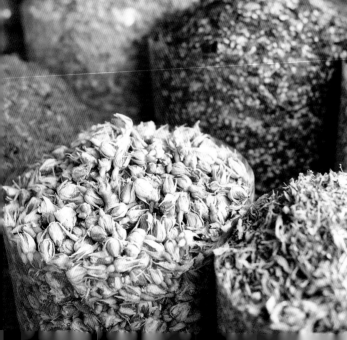

THE ESSENTIAL OILS

Complete Reference Guide

Over 250 Recipes for Natural Wholesome Aromatherapy

KG STILES

BA, CBT, CBP, LMT

Aromatherapist to the Stars

PAGE STREET
PUBLISHING CO.

PAGE STREET
PUBLISHING CO.

For my readers and fans.
You made all the years of incessant
writing and the piles of rejection
letters all worthwhile, thank you!

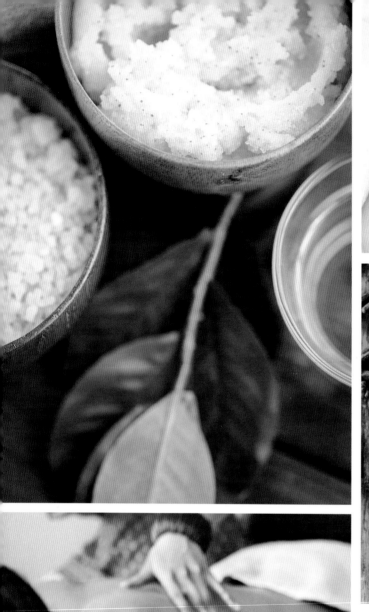
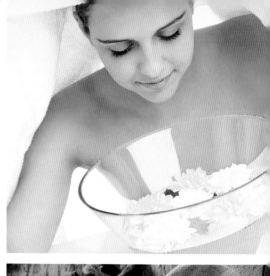
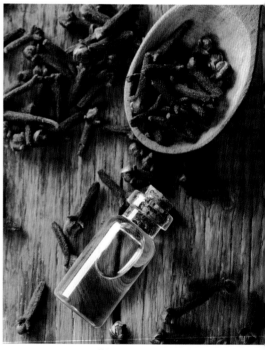
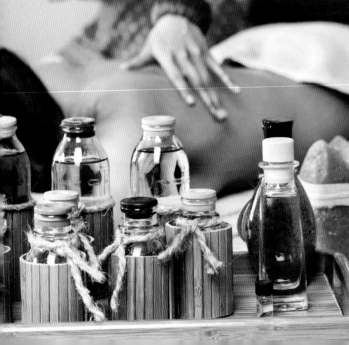
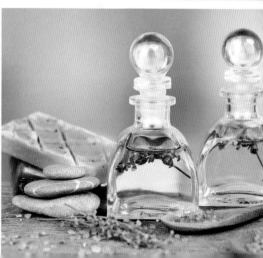

Contents

Introduction ~ 15

PART I

Chapter 1
Background Information on Essential Oils ~ 19

What is Aromatherapy? ~ 20

Brief History of Aromatherapy ~ 22

Aromatherapy Terms ~ 23

Chapter 2
How Aromatherapy Works ~ 26

Chapter 3
How to Use Essential Oils ~ 29

Therapeutic Use of Essential Oils:
Delivery Methods for Best Results ~ 29

Dilution Guide ~ 34

Face Carrier Oils ~ 36

Body Massage Carrier Oils ~ 39

Bath, Compress and Poultice ~ 40, 41 and 42

Masks and Wraps ~ 42

Scrubs and Body Butters ~ 44

Perfume Oil ~ 47

Aromatherapy Spray ~ 47

Food Flavor: Cooking
with Essential Oils ~ 48

Chapter 4
Safe Use of Essential Oils ~ 51

Hot Oils ~ 54

Chapter 5
Aromatherapy Supplies ~ 57

What You Need to Have on Hand for Making Your Products ~ 57

Supplemental Oils to Have on Hand for Concocting Aromatherapy Formulations ~ 60

Chapter 6
Pure, Most Commonly Used Essential Oils ~ 69

Bergamot ~ 69

Eucalyptus ~ 71

Frankincense ~ 74

Geranium, Geranium Roseum
and Graveolens ~ 76

Helichrysum ~ 78

Lavender ~ 80

Lemon ~ 82

Peppermint ~ 85

Roman Chamomile ~ 87

Sweet Marjoram ~ 88

Tea Tree ~ 89

Vetiver ~ 91

Ylang Ylang ~ 93

Chapter 7
Supplemental Oils ~ 97

Ammi Visnaga ~ 97

Atlas Cedarwood ~ 99

Black Pepper ~ 101

Black Spruce ~ 102

Blue Tansy ~ 103

Carrot Seed ~ 104

Cinnamon ~ 105

Clary Sage ~ 107

Clove ~ 109

Cypress ~ 110

Galbanum ~ 112

German Chamomile ~ 114

Ginger ~ 116

Grapefruit ~ 118

Hyssop ~ 120

Ledum ~ 121

Lemongrass ~ 122

Melissa ~ 124

Myrrh ~ 126

Neroli ~ 128

Oregano ~ 130

Palmarosa ~ 131

Patchouli ~ 133

Red Mandarin ~ 134

Rosemary ~ 135

Rose Otto ~ 139

Sandalwood ~ 142

Sweet Orange ~ 145

Thyme ~ 146

Yarrow ~ 148

Additional Oils Used in This Book ~ 151

Chapter 8
Proper Storage of Essential Oils ~ 153

Shelf Life for Essential Oils ~ 154

PART II

Chapter 9
Aromatherapy Blending Guide (and Secrets) ~ 157

Essential Oil Blending Directions ~ 159

Chapter 10
Aromatherapy Formulas ~ 163

Massage Oil Blends ~ 164

Calming Formula ~ 168

Relaxation Formula ~ 164

Restorative Formula ~ 170

Sports Injury Formula ~ 167

Muscle Pain Relief Formula ~ 171

Chapter 11
Healing Blends ~ 173

Headache Relief Formula ~ 174

UV Radiation Burn Relief Formula ~ 197

Headache Relief Formula 2 ~ 176

Mosquito and Insect
Protective Repellent Formula ~ 198

Migraine Relief Formula ~ 177

Allergic Skin Reaction Relief Formula ~ 199

Pain Relief Formula ~ 179

Poison Ivy and Oak Irritation
Relief Formula ~ 200

Muscle Pain Relief Formula ~ 180

Sciatica Pain Relief Formula ~ 183

Warm Bath Treatment ~ 202

Nerve Pain Relief Formula ~ 184

Scar Formula ~ 203

Fibromyalgia Pain Relief Formula ~ 185

Foot Bath for Athlete's Foot
or Toenail Fungus ~ 204

Arthritis Pain Relief Formula ~ 186

Tendinitis Relief Formula ~ 187

Athlete's Foot Formula ~ 205

Leg Cramp Relief Formula ~ 188

Toenail Fungus Formula ~ 207

Constipation Relief Formula ~ 190

Warts Formula ~ 208

Nausea Relief Formula ~ 191

Herpes Formula ~ 209

Burn Care Formula ~ 193

Ringworm Formula ~ 211

Sunburn Relief Formula ~ 194

Ringing Ear Relief Formula ~ 213

Sleep Formulas ~ 214

Chapter 12
Healthy Lifestyle ~ 219

Cleansing and Detoxification Formula ~ 219

Weight Loss Program,
Formula and Treatment ~ 220–225

Stop Smoking Program,
Formula and Treatment ~ 226–228

Steam Inhalation to Support
Respiratory System Formula ~ 231

Oral Health Program ~ 232

Recovery After Illness Formula ~ 235

Rejuvenating and Healing Formula ~ 236

Women's Health Formulas ~ 239

Female Toner ~ 239

Hormone Balance Formula ~ 240

Hot Flash Relief Formula ~ 242

Breast Health ~ 243

Fibroids Formula ~ 245

Breast Health Massage Formula ~ 246

Sitz Bath ~ 247

Chapter 13
Relaxation and Emotional Support Formulas ~ 249

Enthusiasm ~ 249

Lift the Spirits Formula ~ 250

Mood: Lift the Mood Formula ~ 251

Meditation ~ 252

Stress Relief ~ 255

Anxiety Relief ~ 256

Depression Relief ~ 259

Grief and Loss ~ 261

Chapter 14
Spa and Beauty Treatments ~ 263

Complete Skincare
Beauty Treatment Program ~ 263

SKINCARE FORMULAS

Normal to Dry Skincare Formula ~ 265

Oily Skincare Formula ~ 266

Sensitive Skincare Formula ~ 267

Mature Skincare Formula ~ 268

BODY AND FACIAL SKIN TONERS

Facial and Body Toner Formula ~ 270

French Clay Facial Mask ~ 273

REPAIR BUTTERS FOR BODY
AND FACE

Repair Butter Essential Oils Formula ~ 274

Premature Aging Skincare Formula ~ 276

Severely Dry and
Cracked Skin Formula ~ 277

HAIR AND SCALP TREATMENTS

Scalp Reconditioning Formula ~ 280

Hair and Scalp Treatment Program ~ 281

Stop Hair Loss (Alopecia) Formula ~ 282

Scalp Massage Oil ~ 285

LIP BALMS

Dry, Chapped Lips Formula ~ 286

Severely Dry, Cracked, Chapped Lips ~ 288

Cold Sore Formula ~ 289

Healing Bath Salts Formula ~ 291

EXFOLIATING SUGAR SCRUBS

Exfoliating Sugar Scrub Oil Formula ~ 293

pH Balancing Honey Lemon Sugar Facial Scrub Formula ~ 294

SALT GLOW TREATMENTS

Skin Healing and Regeneration Formula ~ 297

Regulating All Skin Types Formula ~ 298

Chronic Skin Conditions Formula ~ 301

Regulating and Balancing, Wound Healing, Problem Skin Formula ~ 302

Moisture Balancing and Healing for All Skin Types Formula ~ 305

Oily Skin Formula ~ 306

Dry and Mature Skin Formula ~ 307

ADDITIONAL BODY TREATMENTS

French Clay Body Mask Formula ~ 308

Healing and Regenerative Body Butter Formula ~ 311

Chapter 15
Love and Romance Blends ~ 315

Aphrodite Perfume Oil Formula ~ 315

Eros Aphrodisiac Formula ~ 316

Audacity Men's Cologne Formula ~ 319

Chapter 16
Babies and New Mommies ~ 321

Pregnancy ~ 321

Childbirth, Labor and Delivery ~ 321

Sleep Remedies and Formulas ~ 322

Baby Massage ~ 323

Teething Solutions ~ 326

Chapter 17
Around the House ~ 329

Clear Stagnant Energy ~ 329

Eliminate Odors ~ 333

Laundry Care ~ 337

Eco-Friendly Cleaning Supplies ~ 338

Chapter 18
Essential Oils in the Workplace and Daily Life ~ 343

Improve Productivity ~ 344

Stimulate Curiosity and Creativity ~ 347

Focus Support and Pay Attention Formula ~ 348

Chapter 19
Cooking with Essential Oils ~ 351

Culinary Wellness Oils and Blends ~ 351

Breakfast and Brunch Recipes ~ 364

Lunch Recipes ~ 368

Appetizers ~ 372

Dinner Recipes ~ 375

Salad Dressings ~ 378

Drinks and Beverages ~ 382

Desserts ~ 393

Chapter 20
Animals and Pets ~ 399

HOW TO USE ESSENTIAL OILS
WITH PETS AND ANIMALS

List of Oils and Their Specific
Uses for Your Furry Friends ~ 400

Flea and Tick Prevention
and Treatment ~ 401

Respiratory Support ~ 402

Chapter 21
Spiritual Blends ~ 405

Essential Oils to Balance Your Chakras ~ 406

5 Elements ~ 416

Planetary Elixirs ~ 427

Angel Therapy ~ 437

Appendix 1
Essential Oils Quick Reference Guides ~ 443

Safety and Dilution Guide ~ 443

Medical Terms: Primary Actions and Effects ~ 444

Psycho-emotional Aromatherapy Chart (Super Oils) ~ 445

Appendix 2
Symptoms Guide: Super Oils to Use ~ 446

Appendix 3
Further Reading, Resources and References ~ 448

Acknowledgments ~ 449

About the Author ~ 450

Index ~ 451

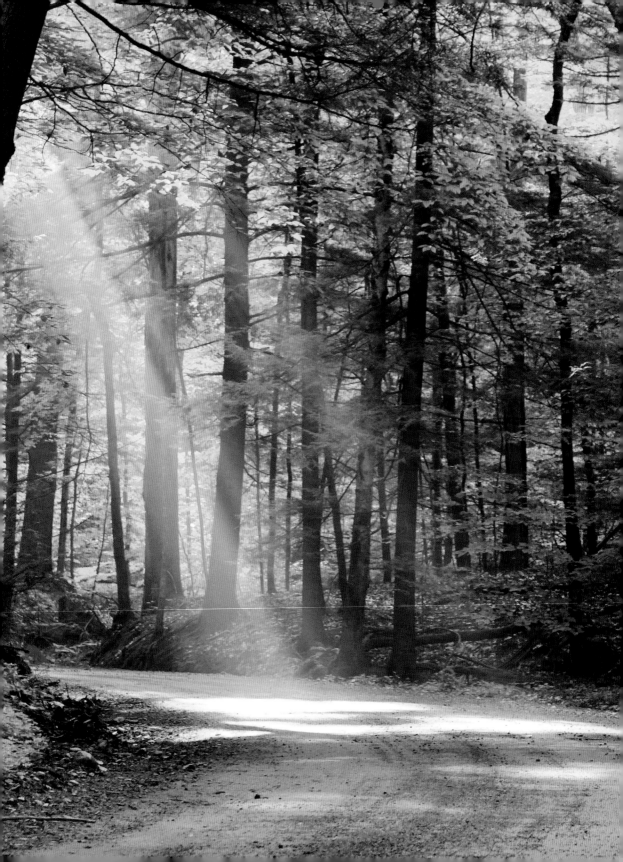

Introduction

My perspective, as a veteran in the metaphysical healing movement, is that everyone is on a healing journey during their lifetime. There's always some challenge that needs a solution. This is very apparent at the collective level where the repetition of patterns of war and strife are prevalent. Perhaps now at this seemingly critical moment in human history in which we've created such a multiplicity of challenges at the world level including global warming, overpopulation, massive poverty, rampant disease, world starvation and species extinction, there is an opportunity for a mass paradigm shift; a transformation in our way of thinking and behaving in which we move from competition to cooperation.

I believe we can look to nature for solutions to our individual and global challenges. Nature and natural life have been adapting to change and evolving for hundreds of thousands of years. If you observe nature you can see that she works holistically and in cooperation through cycles of time to sustain herself. Historically, when things get out of balance, there is massive die-off of species, and natural habitats shift to bring balance once again. I believe we are in one of those major points on planet Earth.

From the metaphysical perspective, everything is working perfectly to bring balance into the crisis point we are faced with on planet Earth. It's attuning to and aligning with natural forces to support them in this natural process of evolution that will help restore balance.

Transformation and healing are always available. It's our willingness to align with natural forces that guides us to see the opportunities available in our own personal life and for planetary evolution. Humans can be the stewards that allow this evolution to take place.

Essential oils can help with this process of transformation and change. On an individual level, when used properly, essential oils can act like trusted allies and friends to help you shift and handle any challenges you may be faced with—whether they be physical, mental, emotional or spiritual—in order to become more integrated and whole.

As a metaphysician and holistic healing practitioner, I've explored using many forms of transformation and healing. Over time I've come to focus solely on working with my clients at the metaphysical and energetic level. Your emotion is literally energy in motion. Resistance to feeling the energy expressed as your emotions creates stress in your body, and physical tension builds. Resistance and the suppression of emotions is at the core of most illness and disease. When you release the blocked patterns of emotional resistance, the natural process of transformation that's always available can occur to bring you back into balance, and healing occurs naturally.

Young children express the inner joy that comes with the experience of being alive. Children are naturally inquisitive and creative. Before age four, the majority of children test at genius level, and by age ten they test at average intelligence. The conditioning and indoctrination children experience results in suppression of their natural talents and abilities.

As I began exploring metaphysical healing, I was introduced to the transformational healing arts at Findhorn, a spiritual community in northern Scotland. Findhorn is one of the largest intentional communities in the world and a working eco-village that was created to inspire and encourage transformation in human consciousness. Findhorn is renowned for growing huge vegetables, produced in cooperation with nature spirits.

While at Findhorn, my communication with the Devic kingdom opened fully. It was like coming home to myself. After Findhorn, I relocated to San Diego, California, a mecca for evolving consciousness and learning about and practicing the healing arts. My own personal healing journey continued as I explored a wide variety of cutting-edge healing modalities. Having a direct personal experience of whatever I taught or used in my practice was essential for me. The same has been true with using essential oils.

Having so many of my own health challenges to heal has been a blessing in that I know firsthand what my client must face and overcome. Though each client is an individual and has their own personal experience, there are similar patterns that surface and must be exposed and released so that natural healing may occur.

Much of the healing journey is about forgiving and releasing the past. We make decisions often in early childhood about what things mean and get locked into perspectives, attitudes and beliefs about ourselves and

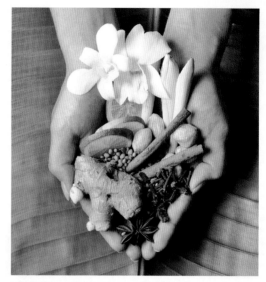

Essential oils are extracted from flowers, leaves, stems, bark, seeds or roots of shrubs, bushes, herbs and trees.

life that can undermine our best attempts at creating a happy life for ourselves. We develop a storyline for our life. When we're affected by these patterns of thinking and behaving, we generate the same chemicals that create the same emotional set points. These emotional set points can hardwire us into feeling depressed or frustrated and angry most of the time. Emotional patterns can become chronic.

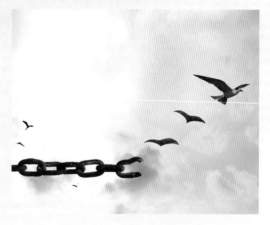

Essential oils can help you break free of the energetic and emotional patterns that bind you.

It's very simple to release these set points, though it can take time to fully cleanse your cup, so to speak, and to experience a paradigm shift and a new way of life for yourself. I'll cover more of this when I speak about the different oils and how they can specifically help you. You'll understand how to use essential oils to help you holistically at all levels of being, body, mind, spirit and emotions.

I'll share some of my own direct personal experiences about how I've used the oils with myself and my clients with outstanding results. I will also pepper in a few of my other preferred methods that will allow you to align with the transformation and healing that is always available to you.

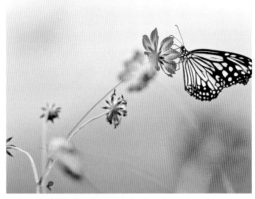

Inhalation of aroma can immediately shift and transform your state of mind from a closed caterpillar to a butterfly, ready to take flight.

You'll find out how I used essential oils in conjunction with a few other holistic healing methods to recover from early childhood issues of abuse, as well as suffering with a ten-year physical disability that included chronic fatigue, chronic patterns of pain and allergies. During that time, I relentlessly spent tens of thousands of dollars searching and trying dozens of allopathic and holistic treatments, none of which ever helped. As a matter of fact, my symptoms of pain and dysfunction just kept getting worse.

Thanks for joining me for a glimpse into the world of essential oils.

KG Stiles

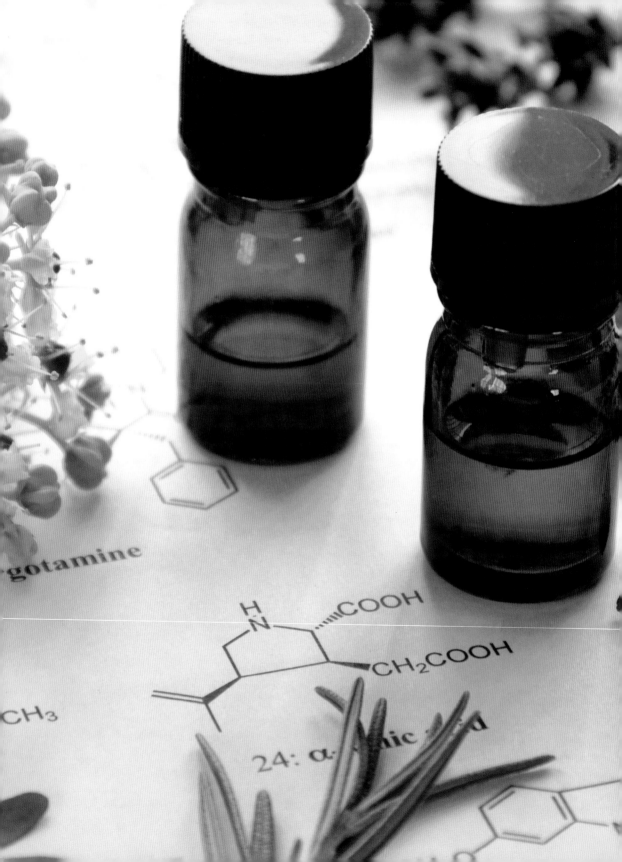

Background Information on Essential Oils

Essential oils are the concentrated volatile or ethereal oils extracted from a single botanical plant source. The part of the plant that yields the maximum amount of volatile oil is what's used in the extraction process, for example flowers, leaves, stems, bark, seeds or roots of shrubs, bushes, herbs and trees.

When the substance of scent is still in the plant, it is called an essence. After distillation from the plant part, the volatile aromatic compound is referred to as an essential oil.

These subtle, highly aromatic plant extracts are found in the specialized cells or glands of plants. Through millennia, these plant excretions have evolved as protection for a plant from predators and to attract pollinators. Surprisingly, aromatic compounds are not found in all plants. Why this is so remains a mystery.

Pure essential oils are most often extracted by steam distillation. Other methods of extraction include cold pressing and expression, solvent extraction, absolute oil extraction and resin tapping. Essential oils are used in manufacturing perfumes, cosmetics, soaps, pharmaceuticals, incense and household cleaning products, as well as to flavor food and drink.

Essential oils have a long history of use as medicinals. Their wide range of use includes treatments for beauty and skincare, cold and flu prevention and treatment, as well as natural remedies to treat a variety of health issues from respiratory conditions to digestive complaints, insomnia and even cancer, and also aid in weight loss. Many of the reports are anecdotal in nature,

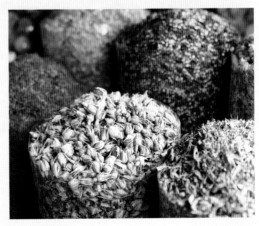

Bundles of rose petals and other plant materials on display and for sale at an open market.

though more and more evidence-based research is being done to corroborate their use. Some medical centers are incorporating essential oils as a part of an integrative health care system.

As the specific compounds and properties of essential oils are studied, there is greater understanding about why certain essential oils have particular actions and effects as natural health remedies.

What is Aromatherapy?

During the early twentieth century, a French chemist by the name of René-Maurice Gattefossé began researching the medicinal properties of essential oils. It is Gattefossé who is credited with having coined the term "aromatherapy."

The story of Gattefossé accidentally burning his arm very badly while conducting an experiment in a perfumery plant is well known. There are different versions about how Gattefossé on "reflex" plunged his arm into a large vat of lavender. Whether he knew it was lavender or thought it was water, the story goes that Gattefossé experienced rapid healing of his burns with very little scarring of tissue.

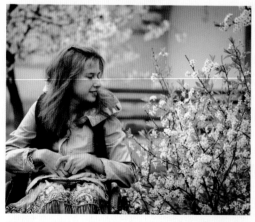

A woman enjoying the benefits of the aromatic scent of flowers in bloom.

In his article "Gattefossé's Burn," aromatherapist Robert Tisserand recounts the actual story that Gattefossé reports himself of the incident in his 1937 book, *Aromathérapie*. According to Tisserand, Gattefossé tells how he was covered with burning substances in a laboratory explosion which he "extinguished by rolling on a grassy lawn." Gattefossé tells how he rinsed both of his badly burned hands with lavender oil which stopped "the gasification of the tissue" that had started. Gas gangrene is a serious and often fatal infection with a 20 to 25 percent mortality rate. Gattefossé further reported that he sweated profusely after the treatment with lavender essence and that his hands showed signs of healing by the very next day.

As essential oils are highly aromatic, many of their benefits are obtained simply through inhalation. Our sense of smell is closely linked to memory, mood and emotion. It is well known that aroma reaches and influences our deepest primitive instincts. When essential oils are diffused and inhaled, aromatherapy not only delivers the calming benefits of fragrance, but also delivers many health benefits unique to essential oils.

The use of plants and herbs is the oldest form of healing disease and pain, and the medicinal effects of plants have been recorded in the oldest writings in history, myth and folklore. Records found in ancient Egyptian hieroglyphics and Chinese manuscripts show that priests and physicians were using plant aromatics thousands of years before the birth of Christ to heal the sick and infirm.

In ancient times, certain plant balms and fragrances like frankincense and myrrh were considered more valuable than gold. There are numerous references to plant substances in the Bible. Now, with the advent of modern scientific research, we are beginning to investigate the incredible healing potential found in essential oils.

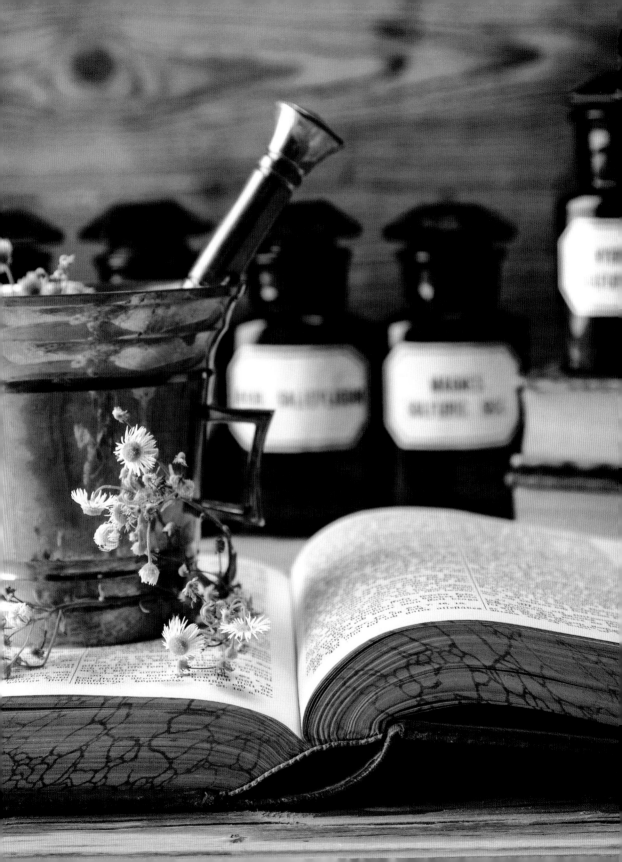

Virtually everything used today in modern drugs can be traced back to a botanical extract. Hippocrates, the father of modern medicine, taught that following traditional healing wisdom and common sense passed down to us for thousands of years in the use of botanical medicines is the best way to health and healing. He recommended a scented bath and daily massage.

Brief History of Aromatherapy

The use of aromatic plants has been around since Neolithic times. It is thought that "smudging" was the earliest form of aromatic treatment, and it is very likely that shamans and priests were the first aromatherapists and perfumers. Medicinal plants have been found inside graves dating back eighty thousand years; however, the use of pure essential oils as we know them today has only been available since the creation of distillation.

The earliest devices for distilling oils were found in the ancient Indus Valley dating to 3000 BC, where terra cotta distillation devices and perfume containers were discovered. Since that time, plant aromatics have been used in every aspect of Indian culture, including

Aromatic medicinal plants have been explored since Neolithic times.

beauty treatments, perfuming, medicinal practices, cleansing and ritual bathing and religious ceremonies. Traditionally, Indian tantric practices have been used to anoint the body with oils to seduce and arouse the passions. The Vedas, the most ancient sacred texts known, contained formulas for plant aromatics. The Rig Veda contained instructions for how to use over 700 aromatic plants, including spikenard, myrrh, sandalwood, ginger, cinnamon and coriander. Humans were seen as part of nature, and the preparation of plant medicinals was considered a sacred art and practice. Ayurvedic medicine is one of the oldest forms of medicine practiced continuously since ancient times.

In 1868, the first synthetic fragrance oils were produced. These synthetic fragrances were considered unsuitable for medicinal use. Chemists began to isolate the active ingredients within aromatic plants and manufacture them synthetically. Manufactured chemical drugs acted more powerfully and were cheaper to produce. As science became more sophisticated, herbs and essential oils were replaced by synthetic drugs.

By the nineteen hundreds, medical doctors became accustomed to using synthetic chemicals, and aromatic oils almost completely disappeared by the early twentieth century.

In the mid-twentieth century, there was a renewed interest in essential oils, and they were used extensively as flavoring, perfumes, cosmetics and household cleaning supplies. Essential oils were commonly used in medicine and in a wide range of pharmaceutical products to mask the strong odor of the chemicals.

In 1964, French ex-army surgeon Jean Valnet published *The Practice of Aromatherapy,* which was written for lay people as well as medical professionals. Valnet had used essential oils for treating wounded soldiers and found them to be highly effective for treating wounds and burns.

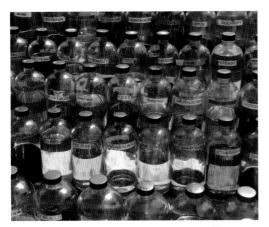

Aromatic oils are enjoying an increase in use for a variety of conditions and applications.

During this same time, Madame Maury, an English biochemist who was influenced by Valnet's research, wrote *The Secret of Life and Youth,* a self-help, holistic approach to beauty using aromatherapy.

Robert Tisserand's book, *The Art of Aromatherapy,* published in England in 1977, was the first book to combine medical and esoteric approaches to aromatherapy.

Since then, there has continued to be a renewed interest in aromatic oils, and aromatherapy is enjoying increased popular interest and use by the general public.

Aromatherapy Terms

ADULTERANT: A substance that was not originally present in the oil at the time of distillation that is added to an essential oil. An adulterant can be artificial or natural.

AROMATHERAPY MASSAGE: A hands-on therapy in which essential oils are applied to the body for emotional and physical benefits.

CARRIER OIL: Vegetable or nut oils such as light coconut oil, jojoba, sweet almond and grapeseed, used to dilute essential oils.

COLD-PRESS EXTRACTION OR EXPRESSION: The cold-pressed method of extraction is one of the best methods for extracting essential oils as there is very little heat applied with this process. Cold pressing or expression applies a mechanical method of extraction in which no external heat is needed for the process. With cold pressing, essential oils are obtained by mechanically pressing the fruit peel. The downside of essential oils produced by cold pressing is that they usually have a very short shelf life. Citrus oils like grapefruit, lemon and orange are obtained by cold-press extraction.

DIFFUSER: A device that disperses essential oils into an area. The three basic types are clay, candle and electric.

DILUTE: Adding a small amount of essential oil to a larger amount of base oil to make it safe for use on the skin.

DISTILLATION: A method used to extract essential oil from the plant. Steam distillation is the most common form of distillation.

ESSENTIAL OIL: A highly aromatic substance found in specialized cells of certain plants. Technically, when this substance is in the plant, it is called an "essence." After distillation of a single type of plant, the aromatic substance is referred to as an essential oil.

EXPRESSION: See Cold-Press Extraction or Expression.

EXTRACTION METHOD: The method by which essential oils are separated from the plant. Common extraction methods include steam distillation, expression and solvent extraction.

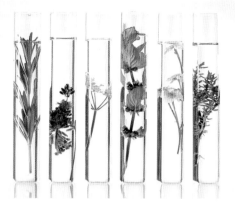
Herbal infused oils carry the plant's aromatic characteristics.

FIXATIVE: A fixative is a plant or animal substance of low volatility that serves to draw together and hold the fragrances of other materials. It may be in the form of a liquid, such as an essential oil or fragrance, that will slow the evaporation process and preserve the aromatic scent of the blend, or it may be in the form of a botanical that will absorb and hold the various aromas. Using a fixative will create a more distinct and longer lasting product. Orris root, amyris, calamus root, angelica root and vetiver root are a few commonly used fixatives.

FOOD GRADE: Considered safe for use in food by the Food and Drug Administration (FDA).

FRAGRANCE: Aroma products labeled as fragrances are not the same as essential oils. Fragrances are derived by synthetic means, while essential oils are completely natural.

GC/MS (GAS CHROMATOGRAPH/MASS SPECTROMETER): A device used by analytic chemists to determine the precise makeup of a given substance. It is used in aromatherapy to determine the precise chemical constituents of an essential oil and whether the oil is pure or adulterated with synthetic chemicals or other products.

HERBAL INFUSED OILS: A process of extraction of volatile oils of a plant which are obtained by soaking the plant in a carrier oil for approximately two weeks and then straining off the oils from the plant material. The resulting oil is infused with the plant's aromatic characteristic actions and effects and used therapeutically.

HERBAL MEDICINE, HERBALISM: Pertaining to natural botanicals and living plants in various forms or preparations. They are valued for their therapeutic benefits and sold as dietary supplements.

HYDROSOL: The name for the water left after steam or water distillation of an essential oil. It is mainly water with only a very small amount of water-soluble plant constituents.

INFUSED OIL: These are oils that carry the medicinal properties of certain herbs. Carrier oil is infused with the medicinal herb, the plant is strained off and the remaining oil can be used directly on the skin.

INSOLUBLE: Unable to be dissolved in a liquid such as water.

LINIMENT: Extract of a plant added to either alcohol or vinegar and applied topically for therapeutic benefits.

NEAT: An undiluted essential oil.

NOTES: As in *top*, *middle* and *base* notes. A type of classification system based on aroma to identify certain oils. Generally, essential oils from citrus peels are top notes; essential oils from flowers, leaves and stems are middle notes; and essential oils from roots are base notes.

OLFACTORY: Relating to, or connected with, the sense of smell.

ORIFICE REDUCER: A device used to reduce the size of the opening of a bottle, making dispensing the essential oil easier and more accurate.

PATCH TEST: A test to assess for sensitivity to an oil. To patch test an essential oil you haven't used before, add one drop of essential oil to a half teaspoon of vegetable carrier oil. Apply to the back of a knee or inside of an arm, and then cover with a bandage and leave it on for twenty-four hours. If any redness, swelling or itching occurs, don't use the oil.

PHYTOCHEMICALS: Chemical compounds or constituents that are formed in the plant's normal metabolic processes. Often referred to as "secondary metabolites," there are many classes of plant distillates. When isolated from the plant, these chemicals are considered pharmaceutical drugs.

PHYTOMEDICINALS: Medical substances that originate from plants.

POULTICE: Therapeutic topical application of plant material or plant extract, usually wrapped in a fine woven cloth for therapeutic benefits.

SEBUM: The oily substance produced by the sebaceous glands, which function to lubricate the skin and seal moisture into the cells. The level of sebum production determines whether your skin is normal, dry or oily.

SINGLE NOTE: An essential oil from a single botanical source without any other ingredients.

SOLUBLE: Able to dissolve in a liquid such as water.

SYNERGISTIC: A characteristic effect in which the sum total is more effective than the individual parts.

SYNTHETIC: An imitation or artificial reproduction of a naturally occurring substance.

VISCOSITY: Relates to the thickness or thinness of an essential oil.

VOLATILE: Describes how quickly a substance disperses (evaporates) into the air. In aromatherapy, top note essential oils may be referred to as "highly volatile," meaning that they disperse quickly out of the bottle and into the air.

VOLATILIZATION: The rate of evaporation or oxidation of an essential oil.

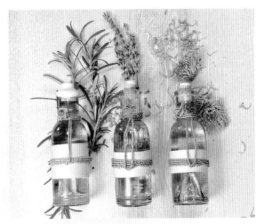

Infused oil carries the medicinal properties of herbs and can be applied directly to the skin.

CHAPTER 2

How Aromatherapy Works

As more and more research is being done that shows the effectiveness of using essential oils as an alternative health care system, there is a growing demand by the public for information.

At the same time, more and more people are taking responsibility for their health, which is fueling a growing revolution in the "Do-It-Yourself" movement. The practice of aromatherapy truly lends itself to this new holistic health culture that wants to freely choose the health care systems we use, spawning a new vision of health care in our future.

With new scientific studies providing evidence of the benefits of using essential oils, there is an increasing demand from people that hospitals and medical centers offer safe alternatives to allopathic drugs, which can produce harmful side effects. As a result, hospitals are beginning to offer integrative health care to patients.

Nurses and staff are receiving training and certification in the effective and safe use of essential oils as a comfort care measure for their patients and are reporting outstanding results.

Essential oils are super-concentrated plant extracts (one drop is equal to three to four cups [121 to 161 g] of raw plant matter). This super concentration means that only a single drop or two of an essential oil is needed for achieving therapeutic benefits, making the use of essential oils extremely cost-effective. In today's world of rising health costs, this is a significant benefit when deciding to use essential oils because a little goes a long way.

Research has shown that most of the therapeutic benefits from essential oils can be experienced simply by inhaling them. This makes the use of essential oils extremely efficient.

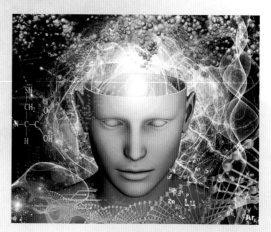

Inhalation of essential oil vapors produces an immediate electro-chemical effect on the brain.

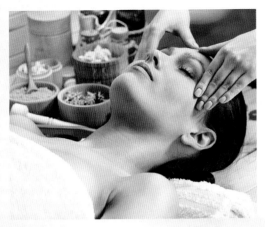

Inhalation of essential oils from an aromatherapy massage can effect an immediate relaxation response.

In the use of essential oils, the meeting of the elements of heat, light, air and moisture activates the release of their scent. Interestingly, scent bypasses your logical brain, which is not at all involved in your process of smell. You actually "feel" the scent of an essential oil.

Research has also shown that essential oils act as powerful chemicals to trigger the limbic part of your brain that controls emotions, memory and mood.

Upon inhaling the scent of an essential oil, the vapors enter through your nose and immediately stimulate your olfactory nerve. The olfactory nerve instantaneously signals your limbic system (control center for emotions), the amygdala and hippocampus (control centers for memory, learning and emotions) which then respond by releasing chemicals such as serotonin that produce a calming effect (refer to chart "The Electro-Chemical Effects of Aromatherapy" [page 32]).

At the same time, your limbic system sends a signal to your cortex (control center for intellectual processes) and to your hypothalamus gland, located at the base of your brain. Also known as the reptilian or old brain, the hypothalamus regulates many body functions including appetite, thirst, temperature, sleep and mood.

Regulating the conversation between your nervous and hormonal systems, the hypothalamus sends a signal to your pituitary gland, the master controller of your entire endocrine system. This cascade of neuro-chemical signals and responses ends at your adrenal glands, which control your fight or flight response, aggression and sexual response.

Essential oils also work through your blood vascular system which delivers them to all of your organs and systems. The vapors entering through your nose go immediately into your lungs where they enter your bloodstream and are delivered to your heart, as well as all of your other organs and tissues. The oils then circulate back to your lungs where they are expelled.

The best delivery method for benefit to the skin, muscles, soft tissues and joints is through skin application using a vegetable carrier oil. As essential oils are extremely concentrated and may cause skin irritation if applied neat to the skin, they should always be diluted for safe skin application.

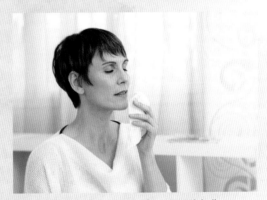

A woman inhaling the scent of an essential oil.

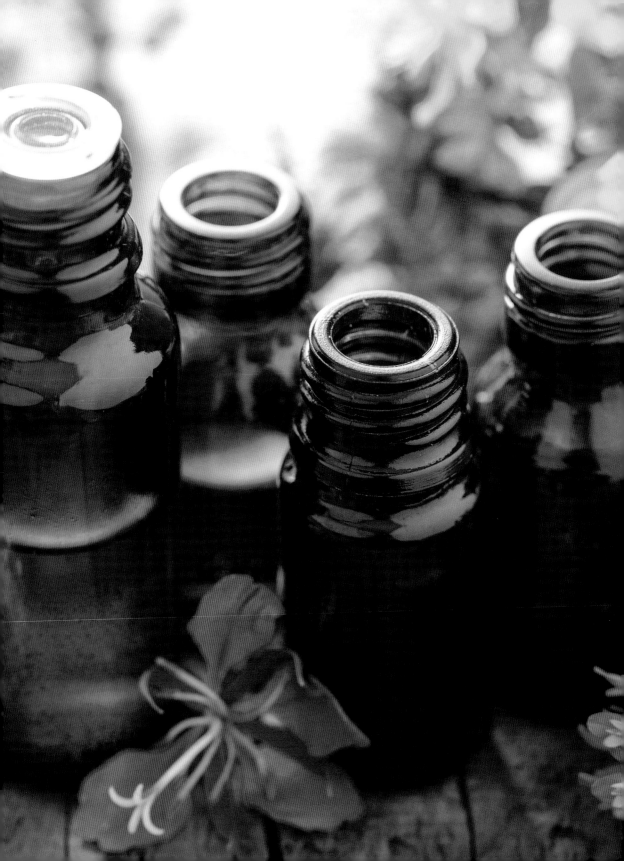

CHAPTER 3

How to Use Essential Oils

THERAPEUTIC USE OF ESSENTIAL OILS: DELIVERY METHODS FOR BEST RESULTS

Pure essential oils have a wide range of therapeutic uses and benefits. The method applied can affect the results. Your choice of delivery method often depends upon your intended goal.

There are three ways to use essential oils: internally, externally and environmentally. Please refer to the chart diagram "Aromatherapy Delivery Pathways" (page 30) illustrating the three ways of using essential oils, as well as their pathways of distribution and the organs and systems being affected.

Direct Inhalation Method

This is one of the quickest, easiest, least expensive and most effective ways to use and benefit from essential oils.

How close together can you use an essential oil or blend? Generally you can use essential oils within half an hour or so of each other; it depends on an individual's absorption and response rate. Increasing your heart rate just prior to direct inhalation will enhance the absorption rate of the oils.

(continued)

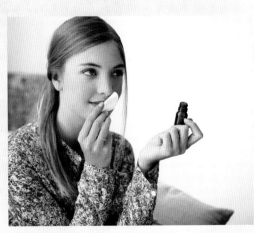

A young woman inhaling scent of essential oil that's been dispensed onto a cotton ball.

Aromatherapy Delivery Pathways

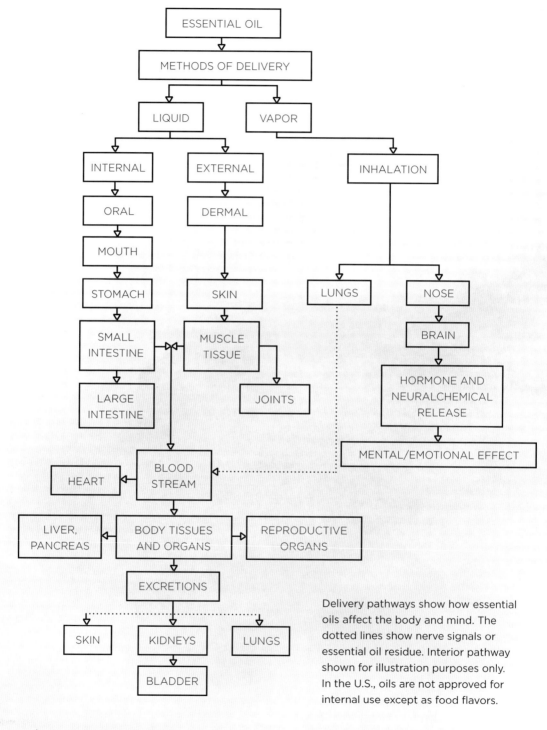

Delivery pathways show how essential oils affect the body and mind. The dotted lines show nerve signals or essential oil residue. Interior pathway shown for illustration purposes only. In the U.S., oils are not approved for internal use except as food flavors.

FOR OPTIMAL RESULTS, FOLLOW THESE GUIDELINES

Dispense 1 to 3 drops of essential oil onto a cotton ball, smell strip, tissue or dram vial of Celtic salts. Close your eyes and inhale as you gently and slowly introduce the oil's aromatic vapors into your system. Take four slow, full deep breaths for up to 10 to 30 seconds to begin. Inhale for a slow count of 1-2-3-4 and exhale for a slow count of 1-2-3-4.

Breathe in slowly and pause briefly on your inhaled breath. Then slowly exhale, letting go of any tension. Repeat this slow, rhythmic breathing pattern for four cycles of breathing. If you feel lightheaded or dizzy at any time, allow yourself to rest before continuing. After direct inhalation, allow yourself to relax for a moment into a feeling of well-being.

The aromatic vapors of the essential oils work through both your hormonal and circulatory systems to produce their effects. Please refer to the chart diagram for "The Electro-Chemical Effects of Aromatherapy" (page 32) and the "How Aromatherapy Works" chapter (page 26) to find out more.

Cold-Air Diffusion

For cold-air diffusion, drops of essential oil are dispensed onto a cotton or wool pad in the diffuser compartment. A small fan then blows cool air through the oils, lifting them into the air for dispersal into the environment. This is a cost-effective way for diffusing your oils into the atmosphere of a room. Cold-air diffusion has the benefits of micro diffusion and is especially good for scenting a room without the cleanup time required with a nebulizing diffuser, especially when using thicker oils.

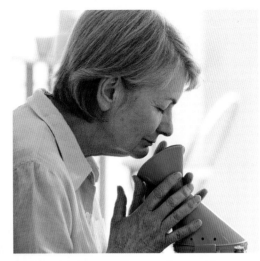

A woman inhales aromatic vapors from a wide-mouthed (electric) diffuser.

Environmental Fragrance

Research has shown that cold-air diffusing certain oils into the environment may:

- Reduce bacteria, fungus, mold and unpleasant odor.
- Relax and relieve tension, as well as clear the mind.
- Assist with weight management.
- Improve concentration, alertness and mental clarity.

Start by diffusing your essential oils for fifteen to thirty minutes per day. As you become accustomed to the oils and recognize their effects, you may increase your time of exposure to them.

The Electro-Chemical Effects of Aromatherapy

How essential oils stimulate the olfactory nerve to affect your hormonal system
(memory, mood and emotions)

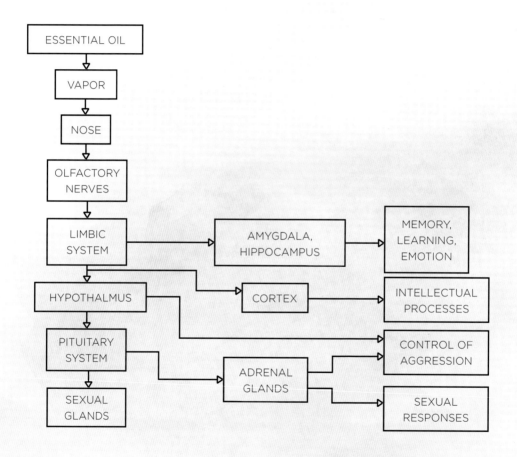

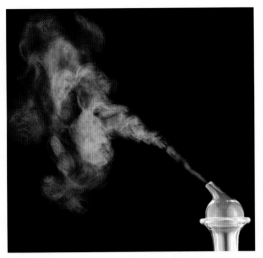

Micro diffusion is one of the most therapeutically beneficial ways of scenting a room.

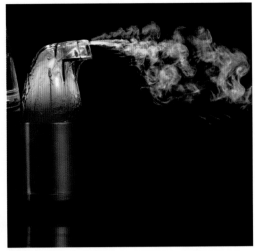

Modern day micro diffusion is a popular way to diffuse oils.

Ultrasonic Micro Diffusion

Micro diffusion uses a nebulizing type of diffuser that breaks down essential oils into millions of micro particles. This type of diffusion disperses oils without the heating that can render oils less therapeutically beneficial.

In illness, you may consider inhaling the oil's vapors near the "mouth" of the nebulizer. A short session of breathing in the oils for four to five minutes should be sufficient; repeat every few hours.

Facial Steam

For your personal skincare, a facial steam with select essential oils plays a key role in any deep cleansing and healing skincare routine. A facial steam uses the trapped vapors from hot water to cleanse the skin. It adds moisture to the skin and loosens toxins from the skin's pores. A facial steam is also very therapeutic for all of your five senses, as well as for relaxing your body and mind.

Extraordinarily easy to do, a facial steam takes very little time to perform. Once a month for five to fifteen minutes is all that's required to get excellent results.

All you need for an at-home facial steam is a small ceramic or stainless steel bowl to which you add hot water (up to 102°F [39°C]), adding your essential oils in a suitable carrier like cream or honey. With a towel draped over your head and eyes closed, you will lean over the bowl of steaming water face forward. The towel will catch the steam from the hot water so that it penetrates the facial skin.

 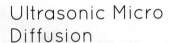

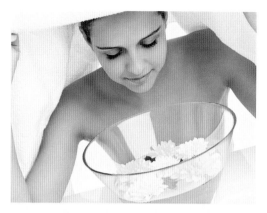

A young woman enjoys an essential oil facial steam.

The amount of time you take to do your facial steam treatment is specific to you and depends upon your comfort level with the steam, but generally takes between five to fifteen minutes.

You can also use your essential oils in facial steaming machines that are commonly used at spas, which you can also purchase for at-home use.

Before performing a facial steam you will usually want to cleanse your face to remove any excess oil, dirt or makeup, which can clog pores, in order to make the most of your facial steam experience.

Once you've completed your facial, towel dry your skin and wipe your face with a facial toner to remove any sweat and cool down the skin. (Refer to the Spa and Beauty Treatments section of this book on page 263 for guidelines on making your own facial toner with essential oils.)

PLEASE NOTE: Essential oils are not water soluble. You must use a dispersant when adding them to a facial steam. Hot water may cause essential oils to penetrate your system more quickly or cause irritation to sensitive or damaged skin, like blemishes, sores or rashes.

Respiratory Steam

Although facial steams are often performed primarily for cosmetic reasons, they can also offer extraordinary medicinal benefits for your respiratory system. You can use steam to effectively soothe cold or flu symptoms like sore throats, nasal congestion and other respiratory symptoms.

CAUTION: If you have serious respiratory issues like asthma, it is recommended that you consult with a health professional or doctor before using a steam that contains any aromatic herbs or essential oils to ensure they won't cause irritation or other breathing complications.

DILUTION GUIDE

The first step in making aromatherapy products is to understand the concept of dilution.

The principle idea is to dilute essential oils for safe skin application. Remember, each drop of pure essential oil is very concentrated. One drop of pure essential oil is equivalent to about 3 to 4 cups (26 to 104 g) of dried plant matter. As pure essential oils are very concentrated, some essential oils can cause skin irritation if used undiluted. Additionally, some people may have sensitivity to certain chemical properties in an

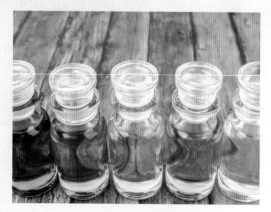

The first step in making aromatherapy products is to understand the concept of dilution.

essential oil. When first using an essential oil never used before, it is advised to do a simple skin test.

See page 163 in Chapter 10 for "Aromatherapy Formulas."

Safe Skin Application

How much essential oil should you put into your carrier for safe skin application?

Generally, effective blends for adults are made using a dilution ratio of 1, 2 or 3 percent of essential oil to carrier. Perfume oils usually have a higher dilution ratio of 5 to 10 percent.

1% DILUTION: 5–6 DROPS ESSENTIAL OIL PER 1 OUNCE (30 ML) CARRIER OIL

Use for children under age twelve, seniors over sixty-five, pregnant women and people with long-term illnesses or immune system disorders. A 1-percent dilution is a good place to start with individuals who are generally sensitive to aromas, chemicals or other environmental pollutants.

2% DILUTION: 10–12 DROPS ESSENTIAL OIL PER 1 OUNCE (30 ML) CARRIER OIL

Use for general health and skincare, natural perfumes, bath products and for your everyday blends.

3% DILUTION: 15–18 DROPS ESSENTIAL OIL PER 1 OUNCE (30 ML) CARRIER OIL

Use for specific application blends and acute health conditions such as cold, flu or pain relief and for sports blends.

5% DILUTION: 28–30 DROPS ESSENTIAL OIL PER 1 OUNCE (30 ML) CARRIER OIL

Use for sports massage blends, natural perfumes and short-term treatment for specific, acute health conditions.

10% DILUTION: 58–60 DROPS ESSENTIAL OIL PER 1 OUNCE (30 ML) CARRIER OIL

Very expensive essential oils like rose, helichrysum and neroli pure essential oils are often made available in a 10-percent dilution of carrier oil. Essential oil blends for natural colognes, perfumes and other specific applications may also be found in 10-percent dilutions. If you're using a 10-percent dilution of any of the pure essential oils, add them directly to your bottle of carrier oil before application.

When making larger quantities of blends of 3 ounces (90 ml) or more, you can try using less essential oil than recommended above. You may find the need for doubling amounts of essential oils is not necessary for effectiveness when making larger quantities of blended oils.

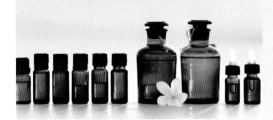

For safe skin application, essential oils should always be diluted in a suitable carrier.

FACE CARRIER OILS

Essential oils are diluted in suitable carriers like oils, lotions, creams, salts and clays to make your products. Generally, whatever will absorb an essential oil and is safe for skin application can be used as a carrier to make your health and beauty treatments.

Water is not an acceptable carrier for essential oil that is being applied directly to the skin, since oil and water do not mix. For general safe use on the skin, it is always best to dilute your essential oil in an oil-based carrier or other suitable carrier; it should be one that will absorb and carry your essential oil.

A 5-milliliter, euro-dropper bottle contains approximately 100 drops of liquid. A 1-percent dilution of essential oil would be 1 drop to 99 drops of carrier oil. Please refer to the "Safety and Dilution Guide" on page 443.

Choose oils that are skin nourishing and healing like pure fractionated coconut oil or jojoba. Both of these oils act as excellent carriers of essential oil. Coconut oil has the added benefit of being fully metabolized by the body, helping it to be absorbed through the fatty tissues beneath the skin and into the blood stream. Diluting your essential oil in a carrier also helps you avoid any possible skin irritation.

Fractionated Coconut Oil
(COCOS NUCIFERA)

Also called light coconut oil, I highly recommend using this oil as the ideal carrier for most of your topical essential oil body and face applications.

Light coconut oil is one of the most effective natural body moisturizers available. I've used light coconut oil in all my personal skincare products for many years and absolutely love the results I experience for myself and my customers. It makes a great base for sensitive skincare products, and its "light" texture makes it suitable for all skin types, especially for dry, itchy, inflamed or sensitive skin. Excellent for nail and cuticle treatments, use light coconut oil as a base for essential oils, on your skin as a moisturizer, after exposure to the sun and at night before bed to nourish your skin. Its cooling and moisturizing action serve to protect your skin while helping it retain moisture.

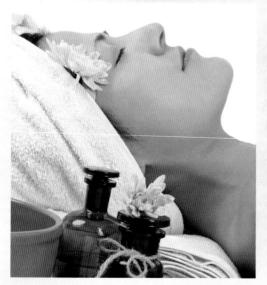

Aromatherapy facial skincare is now quite popular in spa treatments.

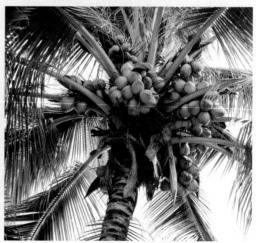

Coconuts have been used traditionally in cosmetics in the tropics.

Light coconut oil's softening and lubricating effects on the skin are excellent for treating conditions that a "totally natural" carrier oil might actually exacerbate. For instance, when using essential oils to treat damaged skin, a totally natural carrier oil could potentially introduce molds, bacteria or fungi to the skin, making the condition worse, whereas using a refined and sterilized carrier oil like light coconut oil can actually prevent further problems and promote beneficial results.

UNIQUE QUALITIES OF FRACTIONATED COCONUT OIL

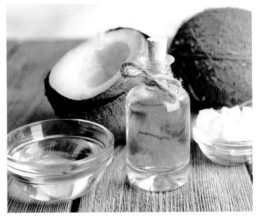

Coconut oil is closest in molecular structure to skin's own natural sebum.

1. Coconut oil is fully metabolized by the body and, unlike most oils, not absorbed into the fat cell tissues of the body. This makes it an ideal carrier for essential oils to move through the fat cells beneath the dermis and into the blood vessels serving the muscles and soft tissues.

2. Light coconut oil remains liquid at room temperature. You may be familiar with the pure, whole coconut oil which solidifies at room temperature, but may not have yet experienced light fractionated coconut oil which uses a simple, non-chemical, physical process to separate the smaller fatty acid triglycerides from the whole coconut oil to produce fractionated coconut oil.

3. Along with jojoba oil, light coconut oil shares the distinction of being closest in molecular structure to your skin's own natural sebum, making it more readily absorbed into your skin and ideal for use in natural skincare and for massage therapy.

4. Its light consistency will not clog skin pores, making it suitable to use on dry, oily, sensitive or problem skin.

5. Light coconut oil has such a light consistency that it easily washes out of most fabrics, table linens, sheets and towels, making it ideal for massage therapy.

6. Due to its molecular structure, light coconut oil is not subject to oxidation. This means that it has an almost infinite shelf life with almost no possibility of going rancid.

7. Its anti-fungal properties make light coconut oil especially suitable for use in your fungicidal essential oil blends, for example, athlete's foot treatment.

8. Light or fractionated coconut oil is produced by heat, rather than cold pressing, which deodorizes the oil. Being odorless, light coconut oil makes an ideal carrier for aromatic oils. You can use it for making perfume oils and 10-percent dilutions of more expensive pure essential oils. This allows you to enjoy the pure scent of the oil without interference from the scent of your carrier oil.

9. Light coconut oil adds a silky, smooth, light quality to other more expensive carrier oils like jojoba.

10. Its consistency is so light you can use it in a spray bottle for misting on skin applications, and it won't clog your atomizer pump.

Of course when you prefer using a natural oil, there are some excellent choices for you.

Organic Jojoba Oil
(*SIMMONDSIA CALIFORNICA*)

Jojoba oil is more like a wax in its consistency and composition than an oil, and closely resembles your skin's own natural sebum. Because of its close resemblance, jojoba readily penetrates through your skin cell tissue and won't clog pores, making it an excellent choice for beauty and skincare treatments.

UNIQUE QUALITIES OF JOJOBA OIL

1. Because of its compatibility with your skin tissue, jojoba oil is highly nourishing for all skin types.

2. Its anti-inflammatory properties have a soothing effect on irritated or inflamed skin cells and connective tissues.

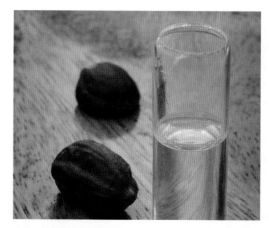

Jojoba oil is produced from the seeds of the plant and is excellent for use in cosmetics and aromatherapy products.

3. Jojoba oil's regulating action makes it excellent for use in reconditioning skin, hair and scalp.

4. As a natural antioxidant, jojoba oil is one of the longest-lasting carrier oils, after light fractionated coconut oil.

Rosehip Seed Oil
(*ROSA RUBIGINOSA*)

High in gamma linoleic and other acids known to nourish and heal skin, rosehip seed oil has an excellent reputation for treating severe skin conditions like dry, cracked and aging skin, as well as treating traumatized skin issues like burns, ulcers, wounds and uneven or excessive pigmentation. You can add rosehip seed oil to your less expensive carrier oils to get all the benefits of rosehip oil without the higher cost.

CAUTION: Avoid using with excessively oily skin types prone to acne outbreaks.

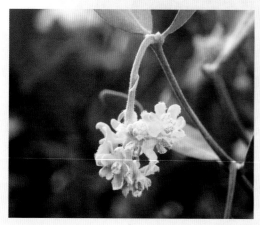

A natural antioxidant, jojoba oil is one of the longest-lasting carrier oils.

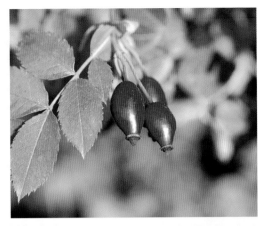

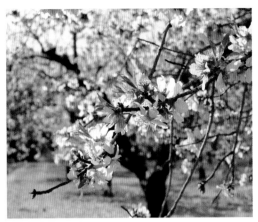

Avoid using rose hip oil with excessively oily skin types prone to acne outbreaks.

Sweet almond oil is recommended for treating dark circles and bags under your eyes.

BODY MASSAGE CARRIER OILS

My top two carrier oils for body massage therapy are fractionated light coconut oil and jojoba for the same reasons that I recommend them for face massage.

Sweet Almond Oil
(PRUNUS AMYGDALUS VAR. DULCIS)

Rich in protein and other vitamins and minerals, sweet almond oil is suitable for all skin types and helpful for relieving dry, itchy skin, as well as for soothing inflammatory conditions like arthritis, fibromyalgia, injuries and burns. Sweet almond oil has been recommended as a remedy for treating dark circles and bags under your eyes.

Sesame Oil
(SESAMUM INDICUM)

Skin nourishing sesame oil is excellent for stimulating circulation and warming the body and internal organs. Sesame oil contains the antioxidant and anti-inflammatory compound sesamol that can promote heart health by preventing atherosclerotic lesions. A great conductor of electro-magnetic flow, sesame oil promotes balance and harmony of the mind and emotions. It is good for all skin types and useful for soothing a wide range of inflammatory conditions. Sesame is good for the skin both topically and internally. Sesame seeds contain anti-cancer compounds including phytic acid, magnesium and phytosterols.

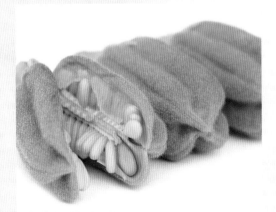

Sesame oil's stimulating and warming action makes it excellent for circulation and treating internal organs.

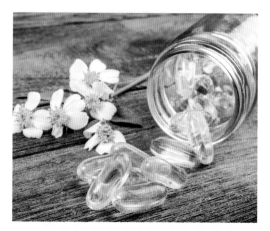

An antioxidant and natural preservative, vitamin E can be used to extend the life of your massage oils and aromatherpy products.

Vitamin E Oil

(ALPHA-TOCOPHEROL)

An antioxidant and natural preservative, vitamin E oil can be used to extend the life of your massage oils and prevent rancidity. Studies have shown immunity levels improve when vitamin E is consumed. Another important benefit of vitamin E is that it reduces cholesterol and the risk of developing cancer.

Wheat Germ Oil

(TRITCUM VUGARE)

Another natural preservative for extending the life of your massage oils, wheat germ oil is an excellent source of minerals, protein, vitamin A, vitamin D, B vitamins, antioxidants and fatty acids. These nutrients are known to moisturize and heal dry, cracked and prematurely aging skin, as well as to help prevent scarring.

BATH

Hippocrates—considered one of the most influential figures in the history of medicine and referred to as the "Father of Western Medicine"—is credited as having said, "The way to health is to have an aromatic bath and scented massage every day." First and foremost, Hippocrates respected the healing forces of nature working within every living organism. Unlike his predecessors, Hippocrates believed that illness was a natural phenomenon that forces us to discover the imbalances occurring within our own life. His holistic approach to illness entailed a rigorous examination of his patient's daily habits and routines to understand what might be leading to an imbalanced health condition, manifesting as a disease.

Research shows that a warm bath is the most effective way to boost your serotonin levels and cleanse and detoxify your body and entire energy system.

Serotonin has been called the happiness hormone. It regulates your mood, appetite and sleep. Serotonin also improves your cognitive functions like memory and learning.

Healing baths and aromatic plants have been used since antiquity for ritual purification, cleansing and healing practices and to restore

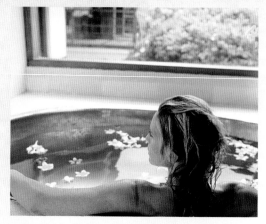

Research shows a warm bath is the most effective way to boost your serotonin levels, and cleanse and detoxify your body and entire energy system.

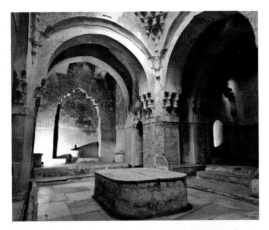

Healing baths and aromatic plants have been used since antiquity for ritual purification, cleansing and healing practices.

the human energy system—body, mind, spirit and emotions. As human beings, we are primarily made of water and have a natural affinity with water as a healing agent. Water represents your emotions. When your emotions flow, your energy stays in motion. The meridian energy system for cycling prana (or life force energy) becomes clogged when you resist and suppress feeling your emotions. Taking a warm water bath naturally frees your emotions.

Natural sea salts are frequently recommended for use as the carrier for essential oil in your healing baths. Salt has been prized for its healing properties since ancient times. During the Middle Ages, salt was at the heart of the spice trade industry, highly traded as a commodity and considered as priceless as gold. Sea salts are rich in minerals and charged with electrical healing properties that you can especially benefit from in a warm bath. Sea salts are inexpensive and readily available in your local health-food store in the bulk spice section.

Enjoying the daily holistic habit of a scented bath promotes regular restful sleep, increased energy and natural weight loss, as well as an enlivened sense of well-being and renewed passion for your life.

If you're someone who wants to live your genius and grow personally and professionally,

as well as leave behind feelings of stress and over-exhaustion, I invite you to commit to a forty-day program of daily scented baths. This will allow you to reboot and rebalance your life and experience firsthand the dramatic changes that can occur. I've now taken a daily aromatic bath for more than four years, and I would not be without it.

Radical self-care is critical if you are to thrive in today's fast-paced environment and create a work–life balance that allows you to live your best life. It has never been more important than now to take extraordinary care of yourself. Come back to yourself and enjoy being alive in the moment with a daily aromatherapy bath. Find out the exact essential oils recipe to use and instructions for your forty-day program for a daily aromatic bath in the "Spa and Beauty Treatments" section on page 263.

COMPRESS

An essential oil compress can be applied directly to an area of the body, including an injury, wound or rash to:

1. Stem the flow of bleeding.

2. Relieve pain.

3. Speed recovery.

4. Promote healing.

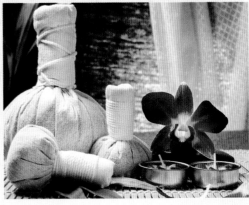

An essential oil compress can be applied directly to an area of the body.

Drops of essential oils are added to a bowl of hot or cold water and then absorbed in sterilized material, like a cotton wash cloth or gauze. This is then applied with pressure to a part of the body to control bleeding or to supply heat, cold, moisture or therapeutic medicinal benefits in order to alleviate inflammation and pain or to reduce infection.

Compresses are excellent for topical application to ease pain from strained muscles, headaches, poison oak, menstrual cramps and more.

POULTICE

A poultice is a soft, moist mass of material, typically made of absorbent plant material or flour that is applied to an area of the body and kept in place with a cloth or bandage. Commonly used as a "drawing salve," a poultice is applied to wounds, cuts or injuries to increase circulation and relieve soreness, inflammation or infection. An essential oil poultice is usually made of heated water to which flour or bran with drops of essential oil has been added. The mixture is then spread on soft cloth and applied over the area requiring treatment.

A common treatment used on horses to relieve inflammation, a poultice can be used on any area of the body where you want to focus your treatment. Poultices can be applied as a

precautionary measure to prevent injury after a hard workout. Effective for treating abscesses and wounds, use poultices where there is excessive discharge or build-up of pus needing to be drawn out.

MASKS AND WRAPS
Facial Masks

A facial mask treatment enlivens your skin cells and provides numerous other benefits. An essential oil facial mask covers your face or part of your face with a carrier like green or pink clay. Other carriers you can try include honey, cream, oats, avocado and egg whites. Your facial mask can take as little as 10–15 minutes, and the time is well worth the pleasure of caring for yourself and getting healthier facial skin.

BENEFITS

- Cleanses and detoxifies skin.
- Renews and nourishes skin cell tissue.
- Balances your skin's pH.
- Improves skin elasticity.
- Reduces fine lines and wrinkles.
- Imparts a radiant, youthful and healthy glow.

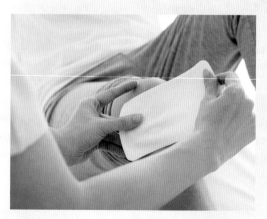

A poultice can be used on any area of the body where you want to focus treatment. Poultices are commonly used to relieve inflammation.

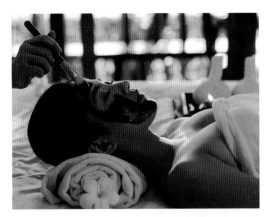

A woman enjoys a facial mask of seaweed and green clay.

Body Wrap

Feel clean inside and out with an essential oil body wrap treatment. An aromatherapy body wrap involves the application of essential oils in a carrier like green or pink clay. Mud can also be used as a base to which you can add seaweed, water, aloe vera and salt. This is followed by wrapping the body or body part being treated with a sheet and then covering the area with blankets to create a warm, cocoon-like effect to activate and assist the cleansing, detoxification and healing process. Heat can also be applied to increase the natural detox of sweating. You can allow at least an hour and a half for a full body wrap experience which includes time for a cleansing shower followed by a 10-minute period of resting afterward to get the most from your treatment.

For the best cleansing results for your skin and internal organs, it's best to do your body wrap in conjunction with a detoxing diet or whole body cleanse.

BENEFITS

- Cleanses, detoxifies and draws out impurities. Can help eliminate harmful toxins from your body and internal organs, as well as provide essential vitamins and minerals to your body's largest and most vulnerable organ, your skin.

- Nourishes the skin.

- Tightens and tones.

- Exfoliates and acts as an astringent, eliminating dead skin.

- Destroys harmful bacteria and fungus.

- Renews skin cell tissues.

- Increases circulation.

- Soothes, moisturizes and softens skin.

- Helps you absorb the beneficial qualities of essential oils.

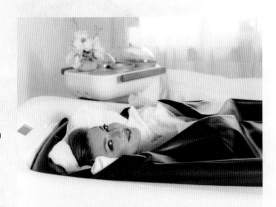

The cocoon-like effect of a body wrap allows for the best cleansing and purification results.

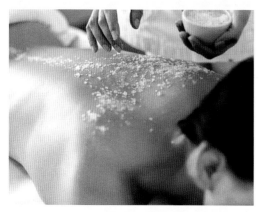

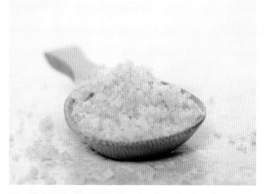

The ritual practice of exfoliation for cleansing and purification was first practiced by the Egyptians.

The moistness of the green clay found naturally in Celtic sea salt allows for fast penetration of essential oils, preserving their scent.

SCRUBS AND BODY BUTTERS

Facial and Body Scrubs

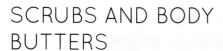

Popularly known to promote a healthy, beautiful and youthful appearance, scrubs have been used for thousands of years by many ancient civilizations to cleanse and exfoliate the skin. The Latin root *exfoliare* actually means to "strip off leaves." The Egyptians were considered the first to use the ritual practice of exfoliation for cleansing and purification, which was seen as a means to sustain life even into the afterworld.

The goal of many of the health and beauty treatments you'll learn about in this book has to do with some type of exfoliation practice. This can be achieved by physically scrubbing the skin with an abrasive type of exfoliant like a natural bristle brush, Celtic salt or sugar, or through some chemical exfoliation process such as essential oils, clay, sea salt and seaweed, which contain compounds known to actively loosen toxins.

CELTIC SEA SALT

Celtic or grey salt, as it is sometimes referred to, is a "moist," unrefined sea salt found along the coastal regions of France. Its light grey to almost light purple color comes from the clay found in the salt flats.

Celtic salt is usually collected by hand using traditional Celtic methods. It has gained great popularity in recent years in the culinary world and is considered by many to be the best quality salt available in the world today.

You can purchase Celtic salt finely ground to use as table salt or for seasoning cuisine; however, for facial and body scrubs, get the plump, coarse-ground variety.

The moistness of the green clay found naturally in the Celtic sea salt allows for fast penetration of your pure essential oils, making it an excellent carrier for aromatic scents when using it in all your scented products.

Another remarkable feature of Celtic salt is how long the scent of your oils will last once absorbed and preserved by the salt which acts as a carrier.

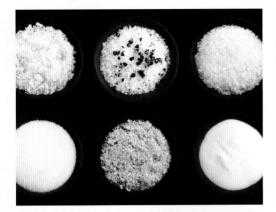

Different grounds of salt and sugar, from fine to coarse, are excellent exfoliants for making scrubs.

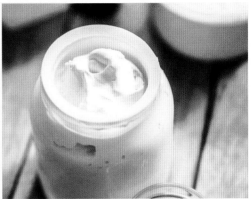

Body butters give your skin a fresh and youthful appearance and keep your skin moisturized.

Though the Celtic salt has a slight, faint scent, it is worth considering for use as a carrier for your more expensive oils like rose and helichrysum. If you'd like to carry the pure scent of an oil or blend with you, as in the case of an appetite suppressant, you may want to keep the salt handy to use as needed. Clients tell me how much they love the steadfast company of their aromatherapy smelling salts.

Body Butters

Although skincare has been around since the dawn of mankind, body butters are a relatively recent addition to a healthy skincare regimen.

Body butter gives your skin a fresh and youthful appearance and has the ability to keep skin moisturized. Body butters also act as a protective barrier from a harsh or toxic environment.

You can choose different types of body butters to use in your recipes. The body butter carries the name of the nut or seed oil it is derived from. You can mix different body butters together as desired to get multiple benefits from one or more of the nuts or seeds.

COCOA BUTTER: Made from the cocoa bean, cocoa butter smells like chocolate and is rich in antioxidants and nutrients. Cocoa butter is one of the most stable fats known and has a slow rancidity rate with a storage life of 2–5 years. Its smooth, velvety texture and pleasant aroma has made it a popular ingredient in many modern-day skincare products. Frequently recommended for prevention of stretch marks, cocoa butter is excellent for treating dry, chapped, cracked or burned skin and as a daily moisturizer to prevent dry, itchy skin and mouth sores.

SHEA BUTTER: Widely used in the cosmetics industry, shea butter comes from the nut of the African shea tree and contains antioxidants as well as vitamins A and E and may have anti-inflammatory properties. Shea butter is used for its moisturizing properties to make skin and hair care products like lip gloss, skin moisturizer creams and hair conditioners.

BEESWAX: Although not a body butter, beeswax makes an excellent carrier for the soul-soothing scent of pure essential oil. I recommend using beeswax that is natural and unrefined as an ingredient in your body butter as needed. It will allow you to control the looseness or density of the body butter recipe you're creating. Beeswax can be used as a base for creams, balms, salves and lotions. The more beeswax you add to your recipe, the denser your product will be.

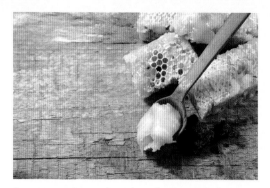

Beeswax can be used as a base for creams, balms, salves and lotions.

CAUTION: Many people have or can develop an allergy to nuts and seeds. It is a good idea to do a patch test with a new product before using it to make sure you do not have a reaction to it. If you have problems with excessively oily skin, the oils in body butters can aggravate the problem.

Skin Brushing

Skin brushing is one of the best ways to eliminate old, dead skin cell tissue and invigorate new skin growth. It keeps your skin healthy and glowing. As skin brushing stimulates your lymphatic system, it encourages detoxification. This cleansing and uplifting ritual of skin brushing is especially effective just before you shower.

You'll want to remember these key guidelines when skin brushing with a body brush for health:

- Always use a natural-bristle brush.
- Be gentle, yet brisk when brushing your skin, covering your entire body and omitting your face and neck in the process.
- Always be sure your brush strokes are from your extremities upward, toward your heart.
- Remember to breathe.
- Relax.

GENERAL DIRECTIONS FOR SKIN BODY BRUSHING

1. Brush from your fingers up to your shoulders.

2. Brush from your toes up to your neck.

3. Include the front and back side of your body as you breathe deeply.

4. Enjoy the wonderful tingling sensations dancing across your skin.

Skin brushing the body with pure essential oil is known to have the following therapeutic effects:

- Invigorates skin.
- Detoxifies the body and mind.
- Stimulates the lymphatic system.
- Improves circulation.
- Exfoliates and regenerates skin tissue.
- Nourishes skin cell tissues.
- Imparts a radiant, healthy glow to your complexion.
- Smoothes and softens your skin.

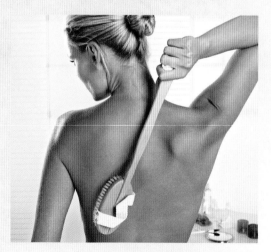

Skin brushing is one of the best ways to eliminate old, dead skin cell tissue and invigorate new cell growth.

PERFUME OIL

Perfume oil is the number one way I use essential oil. I wear perfume oil continuously and frequently mix and match different ones to enjoy the bouquet of scent sensations I can create.

I prefer perfume oils that are made in a 10-percent to 50-percent dilution of pure essential oil to carrier oil. You can also make your perfume oils with alcohol spirits like vodka, though the scent of the essential oil is definitely altered when added to alcohol. Also, alcohol is itself very drying and can cause skin sensitivity for some.

My favorite perfume carrier oil is fractionated coconut oil. I love that it is non-greasy and absorbs quickly into my skin, carrying the therapeutic benefits of the oil directly into my blood stream. But mostly, I love the fact that light coconut oil has no scent of its own and will not interfere with the smell of the pure essential oil I am wearing. Check out the "Face Carrier Oils" section on page 36 to find out more about fractionated coconut oil.

Why Use Perfume Oil?

1. It is a completely natural product. With no additives or preservatives, you know the exact ingredients because you put them there.

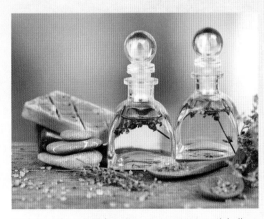

Perfume oil is my #1 favorite way to use essential oils.

2. There is seldom any concern with skin sensitivity or sensitization when using an essential oil diluted in carrier oil, except with "hot" oils. Check out the list of "hot" oils in the "Safe Use of Essential Oils" section on page 54.

3. It is an economical way to use essential oils, and perfume oil is an excellent way to extend your very expensive oils.

4. Perfume oil offers ease of use; carry them wherever you go.

5. You can add them to your sea salt for a luxurious and unforgettable bath experience.

6. It stabilizes volatility of essential oil, extending the life of an essential oil or blend.

7. You can enjoy experimenting and creating a variety of scent sensations.

Join me in the "Love and Romance Blends" section of this book (on page 315) to have fun creating your own variety of perfume oils with a selection of recipes for perfume, aphrodisiac and men's colognes.

AROMATHERAPY SPRAY

An aromatherapy spray is another favorite way of mine to enjoy all the benefits of aromatic oils. Making your own personal aromatherapy spray is quick, simple and easy to do, as well as convenient to use.

You can make your own aromatherapy spray to use as a facial toner, an all-over body freshener or as a room spray and deodorizer. The amount of oil you use depends on the purpose of your aromatic mist.

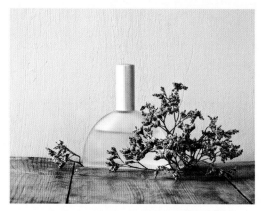

Add your perfume oil to sea salt for a luxurious and unforgettable bath experience.

- FACIAL TONER: 6–10 drops. Shake well and mist onto a cotton facial pad and apply as facial toner.

- BODY FRESHENER: 6–10 drops. Shake well and lightly mist onto skin.

- AIR FRESHENER AND ROOM DEODORIZER: 120–180 drops. Shake well and mist into the air.

Halfway fill a 2-ounce (60-ml) colored glass bottle (containing approximately 600 drops of fluid) with atomizer (spray top) of pure spring or purified water. Add your essential oil or blend. Fill the bottle with pure water, shake well and spray. The pure essential oils will float on top of the water, so you will need to shake your bottle to disperse the oils into the water each time before spraying. You may add an equal amount of alcohol or witch hazel (less drying than alcohol) to essential oils to act as a carrier for your oils to help keep them dispersed in the water. Remember, essential oils are very concentrated, and a little goes a long way.

PLEASE NOTE: Heavier oils can gum up the atomizer spray, especially the higher dilution amounts of oil. If this should happen, simply add more water to your atomizer bottle, shake well and spray.

FOOD FLAVOR: COOKING WITH ESSENTIAL OILS

You can enjoy many of the benefits of essential oils as part of your healthy lifestyle routine by using them as food flavors in all of your cooking and baking needs. Essential oils will lend a unique and distinguishing note to all of your cuisine, including your teas, soups, stews, gravies, sauces, salad dressings, baking and more.

Pure essential oils have been approved and are generally regarded as safe (GRAS) by the FDA to use as food flavors. Cooking with pure essential oils and using them as food flavor is the safest way to use essential oils internally and the only method I personally use and recommend.

Using essential oils as food flavors is very simple and easy to do, and with a little experimentation and practice, you'll be able to incorporate oils into every aspect of your everyday lifestyle, including all of your culinary dishes. By doing so, you'll benefit from the healing properties of the oils to support your overall health and well-being.

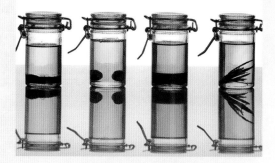

Essential oils will lend a unique and distinguishing note to all of your cuisine.

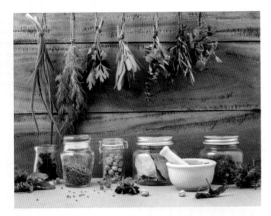

Maximize the therapeutic benefits of essential oils by adding them, when possible, at the end of the cooking process.

Flavoring Your Food

To get you started, here are a couple of ways you can use your essential oils as food flavors. Check the "Cooking with Essential Oils" section of this book on page 351 for exact recipes and to dive more deeply into cooking with essential oils. To maximize the therapeutic benefits of your essential oils, when possible, add them at the end of the cooking process.

TO FLAVOR DRY INGREDIENTS

Fill a 1-quart (.95-L) glass jar that has a lid with the amount of dry ingredients you wish to flavor.

You can add essential oils to any kind of dry, porous ingredients that will absorb flavor. Select your favorite dry ingredients to use, or any of the many varieties of flour products, teas or sugars available.

Next, choose one or more essential oils you'd like to flavor your dry ingredients with. (Citrus and spice oils are especially good for flavoring dry ingredients.) Dispense 1–4 drops of each essential oil onto a paper towel and place the paper towel on top of your dry ingredients inside the jar. Then seal the jar tightly with the lid. You can experiment to find out the exact number of drops of oil that works best for you to get the desired flavor strength you will enjoy.

Place your jar inside a darkened and cool area like a cupboard. Your dry ingredients will absorb the scent of the oils within 1–3 days or maybe longer, depending upon how porous your dry ingredients are.

Use your flavored dry ingredients as you normally would.

TO FLAVOR LIQUID INGREDIENTS

Fill a 1-pint (475-ml) glass jar with the liquid ingredient you wish to flavor (such as honey or maple syrup). Choose the essential oil you would like to flavor your liquid with. For instance, if you're using honey, I like to use floral or citrus oils like lavender or sweet orange as flavorings. Dispense one drop of essential oil onto the top of your honey and seal the jar with the lid tightly. Place in a cool, darkened area for one day. The oil's aroma should completely dissolve into the honey, giving it perfect flavor. If there is any oil on top, which can happen if your liquid ingredient is cool and stiff, simply stir the remaining essential oil into your wet ingredient. You can also stir the oil in at the beginning, though I find there's a better synergy that happens between the liquid ingredient and the essential oil if left to naturally blend together. Experiment and find out exactly the number of drops of essential oil to use and what works best for you.

Use your liquid flavoring as you normally would for your cooking and baking needs.

For more recipes, see page 351.

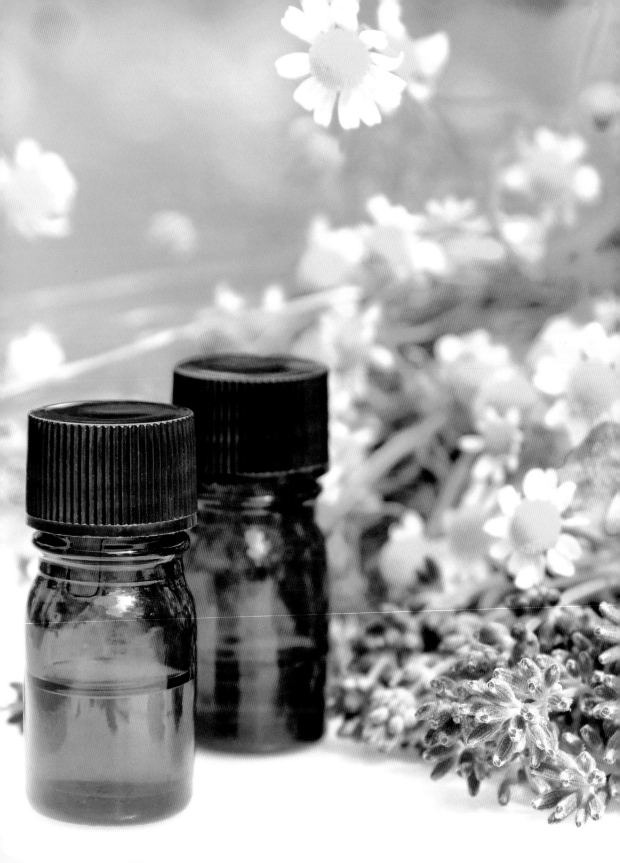

CHAPTER 4

Safe Use of Essential Oils

Never apply essential oils neat or undiluted on your skin. Always dilute your essential oils with a suitable vegetable carrier oil. I recommend cold processed, unfiltered or naturally filtered oils and preferably unscented, so you smell only your essential oil or blend of oils. Vegetable carrier oils like fractionated coconut oil or jojoba are both excellent choices. Stop using essential oils immediately if there is any skin irritation.

When using a pure, undiluted essential oil for inhalation, always keep a bottle of carrier oil, such as jojoba, handy. If pure essential oil comes in contact with your skin, dilute immediately with your carrier oil to avoid discomfort or possible skin irritation. Keep undiluted oils out of the reach of children.

Keep bottles of essential oils tightly closed and store them in a cool location away from light. If stored properly and unopened, most essential oils will maintain their potency for years; however, quicker evaporating citrus oils and conifers have a shorter shelf life because of oxidation which causes them to lose therapeutic qualities. (See "Proper Storage of Essential Oils" [on page 153] for more information.)

Essential oils should be used sparingly. Remember one drop of an essential oil equals about 1–4 cups (26–104 g) or more of dried plant matter.

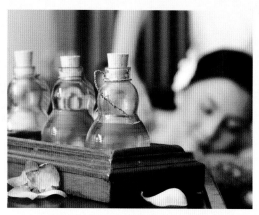
Always properly dilute your essential oils within the recommended safety ranges.

Never smell essential oils straight out of the bottle. The reason for this is twofold. First, you don't want to overwhelm your olfactory senses with a large quantity of essential oil when smelling straight out of the bottle. The second reason, and most important, is that the orifice reducer may likely have old essential oil that has oxidized. You will not be smelling fresh oil, but rancid oil with no therapeutic benefit. It's always best to dispense a drop of oil on a smell strip and inhale to experience your oil.

SENSITIZATION: Please use caution in applying essential oils to broken skin as this can cause severe irritation and may lead to an immune system reaction known as "sensitization."

Skin sensitization is a type of allergic reaction that may occur when first exposed to an essential oil. However, in some instances, there may be little or no noticeable effect on the skin at the time of application, though exposure to the same or similar material in future applications may result in cross-sensitization and trigger a severe inflammatory reaction by the immune system. Skin reactions may appear as hot red welts, redness or rash, and can be quite painful to some individuals.

HOW TO REDUCE THE RISK OF SENSITIZATION

- Always properly dilute your essential oils within the recommended safety ranges. All essential oils have a maximum dilution rate set by the International Fragrance Association (www.ifraorg.org). These can also be found in Robert B Tisserand's trusted reference book, *Essential Oil Safety.*

- Start with the lowest dilution percentage of essential oil to carrier and increase in small amounts.

- Avoid daily application of the same essential oil for prolonged periods of time.

- Avoid known sensitizers.

- Avoid using oxidized oils, especially from the Pinaceae family (such as pines and cypress species) and Rutaceae family (such as citrus oils).

Keep essential oils out of the reach of children. Handle and care for your essential oils as you would any product for therapeutic use.

SELF-SELECTION: When using essential oils in dilution with your child, I recommend you use self-selection. If your child gives any indication they dislike an aroma, the aroma is too strong. If there is any skin sensitivity, please discontinue use. You may dilute your essential oils further and try again at another time. Be respectful and allow your child to self-select.

PHOTOSENSITIZING OILS: Avoid direct sunlight and essential oils. Some oils are known to be "photosensitizers." Most common are bergamot and other cold-pressed citrus oils. Photosensitizing oils should not be used on skin that will be exposed to sunlight or ultraviolet light for 4–6 hours or longer as this may increase your chance of sunburn and cause uneven skin pigmentation—also known as berloque dermatitis.

Essential oils rich in menthol (such as peppermint) should not be used on the throat or neck area of children under thirty months of age. Please note: Menthol is found in high concentrations of many over-the-counter pharmaceutical vapor rubs in common use for congestion.

Keep pure essential oils away from the eye area and do not put into the ears.

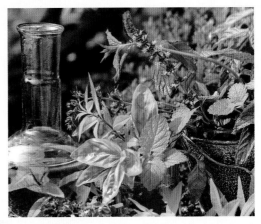

Be respectful and allow your child to self-select oils.

PREGNANT WOMEN: Generally, I recommend exercising caution when using pure essential oils during the first trimester. Though if suffering from severe morning sickness early in pregnancy, the smell of peppermint or spearmint oil can be safe to use and may relieve the nausea. If the skin should become itchy or inflamed during pregnancy, please exercise caution as essential oils in massage or in the bath might make the condition worse.

Mothers of newborn babies should not use, or at least limit the use of, pure essential oils. One of the key reasons for this is because it can interfere with a mother's natural smell and thus interfere with the all-important bonding that occurs between a mother and her child.

Epileptics and people with high blood pressure should consult their health care professional before using essential oils. Avoid hyssop, fennel and wild tansy oils.

You may wish to skin test a small area first if you suffer from hay fever or allergies. Skin tests should always be done for very young children and the elderly.

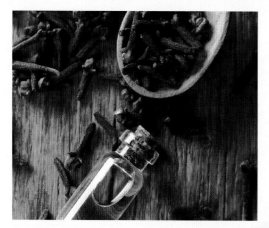

Hot oils are those that have a higher than usual potential for skin irritation.

Hot Oils

Special care should be taken when using "hot" oils. Hot oils are those that have higher-than-usual potential for skin irritation and are often high in phenols which contain carvacrol, eugenol and thymol compounds. Always use hot oils in extremely weak dilutions of less than 1 percent for skin application. Commonly used hot essential oils that may be potential skin irritants include:

- Basil (*Ocimum basilicum*)
- Black pepper (*Piper nigrum*)
- Cinnamon (*Cinnamomum zeylanicum*)
- Clove (*Eugenia caryophyllata*)
- Ginger (*Zingiber officinale*)
- Oregano (*Origanum vulgare*)
- Scotch pine (*Pinus sylvestris*)
- Siberian balsam (*Abies sibirica*)
- Silver fir (*Abies sibirica, alba, balsamea*)
- Thyme (*Thymus vulgaris*)
- Wintergreen (*Gaultheria procumbens*) *not recommended for use

In Some Cases:

- Tea tree (*Melaleuca alternifolia*)
- Ylang ylang (*Cananga odorata*)
- Peppermint (*Mentha x piperita*)

SKIN TEST: Apply pure essential oil in a weak, 1-percent dilution of carrier oil on a cotton swab and lightly touch the skin in an area either under the arm, inside the elbow, behind the knee or on the wrist. Cover the area with a bandage and leave unwashed for 24 hours. If there is any reaction such as itching or redness, you may wish to discontinue using the oil. Sometimes a reaction to an essential oil can indicate a need for an internal cleansing program before using an essential oil. Essential oils can react with toxins built up in the body from chemicals in food, water and the environment. However, sensitivity can also simply be a sign that you are sensitive to one or more of the chemical properties in the essential oil, and you should not use that essential oil.

If any of these essential oils is applied in a weak dilution on the skin and a hot, red weal or skin reaction occurs, this is the result of skin irritation that requires immediate attention. Always have a vegetable carrier oil like pure fractionated coconut oil or jojoba available to apply onto the skin in such cases.

Applying carrier oil will have the immediate effect of calming the skin irritation. Do not wash or rinse the area with water as this will drive the essential oils further into the skin and increase, not diminish, the discomfort.

If you accidentally get essential oil in your eye, use a cotton tissue or swab at the corner of your eye to wick (absorb or draw out) the oil from the eye.

Essential oils are flammable. Please keep them out of the way of fire hazards.

INTERNAL USE: Essential oils should never be used internally for medicinal purposes without trained, professional medical guidance and direct supervision.

Essential oils are approved by the FDA and generally regarded as safe (GRAS) to use as food flavors. You can safely enjoy all the therapeutic effects of essential oils when using them as food flavors.

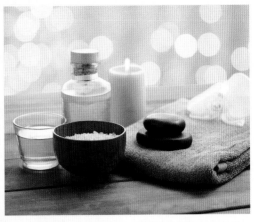

Always have a vegetable carrier, like light coconut oil, available to apply if there is any skin irritation.

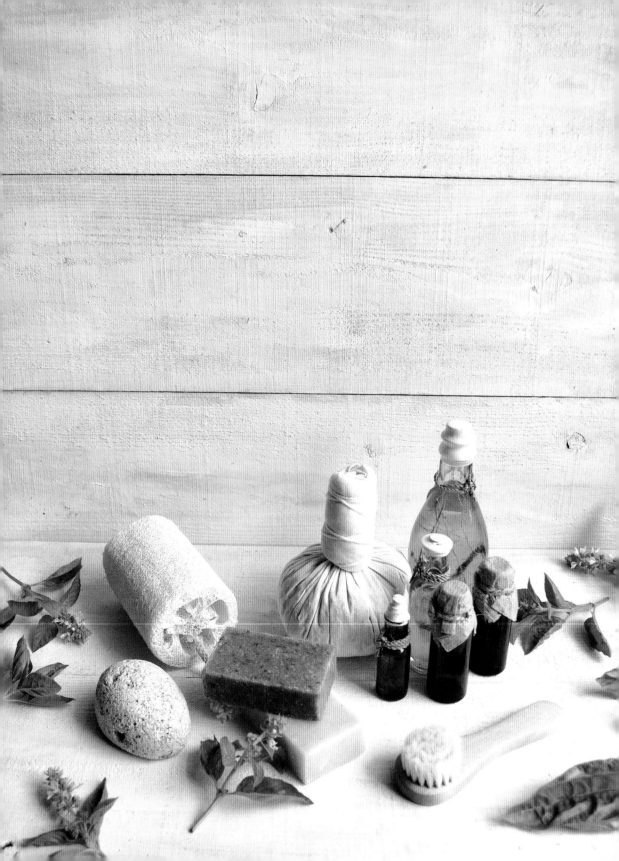

CHAPTER 5

Aromatherapy Supplies

What You Need to Have on Hand for Making Your Products

This is the shopping list of aromatherapy supplies I suggest you have on hand. You will learn about the therapeutic use of each of the oils, as well as how to use them in formulating your own therapeutic blends and aromatherapy treatments.

When selecting pure essential oils, the minimal requirements for choosing your oils should include:

1. Generic name of the essential oil.

2. Botanical species of the plant.

3. Part of the plant that produced the oil.

4. Method of extraction used.

5. Location where the oil was produced.

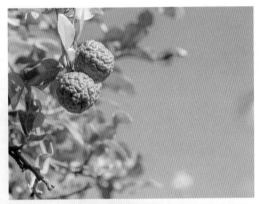

Bergamot (*Citrus bergamia*): cold-pressed peel, Italy (page 69)

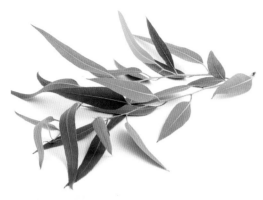

Eucalyptus (*globulus* and *radiata*): steam-distilled leaf, Australia (page 71)

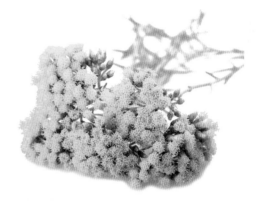

Helichrysum Italian Everlasting (*Helichrysum italicum*), Immortelle: steam-distilled flowers, Italy (page 78)

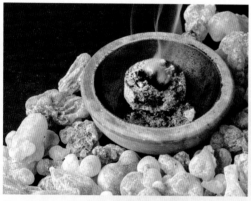

Frankincense (*Boswelia frereana*): steam-distilled resin tears, Somalia (page 74)

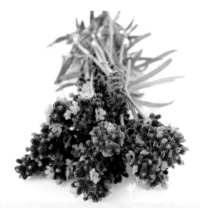

Lavender (*Lavandula angustifolia*): steam-distilled flowers, High Altitude France, Bulgaria or Italy (page 80)

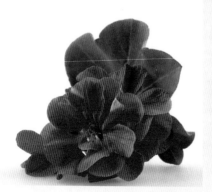

Geranium Roseum and Graveolens (*Pelargonium roseum* and *graveolens*): steam-distilled leaves, Madagascar and Albania (page 76)

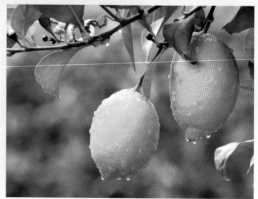

Lemon (*Citrus limonum*): cold-pressed peel, Italy (page 82)

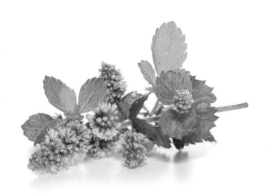

Peppermint (*Mentha x piperita*): steam-distilled flowering tops, USA (page 85)

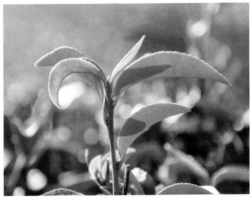

Tea Tree (*Melaleuca alternifolia*): steam-distilled leaf, Australia (page 89)

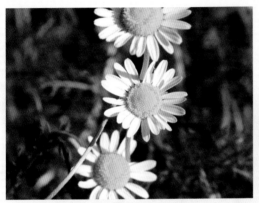

Roman Chamomile (*Chamaemelum nobile*): steam-distilled flower, USA and France (page 87)

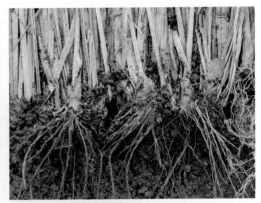

Vetiver (*Vetiveria zizanioides*): hydrodiffused root, Haiti (page 91)

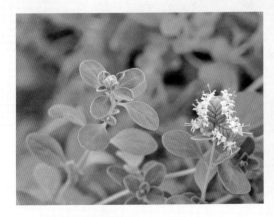

Sweet Marjoram (*Origanum marjorana*): steam-distilled flowers and leaf, Egypt (page 88)

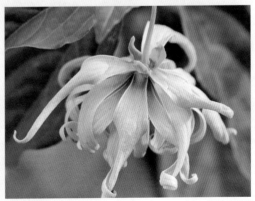

Ylang Ylang (*Cananga odorata*): steam-distilled flowers, Madagascar (page 93)

Supplemental Oils to Have on Hand for Concocting Aromatherapy Formulations

Very expensive oils like rose can be purchased in a 10-percent dilution of carrier oil. The intensity of these pure oils makes them useful in dilution with great effect.

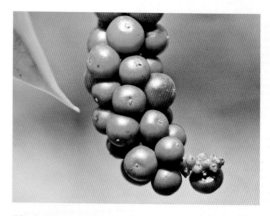

Black Pepper (*Piper nigrum*): steam-distilled fruit, Madagascar (page 101)

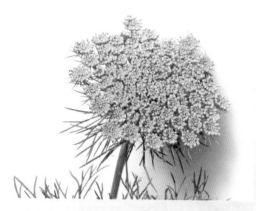

Ammi visnaga (*Ammi visnaga*): steam-distilled herb, Morocco (page 97)

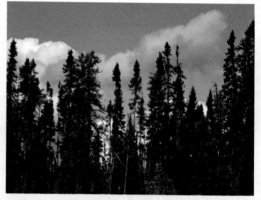

Black Spruce (*Picea mariana*): steam-distilled needle, Canada (page 102)

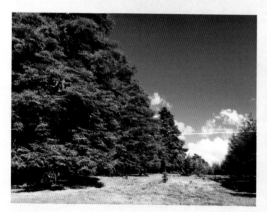

Atlas Cedarwood (*Cedrus atlantica*): steam-distilled wood, Morocco (endangered) (page 99)

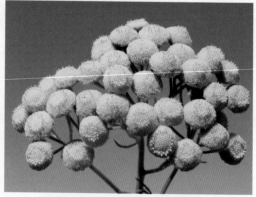

Blue Tansy/Moroccan Blue Chamomile (*Tanacetum annuum*): steam-distilled flower tops, Morocco (page 103)

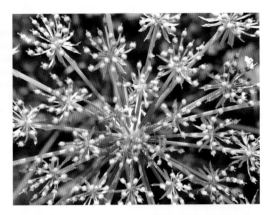

Carrot Seed (*Daucus carota*): steam-distilled seed, France (page 104)

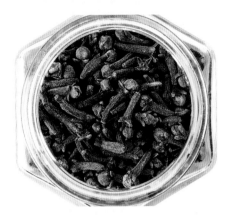

Clove (*Eugenia caryophyllata*): steam-distilled bud, Madagascar (page 109)

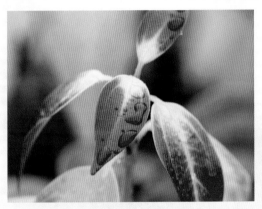

Cinnamon (*Cinnamomum zeylanicum*): steam-distilled leaf, Madagascar (page 105)

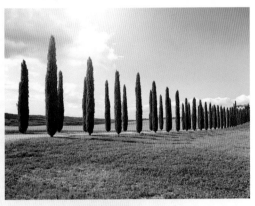

Cypress (*Cupressus sempervirens*): steam-distilled leaf, Crete (page 110)

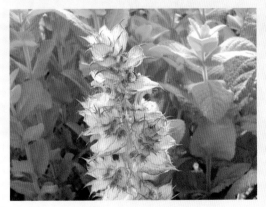

Clary Sage (*Salvia sclarea*): hydrodiffused flower, USA (page 107)

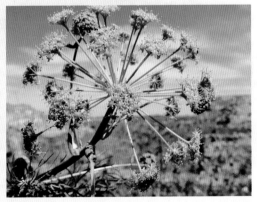

Galbanum (*Ferula galbaniflua*): steam-distilled gum resin, Iran (page 112)

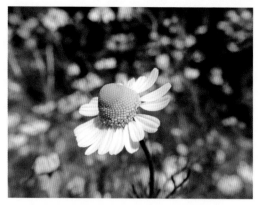

German Chamomile (*Matricaria chamomilla*): steam-distilled flower, Bulgaria (page 114)

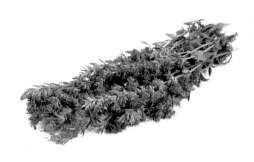

Hyssop (*Hyssopus officinalis*): steam-distilled whole plant, Bulgaria (page 120)

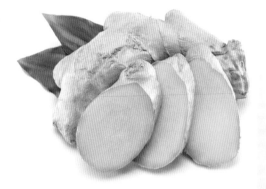

Ginger (*Zingiber officinale*): hydrodiffused fresh root, Sri Lanka and Madagascar (page 116)

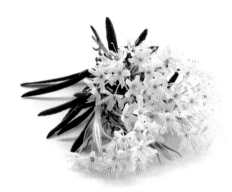

Ledum (*Ledum groenlandicum*): steam-distilled herb, Canada (page 121)

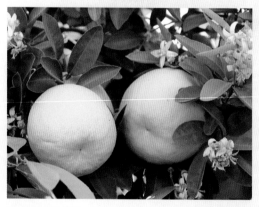

Grapefruit (*Citrus paradisi*): cold-pressed peel, USA (page 118)

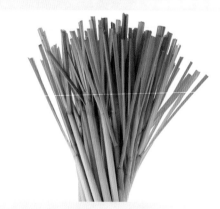

Lemongrass (*Cymbopogon citratus*): hydrodiffused grass, Haiti (page 122)

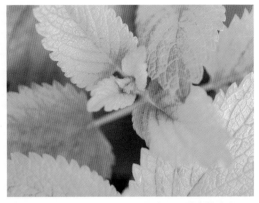

Melissa (*Melissa officinalis*): steam-distilled flowers and leaves, England and France (page 124)

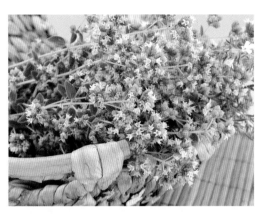

Oregano (*Origanum vulgare*): steam-distilled herb, Turkey (page 130)

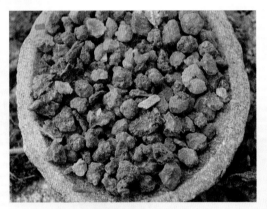

Myrrh (*Commiphora myrrha*): steam-distilled gum resin, Ethiopia (the BEST) and Somalia (page 126)

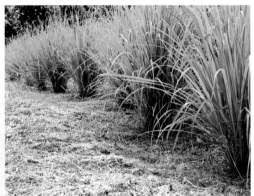

Palmarosa (*Cymbopogon martinii*): steam-distilled herb, Nepal (page 131)

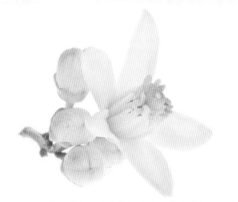

Neroli (*Citrus aurantium*): steam-distilled flower, Tunisia (page 128)

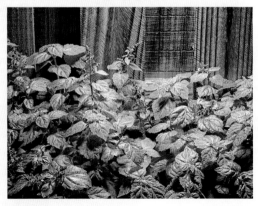

Patchouli (*Pogostemon cablin*): steam-distilled leaf, Indonesia (page 133)

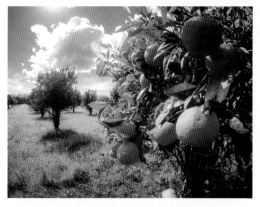

Red Mandarin (*Citrus deliciosa*): cold-pressed peel, Italy (page 134)

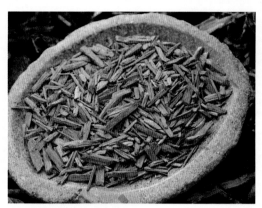

Sandalwood (*Santalum album*): steam-distilled heartwood, Mysore, India (endangered) (page 142)

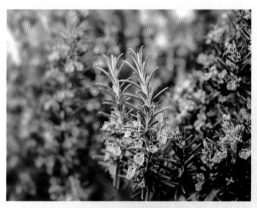

Rosemary (*Rosmarinus officinalis ct. verbenone* and *cineole*): steam-distilled flowering herb and leaf, Italy (page 135)

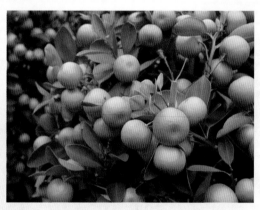

Sweet Orange (*Citrus sinensis*): cold-pressed fresh peel, Italy (page 145)

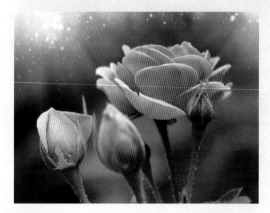

Rose Otto (*Rosa damascena*): steam-distilled flowers, Turkey and Bulgaria (page 139)

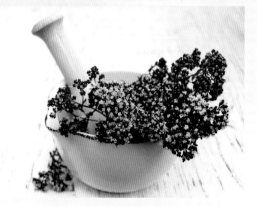

Thyme (*Thymus vulgaris*): steam-distilled herb, Germany and France (page 146)

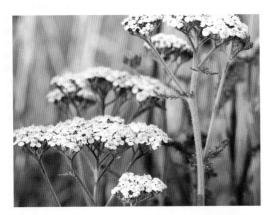

Yarrow (*Achillea millefolium*): steam-distilled flower, Bulgaria (page 148)

ADDITIONAL SUPPLIES TO CONSIDER HAVING ON HAND

- Seven 1-ounce (30-ml) bottles of vegetable carrier oil (for making aromatic medicine and blends)

- Ten 5-milliliter colored glass, euro-dropper bottles (for making aromatic medicine and blends)

- 1 bag cotton balls

- 1 packet smell strips

- Natural bristle skin brush

- Cotton washcloth

- Cotton hand towel

- Cotton bath towel

- Robe

AROMATHERAPY JOURNAL: Highly recommended for recording personal notes about your experiences with essential oils, as well as the various recipes and blends you formulate.

As some of the pure essential oils are very expensive, you may wish to buy them in a 10 percent dilution to use in your aromatherapy products. Please be sure to add a 10 percent dilution of an oil directly to your carrier before application, not to a synergy blend as they will not synergize with the other essential oils.

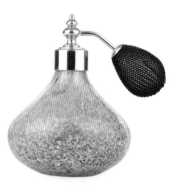

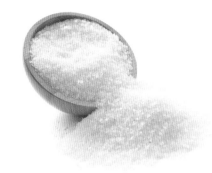

An ornate glass misting bottle adds elegance to any DIY aromatherapy spray.

Detoxifying and purifiying salt for making aromatic bath salts.

For Making Aromatherapy Sprays

- 2 or more 2-ounce (60-ml) colored-glass atomizer misting bottles
- 1 quart (945 ml) or more, purified water
- Optional: Witch hazel or alcohol

For Making Smelling Salts

- ¼ cup (130 g) Celtic (grey) salt
- ⅛-ounce (4-ml) vial(s) with cap for smelling salts

For Making Aromatic Bath Salts

- Sea salt
- Epsom salts
- Celtic (grey) salts
- Baking soda

For Making Facial and Body Masks and Scrubs

- 1 cup (200 g) sugar
- 1 cup (236 ml) honey
- 1 cup (236 ml) cream
- 1 cup (230 g) French green or pink clay
- 1 avocado
- 1 egg

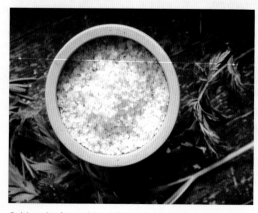

Celtic salts for making DIY smelling salts.

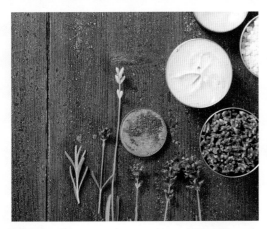

DIY aromatherapy products are fun and simple to make and can ease your life.

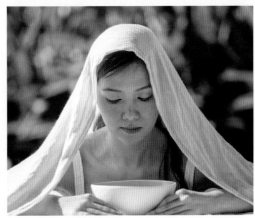

Woman enjoying simple DIY facial of respiratory steam.

For Making Lip Balms, Butters, Creams, Healing Salves and Ointments

- 1 or more ¼- or ½-ounce (7- or 15-ml) colored-glass jars with lid
- One 4-ounce (118-ml) colored-glass jars with lid
- One 2-ounce (60-ml) colored-glass jars with lid
- ¼ cup (57 g), or more, beeswax
- Light coconut oil
- ¼ cup (55 g) shea butter
- Aloe vera gel
- Vegetable glycerin

For Facial and Respiratory Steams

- Stainless steel or ceramic bowl

For Aromatherapy Blends

- 1 dozen or more 5-milliliter, colored-glass, euro-dropper bottles

Optional Supplies

- Footbath or basin for foot soak
- Diffuser
- Humidifier

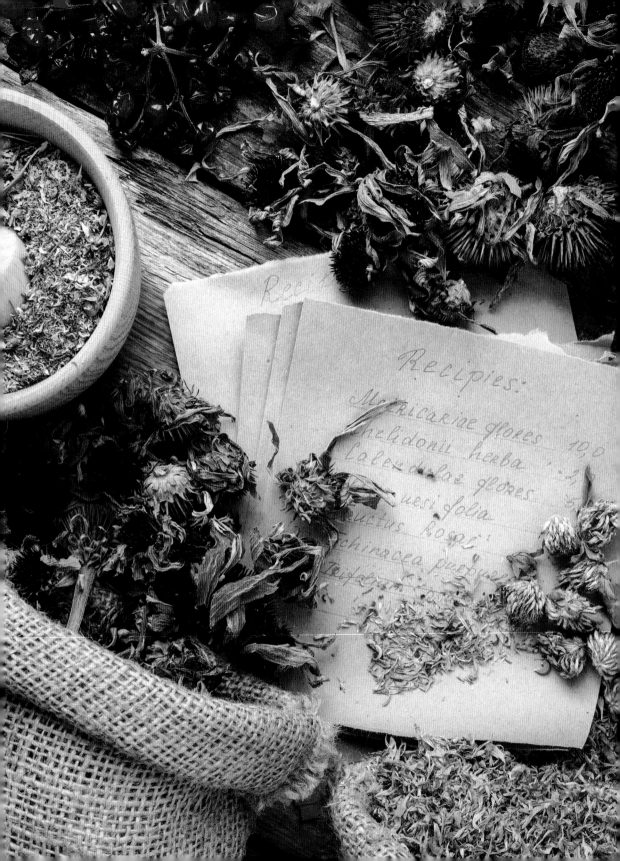

CHAPTER 6

Pure, Most Commonly Used Essential Oils

BERGAMOT ESSENTIAL OIL

(*CITRUS BERGAMIA*): COLD-PRESSED PEEL— SPIRITUAL AND EMOTIONAL HEALER

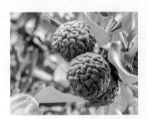 As bergamot oil requires special soil and climate, the best location for growing and distilling is the Calabria district of southern Italy.

A fresh, lightly sweet and fruity citrus oil with spicy, floral overtones, bergamot has a warm, friendly and inviting scent. Folklore has it that bergamot was brought to Italy by Christopher Columbus from the Canary Islands and first grown in Bergamo from where its name originated.

Bergamot's regulating properties act to promote balance and harmony to all the body's functions. Of all the citrus oils, bergamot is the one that is most supportive and comforting.

Psycho-emotionally, bergamot oil acts as a spiritual and emotional healer. Its anti-depressant, antispasmodic and regulating action can uplift and brighten the mood and balance even the most extreme emotional states like anxiety, depression, despair and worry. Its refreshing influence has been shown to calm even the most extreme emotions, as well as relieve mental and emotional fatigue.

Paolo Rovesti, a professor at the University of Milan in Italy, conducted research at several psychiatric clinics on the emotional, mental and psychological effects of essential oils, showing their benefits for depression, anxiety and hysteria.

He reported that the most important psychological benefits of bergamot oil were for relieving fear and calming anxiety. Other oils he researched included combinations of jasmine, neroli, lemon verbena, lime, rose, violet, marjoram, cypress and petitgrain. Rovesti reported great success with these treatments and concluded that essential oils, "bring a person into a place of relaxed alertness."

A randomized controlled study of 109 preoperative patients reported that those exposed to the scent of bergamot essential oil were less anxious. Though the mechanism for why bergamot oil reduces anxiety is not completely understood, it is thought to be due to the release of neurotransmitters that interfere with the normal response to stress.

(continued)

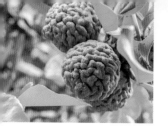

BERGAMOT ESSENTIAL OIL

(*CITRUS BERGAMIA*): COLD-PRESSED PEEL—
SPIRITUAL AND EMOTIONAL HEALER

Another study with animals showed bergamot oil to affect the hypothalamic-pituitary-adrenal activity by reducing the corticosterone response to stress, bringing about a balancing effect on the activity of the hypothalamus gland. The hypothalamus is the seat of our more intense emotions such as terror and rage. The hypothalamus gland works in synchrony with the pineal and pituitary glands to help regulate and balance your hormonal cycles, including your natural sleep and wake cycles. It is thought that this effect to balance the natural sleep cycles may make bergamot helpful for relieving symptoms of jet lag.

Highly valued in the perfume industry, bergamot oil is often used in blends like Eau de Cologne. However, due to safety concerns in recent years, an artificial bergamot oil has been developed for use in the perfume and skincare industry, and natural perfume oils have all but disappeared from use.

A very versatile oil, bergamot shares the antiseptic properties of other citrus oils without the sharp scent. Natural bergamot's antiseptic, cicatrizant and regulating properties were once enjoyed in many skincare formulas, as it is known to be effective for treating skin conditions like acne, cold sores, skin rash, eczema, herpes and shingles.

Bergamot's digestive and regulating properties have been reported to make it helpful for relieving many digestive system complaints.

Metaphysically, the lymphatic system and immune function are related to a strong sense of self-worth and a feeling of "I can do it." When you doubt your ability to take care of yourself and lack confidence, your immune function

can be affected. Energetically, your psychic defenses to protect against foreign invaders are lowered. Bergamot oil may be helpful for building morale and self-esteem and can help you to rebuild strength and regain self-confidence.

Its natural deodorant and disinfectant properties make bergamot useful as a cleanser and freshener. Bergamot is often used as a breath freshener. Use in your aroma lamp to brighten and cheer a stale or smoke-filled room.

Traditionally, bergamot oil is used as a flavoring in Earl Grey tea.

Bergamot blends well with many different oils including black pepper, lavender, geranium, ylang ylang, rosemary and vetiver.

Dispense 1 to 3 drops of bergamot oil on a cotton ball or smell strip, close your eyes and inhale. Note in your journal the aroma qualities you can discern and the effects the oil has on your body, mind, spirit and emotions.

CAUTION: Though bergamot is helpful for treating a variety of skin conditions, care should be taken when using it in skin applications. As bergamot is phototoxic, please avoid exposure to direct sunlight or sunlamps for a minimum of 3 to 12 hours after use as *Berloque Dermatitis* (permanent pigmentation) of the skin may result. In the 1950s and 1960s several cases were reported following increased use of perfumes containing bergamot oil. However, since the introduction of artificial bergamot oil there has been a reduction of the natural oil in perfumes, and Berloque Dermatitis is now rare.

EUCALYPTUS ESSENTIAL OIL

(*EUCALYPTUS GLOBULUS* AND *RADIATA*): STEAM-DISTILLED LEAF—
RESPIRATORY SUPPORT

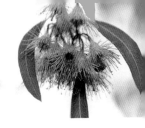

Traditionally, the best place for growing and distilling eucalyptus is Australia.

A popular and well-known oil that most people can recognize, along with mint, rose and lavender, eucalyptus oil has a reputation as a powerful decongestant. Its fresh, sweet and camphoraceous scent is long lasting.

The *globulus* species is probably the most well-known and commonly used eucalyptus oil. However, the *radiata* species has the gentler scent of the two and is safe for children. Its powerful antimicrobial action can be enjoyed daily. The primary difference between the two oils is the presence of piperitone—also found in peppermint oil—which gives the radiata a more pleasant and soothing aroma. Otherwise, the aroma and the uses of the two oils are very similar.

Eucalyptus's stimulating, pungent and camphoraceous notes bring to mind the smell we associate with medicine. In fact, many traditional medicines contain eucalyptus. Its tonic and regulating properties help to strengthen and enliven the body and have a stabilizing and balancing effect.

Eucalyptus is prized for its strong antibacterial and antiviral properties. It may be helpful for preventing, as well as treating, the common cold and flu and their associated symptoms.

As an antipyretic (fever reducer), use eucalyptus in a cooling compress to relieve fever. Similar to peppermint, use only a small amount as too much can have a chilling effect. Its antispasmodic action makes eucalyptus helpful for relieving any associated symptoms like body aches or pains.

One of the most powerful respiratory support oils in aromatherapy, eucalyptus's decongestant properties stimulate oxygen uptake in the cells and circulation of the blood and lymph. This increased oxygen in the lungs promotes the cleansing and repair of your blood capillaries and vessels. For this reason, eucalyptus oil is an excellent blood cleanser and helpful for regenerating damaged lung cell tissue.

Its strong expectorant properties are what give eucalyptus its reputation for breaking up congestion and removing excess mucous from your nasal passageways. This, coupled with its potent anti-inflammatory properties that help relieve swollen and painful nasal passageways, make eucalyptus the standout choice for treating respiratory issues.

(continued)

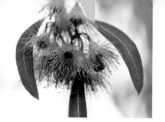

EUCALYPTUS ESSENTIAL OIL

(*EUCALYPTUS GLOBULUS* AND *RADIATA*): STEAM-DISTILLED LEAF—
RESPIRATORY SUPPORT

To treat congestion and bronchial problems, eucalyptus oil is most effective when used as an inhalant (such as steam inhalation or diffusion into the air). You can also add eucalyptus oil to a vegetable carrier oil or salve and apply to sinus points, the chest and upper back areas.

A powerful antiseptic agent, eucalyptus oil's antimicrobial properties make it effective for treating a broad spectrum of infections. Eucalyptus oil has been reported effective for symptomatic relief of tuberculosis and malaria. It may also be useful for treating cold sores, skin ulcers, shingles and insect bites.

A study published in the *Iranian Journal of Pharmaceutical Research* concluded that the anti-Staphylococcus activity of eucalyptus essential oil suggests that it has potential for clinical use.

Staphylococcus aureus (staph) is a pathogen that causes serious infections in humans. Staphylococcus is known as one of the most resistant bacterium against typical antibiotics. It causes tremendous problems in medical centers and is a growing concern in society.

The report goes on to say that, "Nowadays, scientists and clinicians are looking for more efficient drugs, derived from natural and herbal resources, against microbial and viral infections. Plants are considered as rich sources of antibiotic treatment medications, and the eucalyptus leaf with its antimicrobial properties has been used in the treatment of infectious diseases formerly in ancient medicine."

In Japan, scientists revealed findings about using essential oils of eucalyptus, orange thyme and tea tree to destroy bacteria by diffusing them into the air. The scientists said that the use of these essential oils could help people to easily and conveniently kill bacteria lurking in their homes. Further research is planned on the effectiveness of using essential oil against the super bug *Methicillin-resistant Staphylococcus aureus* (MRSA) among other strains of bacteria.

Another research study by scientists Dr. Lindsey Gaunt and Sabrina Higgins of the University of Southampton reported that essential oils like eucalyptus, orange and thyme can destroy the bacteria *Escherichia coli* (E. coli) and Staphylococcus aureus on surfaces.

Many essential oils have been reported to have potential in dental health. In research studies, tea tree and eucalyptus showed antimicrobial effects against common oral pathogens. Eucalyptus oil's germicidal properties may be enjoyed as a gargle or a mouthwash to kill germs, as well as relieve sore throats. Traditionally, eucalyptus has been used as a remedy for sinusitis, bronchitis, asthma, strep throat, colds and flu, hay fever, catarrh, coughs, and sinus and tension headaches due to congestion or poor digestion.

Eucalyptus's analgesic and anti-inflammatory properties are well-known. It is found in many topical preparations for relieving inflammatory conditions like fibromyalgia, nerve pain, muscle cramps and joint pain.

Eucalyptus has been reported to have a lowering effect on blood sugar, along with coriander, fennel, geranium and juniper berry.

Psycho-emotionally, eucalyptus has a rejuvenating effect on your emotions and thought processes. Use it to promote clarity and the flow of fresh, new ideas. When you're feeling confused or overwhelmed with too many details, eucalyptus can get things flowing again for you.

Excellent for eradicating household odors, use eucalyptus as an air freshener or underarm antiperspirant to control body odor.

Eucalyptus oil blends well with basil, Himalayan cedarwood, cypress, frankincense, lavender, lemon, rosemary, tea tree and thyme.

Dispense 1 to 3 drops of eucalyptus oil on a cotton ball or smell strip, close your eyes and inhale. Note in your journal the aroma qualities you can discern and the effects the oil has on your body, mind, spirit and emotions.

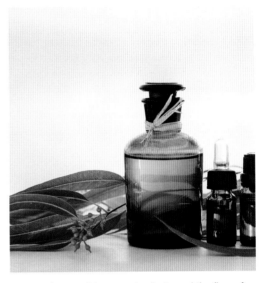

Use eucalyptus oil to promate clarity and the flow of fresh, new ideas.

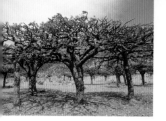

FRANKINCENSE ESSENTIAL OIL

(*BOSWELLIA FREREANA* AND *CARTERII*): STEAM-DISTILLED RESIN TEARS—
SPIRITUAL AND EMOTIONAL SUPPORT

Oman, India is considered by many aromatherapists and perfumers to be the best location for growing and distilling frankincense; however, oil produced in Somalia—where the Roman Catholic Church buys most of its stock—is considered of the finest quality.

Frankincense is "tapped" by slashing the bark of the thin and haggard-looking, but robust trees. This process called striping allows the tree's resin to bleed out and harden into tears. There are several species of frankincense trees used for distilling the oil.

Many of the characteristic properties of frankincense oil are found in each species. *Frerana* is most often preferred by aromatherapists and perfumers. In recent years, the *Boswellia carterii* species has been the subject of much research for cancer.

Tapping is done two to three times a year with the final tap producing the best tears due to their higher aromatic chemical content. Generally, the opaquer the resin tears are, the more superior the quality.

There is some concern that frankincense tree populations are in severe decline due in part to over-harvesting, as well as other environmental factors.

The aroma of frankincense is exotic, fresh, sweet, balsamic and resinous with a hint of spice. Its enticing wood aroma is sensual and freeing.

Frankincense has been traded for over 5,000 years. It is one of the sacred and holy oils used since ancient times, when aromatic oils were traded like valuable commodities and considered as precious as gold.

Its remarkable ability to maintain its integrity in any blend has given frankincense a reputation for bestowing this same stability of character, to remain true to oneself, to the one using its fragrance.

Spiritually and psycho-emotionally, frankincense is best known for its enduring emotional and spiritual support. It lends support to help you be strong and recover after grief and loss or post-traumatic stress.

Frankincense is often used in religious ceremonies as a perfume oil and for anointing and consecrating the body for performing holy deeds. Thought to possess miraculous healing powers, frankincense has been reported to heal and cure every possible illness since ancient times.

The anti-tumoral properties of frankincense have become the subject of much study in recent years. The United States National Library of Medicine (NLM) at the National Institutes of Health maintains the database on evidence supporting the use of essential oils for treating cancer. Some of the evidence gathered is related to frankincense and cancer.

Traditionally, frankincense has been used in many cultures for increasing cellular respiration, slowing down breathing and heart rate and releasing problems into God's care. This is the purpose for which it's used in many religious ceremonies.

Frankincense oil is said to promote your spiritual awakening and to enhance your meditation practice. It can be helpful for overcoming negative mental and emotional states, fear about taking action, depression, low self-esteem, insecurity and anxiety.

An analgesic (pain reliever) and anti-inflammatory, frankincense may be helpful for treating rheumatism and sports injuries. Its expectorant and anti-catarrh action makes it useful for treating symptoms of asthma and bronchitis.

Its immune-stimulant properties increase white blood cell (WBC) count and support a healthy immune function. A natural diuretic, frankincense is also known to relieve digestive discomfort and flatulence.

Frankincense's regulating properties may be helpful for balancing menstrual cycles and relieving pre-menstrual symptoms like irritability, headache and cramps.

Its characteristic effects of calming and rejuvenating make frankincense nourishing for all skin types. Its action to tone and balance the skin's natural sebum production make it especially nourishing for oily and mature skin types.

Frankincense oil blends well with many different oils including sandalwood, myrrh, lavender, bergamot, patchouli, lemon, clove, cinnamon, vetiver, orange and ylang ylang.

Dispense 1 to 3 drops of frankincense oil on a cotton ball or smell strip, close your eyes and inhale. Note in your journal the aroma qualities you can discern and the effects the oil has on your body, mind, spirit and emotions.

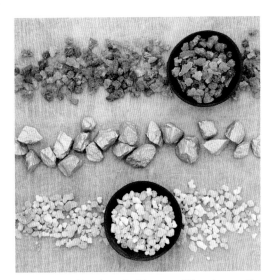

Frankincense blends well with many different aromatic plant oils.

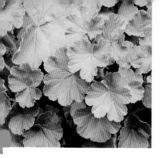

GERANIUM, GERANIUM ROSEUM and GRAVEOLENS ESSENTIAL OIL

(PELARGONIUM ROSEUM AND *GRAVEOLENS*): STEAM-DISTILLED LEAF—HORMONE BALANCE

Some of the best locations for growing and distilling geranium oil are the Reunion Islands, Madagascar and Albania.

The heady and exotic aroma of geranium oil is delightfully fresh, sweet, floral and sensuous. Traditionally, geranium oil has been used by women to relieve many common complaints associated with hormonal imbalance.

Considered by many to be the most desirable essential oil to use for hormonal imbalance for both men and women, the rose (*roseum*) and *graveolens* varieties of geranium oil are used most often.

Although geranium oils from Madagascar are considered the finest available and have been the most researched for their therapeutic effects in recent years, distillations of geranium oils from Albania have also gained popular use and appreciation.

The effects of both the *roseum* and *graveolens* geranium oil are similar. Women have used geranium oil successfully for years to relieve premenstrual tension and menopausal symptoms. Geranium oil helps you navigate smoothly through natural hormonal cycles.

Geranium oil contains about sixty-seven compounds. The main constituents are citronellol (27 percent) and geraniol (13 percent). Clinical evaluations were conducted in Germany on the chemical components of geranium oil to understand the mechanism for why geranium oil is so effective in treating female hormonal imbalance. It was found that the alcohol geraniol had a balancing effect on the autonomic nervous system.

The autonomic nervous system is known to stimulate hormonal production and response. Balance of your autonomic nervous system is absolutely essential for maintaining a healthy and fully functioning human organism—body, mind and emotions.

Common symptoms of autonomic nervous system imbalance include headache, hot flashes, irregular heartbeat, nervousness, depression and anxiety.

According to Dr. Andrew Weil, medical vocabulary for imbalances of the autonomic nervous system practically do not exist in North American medicine. However, both Germany and Japan, two modern-day industrial giants, acknowledge the condition and use the term "vegetative dystonie."

Our modern-day lifestyle promotes living in a chronic state of stress while being subject to an increasing array of foreign and invasive environmental toxins. These two conditions are cited as primary causes of autonomic nervous system imbalance and the resulting hormonal disturbances.

Geranium oil's regulating properties act to have a wonderfully calming and uplifting effect on the human emotions and can be useful in promoting hormonal balance and relieving depression, nervousness, anxiety, confusion, lethargy, energy and mood swings, tearfulness and fear.

As with other adaptogenic essential oils, geranium oil acts to gently balance extreme states. Geranium oil is perfect to use when you're feeling out of sync with your own natural rhythms and need to reconnect with yourself.

Geranium oil's decongestant properties are helpful for relieving congestion of breast tissue and stimulating healthy circulation of blood and lymph flow for detoxifying the body. It can be helpful for promoting relief of constipation and fluid retention, as well as promoting digestion.

Geranium oil's hormonal balancing and detoxification effects can make it useful for overcoming addiction of all kinds. I recommend blending it with petitgrain and black pepper, which are the most helpful oils I've found for breaking bad habits.

An excellent skincare oil, geranium oil's astringent and cicatrizant properties make it effective for preventing signs of aging skin like wrinkling and sagging and can help tone facial muscles. Geranium oil can soften and even eliminate scars and dark age spots by improving blood circulation and the even distribution of melanin beneath the skin. Geranium oil is nourishing and balancing for all skin types including oily, dry or combination skin. Use it to soothe sensitive, problem or irritated skin. It may be useful for a variety of skin issues like ringworm, acne, burns, bruises, shingles, herpes, eczema and dermatitis.

Geranium oil blends well with many different oils including: clary sage, rose, sandalwood, frankincense, lavender and chamomile.

Dispense 1 to 3 drops of geranium oil on a cotton ball or smell strip, close your eyes and inhale. Note in your journal the aroma qualities you can discern and the effects the oil has on your body, mind, spirit and emotions.

CAUTION: Geranium oil can lower blood sugar and should be avoided in cases of hypoglycemia. Due to its hormonal effect, avoid geranium during pregnancy.

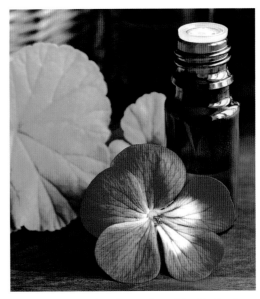

An excellent skin care oil, geranium oil is effective for preventing signs of aging.

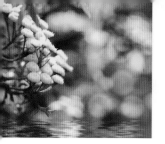

HELICHRYSUM ESSENTIAL OIL

(HELICHRYSUM ITALICUM): STEAM-DISTILLED FLOWERS
(PREMIUM BEST QUALITY) OR FLOWER AND LEAVES (SECOND QUALITY)—
NO. 1 INJURY HEALING, PAIN AND INFLAMMATION

Commonly referred to as Italian Everlasting or Immortelle, the best distillations of helichrysum italicum are grown and distilled in the Mediterranean climate of Corsica and southern France. There are over 600 known species of helichrysum.

Helichrysum italicum essential oil is the most powerful healing and regenerative oil in aromatherapy. Its scent is sweet, warm and radiant with a slight herbal top note. Its character is honey-like, delicate and light.

A gentle healing oil, helichrysum italicum is used primarily for tissue repair and healing. Its highly regenerative nature makes it one of the most powerful oils in aromatherapy for relieving inflammation.

Its reputation for preventing swelling and inflammation and alleviating pain and accelerating the formation of scar tissue is unsurpassed by any other essential oil.

Its powerful anti-inflammatory action makes helichrysum oil your first choice for soothing and healing inflamed tissues.

Helichrysum has been used for centuries in European countries. Some of its common uses include treatment for allergies, colds and cough, skin, liver and gallbladder problems, as well as for inflammation, control of infection and sleep issues.

Over the last decade, research studies have confirmed helichrysum italicum to have antimicrobial and anti-inflammatory properties. It was shown to be effective against bacteria like Staphylococcus aureus, as well as an effective antifungal agent against Candida albicans. It also inhibits the growth of HSV and HIV.

Helichrysum protects newly formed tissue. Studies demonstrated helichrysum italicum to inhibit and mediate the inflammatory cellular response in both humans and animals.

As a free-radical scavenger, helichrysum oil works by way of cell mediation to reabsorb cellular debris from areas of damaged tissue through your blood. This reabsorption process creates less pressure on nerves to relieve pain and swelling.

Helichrysum oil's remarkable anti-hematoma and tissue-regenerating activity are superior to any other essential oil. I've seen helichrysum oil completely heal a massive and swollen contusion that covered the chin of an adult woman who had fallen onto concrete. The contusion was swollen, painful and tender to the touch and a deep black, purplish color. Only two days after the application of pure helichrysum oil (3 to 4 times daily) directly onto the bruise, it was no longer swollen or painful and only slightly visible as a faint yellowish color. My client and I were completely amazed by the rapid healing results she experienced.

A circulatory stimulant, helichrysum promotes circulation in areas of stagnation and blockage and is helpful for stimulating the growth of liver cell formation and enhancing lymphatic flow.

Through enhancing circulation of blood, lymph and nerve supply, helichrysum oil is helpful for mending fractures and broken bones and the formation of new tissue. Use helichrysum to promote healing of bumps and bruises, tendinitis, carpal tunnel syndrome, cuts and scrapes, scars, stretch marks and hemorrhoids.

Helichrysum oil's effect on the circulatory system may help to regulate blood cholesterol and reduce hypertension.

It is excellent as a massage lubricant to speed healing of soft tissue injuries and to relieve muscle aches and pains and joint stiffness.

Helichrysum oil blends well with many different oils including bergamot, clary sage, clove, geranium, lemon, peppermint, sweet orange, mandarin, spikenard, thyme and ylang ylang.

Dispense 1 to 3 drops helichrysum oil on a cotton ball or smell strip, close your eyes and inhale. Note in your journal the aroma qualities you can discern and the effects the oil has on your body, mind, spirit and emotions.

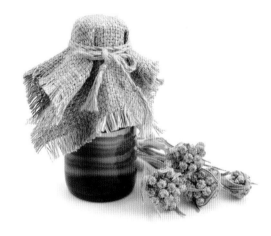

Highly regenerative helichrysum oil has a sweet, warm scent.

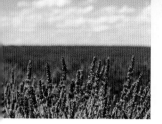

LAVENDER ESSENTIAL OIL

(*LAVANDULA ANGUSTIFOLIA*): STEAM-DISTILLED FLOWERS AT HIGH ALTITUDE—THE UNIVERSAL HEALER

Some of the best locations for growing and distilling lavender oil are France, Bulgaria and Italy.

One of the most well-loved and frequently used oils in aromatherapy, lavender is highly scented. It has a distinctly sweet, clean, fresh and floral-spice scent with herbal and woody notes that are freeing to the senses.

Distilling lavender at a high altitude allows for lower temperatures and lower pressure for distillation of the oil, which allows the volatile phytochemicals to come through and be present in the final product.

Lavender oil was first cultivated in the high mountains of Persia and the south of France where it thrives in barren environments. As a plant adapts to the environmental conditions it grows in, it develops the characteristics and properties that help it to survive in its natural environment. Indigenous healers understood this wisdom of nature. When looking for suitable preventatives and remedies for illness and disease, they looked for plants that grew well in areas with similar conditions as the symptoms of an illness or disease they were treating.

For instance, lavender's hearty and robust characteristics allow it to thrive in harsh, barren environments, giving it a natural power to act as a universal healer. It can be used to treat and balance almost any condition and promote healing. It's no wonder that lavender oil is recommended to be kept on hand at home and at work.

As lavender oil has such a broad-spectrum application, it can be beneficial for treating a wide assortment of wounds, as well as for relieving inflammation. Conditions like fever blisters, herpes outbreaks, rheumatism, sore muscles and back pain respond favorably to lavender oil.

Its analgesic and antispasmodic properties make it useful for relieving common aches and pains like headaches, especially sinus headaches.

Its calmative action makes lavender oil effective as a first aid treatment for motion sickness. It can be blended with peppermint or ginger oil to enhance this effect. This same calming action makes lavender useful for relieving premenstrual tension, alleviating insomnia and promoting restful sleep.

Lavender oil has also been used to treat urinary tract and bladder infections. Its antiseptic properties make it an effective treatment for vaginal yeast infection when used as a douche. Blending it with tea tree or juniper berry oil can enhance this effect.

With a reputation for alleviating hot, inflamed conditions (remember the environment it thrives in), lavender oil is an absolute classic for treating burns. Its regenerative and healing properties stimulate tissue repair.

Though the actual events of the story of Gattefossé's burn (page 20) vary from the popular myth, it still shows the incredible power of lavender oil as one of the best essential oils for treating burns.

Lavender oil is a key ingredient in all of my formulas for treating various types of burns.

Its antidepressant and sedative properties make lavender oil excellent for balancing the mood and extreme emotional states such as depression, shock, rage, panic, nervousness, stress, fear, frustration, jealousy, impatience and irritability. Lavender essential oil has been used to help insomnia.

Its fresh, uplifting scent supports the development and growth of inner freedom from compulsive-type behaviors. As with many essential oils, lavender can be used to help break bad mental habits like a harsh inner critic or negative self-talk.

Lavender oil is excellent for skincare and promotes healing and regeneration for all skin types, especially dry, inflamed or cracked skin. Its anti-inflammatory properties make it useful for treating any hot, inflamed condition like rashes, acne, eczema, boils, dermatitis, leg ulcers and psoriasis.

Lavender is an immune stimulant and has been used to strengthen the body's immune system. Used as a popular preventative for bronchitis, cold and flu researchers are conducting studies to learn if lavender and other pure essential oils may be effective against the super bug MRSA (Methicillin-resistant Staphylococcus aureus), among other strains of bacteria.

Lavender oil's antiviral properties make it useful as a treatment for cold sores and herpes. Blend it with other oils with antiviral properties like thyme and clove oil.

Lavender oil blends well with many different oils including bergamot, clary sage, clove, geranium, lemon, peppermint, sweet orange, mandarin, spikenard, thyme and ylang ylang.

Dispense 1 to 3 drops of lavender oil on a cotton ball or smell strip, close your eyes and inhale. Note in your journal the aroma qualities you can discern and the effects the oil has on your body, mind, spirit and emotions.

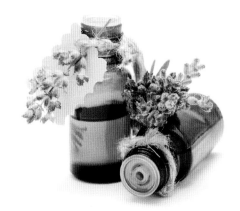

Its antidepressent and sedative properties make lavender oil excellent for balancing the mood and extreme emotions.

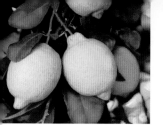

LEMON ESSENTIAL OIL

(*CITRUS LIMONUM*): COLD-PRESSED PEEL—BODY AND BRAIN TONIC

Genuinely reminiscent of the clean, fresh scent of fresh fruit, the aroma of lemon peel is sharp, sweet, fruity, light and fresh. The Mediterranean climate and Italian soil produces the finest lemon oil with a superior scent.

As with all citrus oils, lemon essential oil is extracted by cold-pressing (expressing) the fresh lemon peel. This oil is fluid, and its color is pale yellow. When used in cooking, lemon oil adds an unmistakable tart, tangy and scintillating flavor to all of your recipes.

As pure lemon oil comes from the fresh fruit peel, you should consider only purchasing oil that has been GC/MS tested and grown without the use of pesticides.

Lemon oil's powerful tonic action strengthens and enlivens the body and rapidly fires up your metabolism and fat-burning cells.

Its immuno-stimulant properties stimulate the flow of blood and lymph circulation to effectively promote cleansing and detoxification of the body when you're losing weight.

Research studies on lemon oil's anti-stress and antidepressant action has been well documented. A study conducted on lavender, rose and lemon essential oil showed that lemon oil had the strongest anti-stress effect of the three oils. It was also shown that lemon oil had an antidepressant-like effect and significantly accelerated the metabolic rate governed by the hippocampus, as well as the action of the prefrontal cortex for rational thinking.

Other research conducted to learn about the effect of aroma on the brain discovered that lemon oil activates the center of the hippocampus and triggers left-brain, rational thinking. Inhaling the scent of lemon oil was shown to short-circuit your emotional triggers, which can help prevent cravings for sweets and second helpings.

Lemon oil energizes and refreshes your body and mind and increases your ability to focus and memorize. In times of confusion, or when needing clarity to make decisions, lemon oil can be a great aid.

Japanese scientists studied the effect of lemon essential oil on the ability to focus. They discovered that the typical mistakes were reduced by 54 percent when lemon oil was diffused into the workroom.

These studies demonstrate that lemon oil's tonic action enlivens your brain, relieves fatigue and increases your physical energy and stamina.

Psycho-emotionally, the smell of lemon oil relieves mental heaviness and feelings of being burdened or weighed down by life's responsibilities. Lemon oil is helpful for allaying reactive emotional outbursts that can be detrimental to developing healthy relationships with others.

Lemon oil stimulates the body's immune system by activating white blood cell formation. It can be relied upon for protection against colds and the flu!

A powerful germicide, lemon oil's antiseptic properties act to prevent or inhibit the spread of infections.

Fox News reported that over fifty hospitals across the United States are using pure essential oils; "They claim that not only do essential oils improve the smell of hospitals, relieving patients of 'bad smell association,' but also raise the morale of workers and ward off infections."

Use lemon oil in your aroma diffuser to purify the air or in your household cleaning spray to disinfect surface areas. Lemon essential oil can be effective for destroying airborne bugs in hospital rooms, schools and waiting rooms. Hospitals in Europe routinely diffuse lemon oil into the air to reduce the chance of the spread of viruses and bacteria.

Lemon oil's powerful antiseptic action makes it effective for treating Candida yeast overgrowth. A 2014 study showed that lemon oil could be used as a very effective natural remedy against candidiasis caused by *C. albicans*. Use lemon oil for treating colds and flu, Candida overgrowth, bronchitis or as a gargle for sore throat.

Lemon oils may be useful for treating circulatory problems such as "spider" veins or broken capillaries. Its tonic action is helpful for strengthening the heart and increasing blood circulation.

(continued)

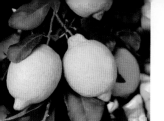

LEMON ESSENTIAL OIL

(*CITRUS LIMONUM*): COLD-PRESSED PEEL—BODY AND BRAIN TONIC

It may be helpful for relieving heartburn and neutralizing a high-acid pH condition in the body. Lemon oil's cleansing action makes it useful in blends for liver regeneration and detoxification.

Recently, research on limonene, a chemical component of lemon oil, was documented to have a range of influences on receptor-mediated processes showing it to be preventative and curative for breast cancer in rats.

Lemon oil has been shown to be effective for controlling acne and treating oily skin and scalp conditions such as seborrhea and dandruff. It may also be helpful for treating itchy and flaky skin conditions like psoriasis.

Lemon oil is a top note and adds lift to any blend. It blends well with many different oils including all the citrus, wood and spice oils.

Dispense 1 to 3 drops of oil on a cotton ball or smell strip, close your eyes and inhale. Note in your journal the aroma qualities you can discern and the effects the oil has on your body, mind, spirit and emotions.

CAUTION: Lemon oil may be a skin irritant, as well as a photosensitizer. Avoid sunlight after skin application for twelve hours.

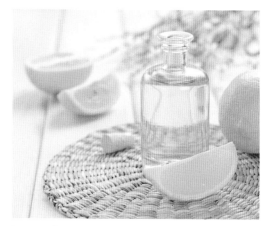

Lemon oil's powerful antiseptic action makes it effective for candida yeast overgrowth.

PEPPERMINT ESSENTIAL OIL

(MENTHA X PIPERITA): STEAM-DISTILLED FLOWERING TOPS—
ENERGY, FOCUS SUPPORT AND ANALGESIC (PAIN RELIEF)

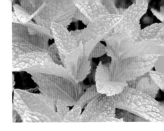

One of the best locations for growing and distilling peppermint oil is the United States.

Everyone can recognize the scent of peppermint oil. Considered a basic necessity for your aromatherapy first aid kit, peppermint oil is a fluid, colorless oil with a clean, fresh, minty scent that is distinctly penetrating. It's similar to smelling peppermint candy.

Peppermint oil is an adaptogenic oil, meaning that it acts to regulate excess conditions and can have a relaxing or invigorating effect depending on the circumstance for which you are using it.

Inhale peppermint oil for almost instant relief of nausea. It is also excellent for staying alert and helping you to focus when prolonged concentration and attention are needed.

Peppermint oil is known to clear brain fog and works better than coffee as a stimulant. Great for helping to improve your ability to focus and sustain attention, use peppermint oil when you need to get going fast. Inhale peppermint oil first thing in the morning instead of having a cup of coffee.

A research study on both peppermint and cinnamon oil showed the effect of each oil on drivers was to relax tension and relieve fatigue while increasing alertness. Additionally, peppermint oil was also linked to minimizing driver frustration.

I've used peppermint oil in my metaphysical healing practice to help clients strengthen their inner will when they were having challenges with following through and taking consistent action to achieve their goals. I recommend using peppermint oil when you are in the planning stages of an important project.

A definite pick-me-up oil, use peppermint to break through negative habits like procrastination or when you're feeling lethargic. Peppermint is also good for memory retention. Use it alone or in a blend with lemon oil when completing a work project or homework assignment or when studying for an exam.

A powerful analgesic pain reliever, use peppermint oil to relieve your sore and achy muscles and joints. Add peppermint oil to a footbath to relieve swollen ankles and feet. Research has shown peppermint oil to be effective for relieving migraines and tension headaches resulting from weak or poor digestion.

Peppermint oil's powerful astringent properties also make it a good blood cleanser. These same astringent properties make peppermint oil a powerful cleanser in your home or work environment. Similar to lemon in its action, peppermint is excellent for cutting and removing grease and grime deposits. It has been used

(continued)

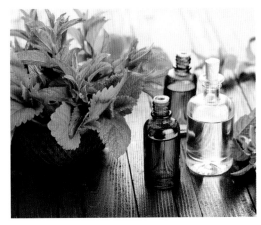

Inhale peppermint oil for almost instant relief of nausea.

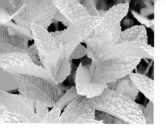

PEPPERMINT ESSENTIAL OIL

(*MENTHA X PIPERITA*): STEAM-DISTILLED FLOWERING TOPS—
ENERGY, FOCUS SUPPORT AND ANALGESIC (PAIN RELIEF)

for generations by energy healers to protect against picking up "bad vibes" and is excellent for anyone who is especially sensitive and prone to picking up environmental psychic toxins.

Peppermint's antiseptic and antibacterial properties are effective for treating minor cuts or abrasions to prevent infection.

Peppermint oil has been reported to repel insects like ants and mosquitoes. In fact, one published research study showed peppermint oil to repel insects like the Dengue-fever-infecting mosquitoes.

Its decongestant properties make peppermint one of my first choices for relieving congestion of any kind, including sinus congestion. Inhale peppermint oil's lovely sweet, fresh, penetrating, candy-cane scent for immediate relief of congested sinus cavities.

Peppermint oil is one of the most powerful vasoconstrictors in aromatherapy. Its anti-inflammatory properties and action to constrict and narrow the blood vessels make it excellent for cooling inflamed, hot conditions like hot flashes and tired and achy legs, hands and feet. Use it topically for relieving acne or as a mouthwash to relieve swollen gums and mouth ulcers.

An antiemetic research finding showed inhalation of peppermint oil was effective for relieving pregnancy related symptoms of nausea and vomiting. Another 2012 review showed both ginger and peppermint to be effective for pregnancy-related nausea.

In a 2014 study, peppermint oil was shown to be as effective for stimulating hair growth as Minoxidil (an over-the-counter hair loss product). The study showed that the topical application of peppermint oil, when compared to saline, jojoba oil and Minoxidil, stimulated the most hair growth and resulted in an increase in dermal thickness, follicle number and follicle depth with no signs of toxicity.

Research studies have also shown that the use of peppermint can reduce some symptoms of IBS (Irritable Bowel Syndrome). Another study for stomach pain supported peppermint's use showing that enteric-coated peppermint oil capsules improved IBS symptoms in children.

Peppermint oil blends well with many different oils, including black pepper, ginger, lavender, lemongrass, rosemary, basil, lemon, cinnamon and juniper berry.

Dispense 1 to 3 drops of peppermint oil on a cotton ball or smell strip, close your eyes and inhale. Note in your journal the aroma qualities you can discern and the effects the oil has on your body, mind, spirit and emotions.

CAUTION: Peppermint cools by constricting your blood capillaries; therefore, please use in extremely weak dilutions. One or two drops in a dispersant added to your bath water is sufficient for experiencing beneficial results. Research indicates that peppermint oil may aggravate GERD (gastroesophageal reflux disease), a type of heart burn. Due to its strong cooling action, peppermint should not be used by children under two and a half years of age.

ROMAN CHAMOMILE ESSENTIAL OIL

(*ANTHEMIS NOBILIS*, SYNONYM: *CHAMAEMELUM NOBILE*):
STEAM-DISTILLED FLOWERS—CALMING AND PAIN RELIEVER

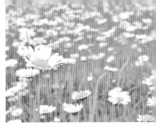

Chamomile oil comes from one of the most well-loved herbs in the Western world. It is considered one of the "Nine Sacred Herbs" of the ancient Anglo-Saxon manuscript, the Lacnunga. It must be noted that the characteristics of the chamomile essential oil and the herb, though having similarities, can prove quite different in some of their effects.

The two plants from which the chamomile oil is distilled are the more popular German chamomile (*Matricaria recutita*), which has been in use for more than 3,000 years, and Roman or English chamomile (*Anthemis nobilis*). Although these two oils belong to different species, they are often used for symptomatic relief of the same health complaints.

Both oils are used to calm emotional upsets and soothe the nerves and nervous conditions like headache and sleep disturbances.

Other common applications include digestive issues and stomach problems like indigestion, gastritis, diarrhea, ulcers, IBS, mouth ulcers and toothache.

Both chamomile oils have analgesic and antispasmodic properties, making them helpful for relieving musculoskeletal conditions like muscle spasms, arthritis, rheumatism, sprains and inflamed joints.

The calming and soothing anti-inflammatory properties of both oils make them useful for treating any type of red, inflamed or irritated skin condition like acne, boils, bumps, cuts, scrapes and bruises, burns, dermatitis, rash, eczema, psoriasis and sensitive, dry, itchy or flaky skin.

Both oils are helpful for treating mild to chronic infections as they stimulate the production of white blood cells and support the immune function.

Psycho-emotionally, Roman chamomile calms the emotions and relieves tension. It can be helpful for relieving anger, oversensitivity, sleeplessness and depression.

Roman chamomile oil is a lovely scented oil on its own. In a blend, use with more gently soothing and emotionally supportive oils like helichrysum, lavender, bergamot, rose, neroli, melissa, sandalwood, frankincense, geranium, red mandarin, spikenard, vetiver and ylang ylang.

Dispense 1 to 3 drops of Roman chamomile oil onto a cotton ball or smell strip, close your eyes and inhale. Note in your journal the aroma qualities you can discern, and the effects the oil has on your body, mind, spirit and emotions.

CAUTION: Roman chamomile may make asthma and some allergies worse, so people with known sensitivities should not use it. If you're unsure if you have a sensitivity, do a skin patch test. Although Roman chamomile can be quite helpful for pregnant moms, never use it during the first three months of pregnancy without the supervision of a qualified health professional as it may induce menstruation and/or premature labor due to its emmenagogue and uterotonic side effects.

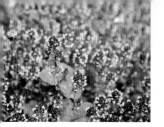

SWEET MARJORAM ESSENTIAL OIL

(ORIGANUM MARJORANA): STEAM-DISTILLED FLOWERS AND LEAVES—
ANTISPASMODIC; RESTORATIVE PAIN RELIEVER

One of the best locations for growing and distilling marjoram essential oil is Egypt.

Smelling just like the fresh herb, sweet marjoram oil has a fresh, warm, radiant, spicy and balsamic scent with camphoraceous and woody notes.

Indigenous to Cyprus and southern Turkey, folklore has it that sweet marjoram was a symbol of happiness to the Greeks and Romans. There is another legend from early Greek mythology that Aphrodite, the goddess of love, grew marjoram and used it as a love potion.

Stories passed down to us from antiquity often have some element of truth to them. In the case of sweet marjoram, objective evaluation of scientific evidence compiled from numerous research databases worldwide and published in more than fifty scientific journals reported sweet marjoram to be effective as an antioxidant, anticoagulant and anti-diabetic aid, as well as having antimicrobial, fertility, gastroprotective and neurologic effects in the central nervous system.

Sweet marjoram is one of the most relaxing and comforting oils in aromatherapy. As an adaptogenic oil, it acts to regulate and balance extreme conditions depending upon the purpose for which it's used.

Its antispasmodic and restorative properties act to calm and restore the nervous system. Sweet marjoram may be used as an effective treatment for relieving symptoms of chronic fatigue and fibromyalgia.

Sweet marjoram may be helpful for releasing long-held mental and emotional patterns of deep tension. Blend with clary sage oil to enhance this effect.

It can be helpful for relieving anxiety and panic attacks, stress, physical and emotional exhaustion, as well as insomnia.

Sweet marjoram oil's stimulant and antispasmodic properties make it an excellent addition to your favorite sports massage blend for relieving muscular aches and pain. It may be especially useful for relieving chronic tension in the upper back and neck areas.

It may be helpful for relieving migraine and tension headaches.

Sweet marjoram oil blends well with clary sage, ginger, helichrysum, cypress, lemongrass, peppermint, lavender, ylang ylang and black pepper.

Dispense 1 to 3 drops of marjoram oil on a cotton ball or smell strip, close your eyes and inhale. Note in your journal the aroma qualities you can discern and the effects the oil has on your body, mind, spirit and emotions.

CAUTION: As marjoram is a stimulant, it should be avoided during pregnancy.

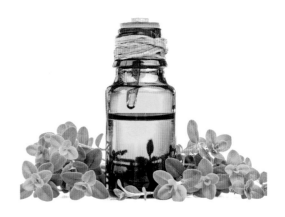

Sweet marjoram oil may be helpful for releasing deep tension.

TEA TREE ESSENTIAL OIL

(*MELALEUCA ALTERNIFOLIA*): STEAM-DISTILLED LEAF—
POWERFUL ANTIFUNGAL

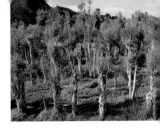

One of the best locations in the world to grow and distill tea tree is Australia.

The smell of tea tree is fresh, penetrating, warm, spicy and camphoraceous with slight herbal notes. Another of the first aid oils to consider having on hand, the pungent, antiseptic and medicinal scent of tea tree oil is well tolerated by most individuals. In recent years, it has become a popular panacea for many common ailments, most especially foot and toenail fungus.

In 1770, Captain James Cook of the H.M.S. Endeavor landed in Australia near where Sydney is located today. Captain Cook drank an infusion of tea from a native shrub he called "tea tree."

Tea tree's reputed antiseptic properties make it the first choice of essential oils by many when treating both chronic and acute bacterial and fungal infections.

The continued studies by research scientists to learn if essential oils are effective against the super bug Methicillin-resistant Staphylococcus aureus (MRSA), among other strains of bacteria, include a project using a hand and body wash containing essential oils of lavender and tea tree. Lavender and tea tree oil contain proven antibacterial agents.

In 1979, French physician Paul Belaiche published his extensive in-vitro research on the antimicrobial effects of essential oils with his successful clinical findings. One of his studies was on the use of tea tree to effectively treat vaginal yeast infections caused by Candida albicans. Dr. Belaiche discovered that in most cases, vaginal yeast infections could be treated effectively without the use of conventional medical treatments that resulted in unwanted side effects.

Another research study showed that tea tree oil is useful for treating Trichomoniasis, a common cause of vaginitis. In 1962, an American study of 130 women treated using tea tree oil recovered from this infection.

Research on treating oral pathogens in dental health showed tea tree to have beneficial effects on gingivitis but not plaque. Tea tree oil was shown to have significant antimicrobial effects against common oral pathogens.

(continued)

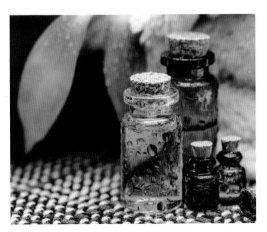

Tea tree oil is the first choice by many when treating chronic and acute bacterial and fungal infections.

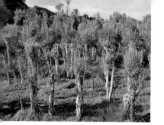

TEA TREE ESSENTIAL OIL

(*MELALEUCA ALTERNIFOLIA*): STEAM-DISTILLED LEAF—
POWERFUL ANTIFUNGAL

As an immune stimulant, tea tree oil promotes and strengthens the body's immune system by stimulating the formation of white blood cells. A study showed that, if given oral tea tree oil, rats infected with a pathogenic protozoa lived longer. The oral dosage of tea tree also modified the immune response, but did not cure them. An animal study using topical tea tree oil mixed with DMSO (a solvent that allows whatever it's mixed with to penetrate the skin) showed the mixture to inhibit the growth of established skin cancer cells.

Antiviral properties make tea tree effective for preventing and inhibiting viruses like cold sores and herpes outbreaks. Its anti-infectious properties make tea tree helpful for balancing sebum production and relieving skin conditions like acne. It is also effective for treating bladder infections, bronchitis and sinusitis.

As a decongestant and analgesic pain reliever, tea tree oil is helpful for relieving cold and flu symptoms.

Psycho-emotionally, tea tree oil promotes self-confidence in one's ability to negotiate disagreements with others without feeling threatened.

It is also reported to be helpful for relieving insect, scorpion and snake bites.

Tea tree blends with many oils, including Himalayan cedarwood, black pepper, ginger, lavender, myrrh, thyme, oregano, eucalyptus, rosemary and lemon.

Dispense 1 to 3 drops of tea tree oil on a cotton ball or smell strip, close your eyes and inhale. Note in your journal the aroma qualities you can discern and the effects the oil has on your body, mind, spirit and emotions.

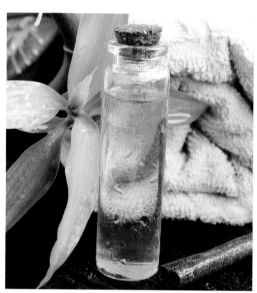

Tea tree oil is made from the leaves of the tea tree, not to be confused with tea plants used for black and green teas.

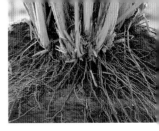

VETIVER ESSENTIAL OIL

(*VETIVERIA ZIZANIOIDES*): WILD-CRAFTED, HYDRODIFFUSED ROOT
(STAINLESS)—GROUNDING AND STABILIZING

One of the best locations in the world to grow and distill vetiver is Haiti.

A thick, resinous oil, vetiver's aroma is sweet, earthy, balsamic, smoky and woody with exotic, spicy and sensual overtones. There is a rare and mysterious quality to the fragrance of an artistically distilled vetiver oil. Its deep and rich allure is captivating.

If you're a nervous or high-strung and emotionally sensitive soul, then look to vetiver to calm and settle you. Though vetiver has notable physical properties and effects, for me its strength lies in its distinctive psycho-emotional effects.

There's a purity of intent to reassure and comfort you that comes through when you inhale the earthy scent of vetiver. It's like the reassuring hug from your grandmother that lets you know everything is okay. When you're feeling uncertain, inhale the scent of vetiver oil. It will help you feel still and quiet inside.

I prefer the wild-crafted, hydrodiffused specimen from Haiti. Other distillations using cast iron just do not convey the essence of what the plant offers aromatically.

The hydrodistilled specimen in stainless steel is an excellent example of how this oil should smell: sweet, earthy, rich and lovely. The traditional iron-distilled vetiver oil most commonly in use has a burnt after-odor that distracts from the full-bodied depth and loveliness of the vetiver plant when artfully distilled.

The strong and hearty roots of this tropical grass reach deep into the earth. Many countries plant vetiver for protection against soil erosion. Vetiver can tolerate and survive even the severest conditions. Vetiver oil imparts this same ability to strengthen, ground and support you through life's severest trials.

Harvesting the roots for a single pound (454 g) of material for the distillation of an essential oil can require the removal of 1,000 pounds (454 kg) of earth or more.

I absolutely love vetiver oil and have frequently relied upon it in my aromatherapy practice. Its regulating properties make it very versatile for relieving a variety of issues. For instance, its sedative and relaxant properties help to deepen cellular respiration and make it useful for promoting rest and relaxation and helpful as a sleep aid.

Its well-documented action as an immune and circulatory stimulant in controlled experiments explains its ability to promote the production of red blood cells and why it is so useful for relieving stress and tension held deep within the physical body.

Vetiver is especially helpful when feeling vulnerable and needing help dealing with long-term, stressful situations. Its restorative and revitalizing properties act to stabilize and promote relief of chronic stress, anxiety or panic.

(continued)

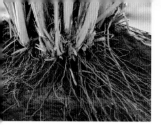

VETIVER ESSENTIAL OIL

(*VETIVERIA ZIZANIOIDES*): WILD-CRAFTED, HYDRODIFFUSED ROOT (STAINLESS)—GROUNDING AND STABILIZING

"Do not be afraid to love. Without love, life is impossible." —Thich Nhat Hanh

A common issue for many clients that has become a general concern in our modern world is the tendency to close off the heart's energies as a way protect against feeling vulnerable. Your heart is your organ of love and is for giving and receiving love. It is through your heart that you can connect to and share with others in mutually beneficial and satisfying ways. Vetiver oil helps you to gently reopen your heart and allow the sharing of love, so that you get the love and support you need to face life's challenges. You don't have to go it alone!

Vetiver oil strongly resonates with the Muladhara or root (first) chakra—the energy center for your survival instincts that connects you with a sense of belonging, community roots and feeling at home on Mother Earth. Vetiver oil reconnects and energizes your natural, instinctual sense of self and can be helpful for relieving symptoms of old, unprocessed grief, shock and trauma.

If you have hidden, subconscious patterns that block you from feeling connected, vetiver oil's tranquil and evocative beauty can help soften any resistance to facing repressed fears or shadows about survival.

Interestingly, a strong dislike or aversion to vetiver's aroma may be the result of negative associations with natural animal instincts or an imbalanced Vata Dosha. In Ayurveda—an ancient system of healing codified and practiced in India for thousands of years—the doshas are derived from the Five Elements and their related properties. Vata is composed of Space and Air, Pitta of Fire and Water and Kapha of Earth and Water.

Its analgesic, antispasmodic and anti-inflammatory properties make vetiver useful for relieving muscle aches and pains and joint stiffness.

Vetiver oil's cicatrizant properties make it helpful for skin cell rejuvenation and healing, as well for hair, skin and scalp reconditioning.

Vetiver oil works well as a stand-alone oil or blends well with a variety of oils. It is especially helpful when blended with citrus oils to relieve symptoms of panic that arise when cleansing and detoxifying from substance abuse or addiction.

Use vetiver oil when you need to anchor a blend or need a lower base note. Try blending with bergamot, petitgrain, clary sage, clove, geranium, lemon, peppermint, sweet orange, mandarin, spikenard, thyme, ylang ylang and galbanum.

Dispense 1 to 3 drops of vetiver oil on a cotton ball or smell strip, close your eyes and inhale. Note in your journal the aroma qualities you can discern and the effects the oil has on your body, mind, spirit and emotions.

YLANG YLANG ESSENTIAL OIL

(*CANANGA ODORATA*): STEAM-DISTILLED FLOWERS—
BEAUTY OIL; NEUTRALIZES NEGATIVITY

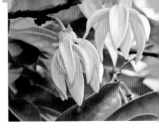

The ylang ylang tree originated in the Philippines and was developed for the aromatherapy trade as a perfume oil. Today, one of the best locations for growing and distilling ylang ylang is the Reunion Islands, Madagascar.

Pronounced "eelang," ylang ylang is sweet, floral, balsamic, exotic and sensual and in the Malayan language means "flower of flowers." It is one of the best essential oils for promoting a balanced nervous system and neutralizing negative mental chatter. It is one of the best oils in aromatherapy to enhance beauty at all levels—body, mind, heart and soul.

A decidedly sensuous aroma, ylang ylang oil's soft and sweet scent has a mesmerizing and intoxicating quality. It is what I imagine a perfect dream from your angels might smell like.

It is customary in Indonesia for newlyweds to find the pale yellow blossoms of the ylang ylang tree scattered on their marriage bed as a blessing for lasting love and happiness.

The cultivated ylang ylang tree develops its fragrance more fully than one that is left to grow alone on its own. Left unattended, the blossoms of the ylang ylang tree can have little or no scent. Trimming trees every couple of months allows the fragrance to develop fully. As with other delicate flowers like jasmine and rose, the blossoms must be harvested early in the morning and immediately prepared for steam distillation.

Ylang ylang is often distilled in what is called "fractions" or parts, meaning the distillation process is halted during different stages of distillation. At each completed stage of distillation the oils gathered are taken out of the collection chamber. Then the distillation process is continued.

As with all oils, the quality of distillation varies among distillers and is influenced by crop conditions for that season and the moment chosen for harvesting and distillation. The distiller's art for the production of exquisite oils is rare and reflected in the price of an oil.

There are at least three fractions of ylang ylang collected during distillation. A fraction is a part of a distallation or a stage in the distillation process. The first distillation is the lightest. It is considered the most ethereal fragrance and is often most prized by perfumers. The stages of distillation are determined according to principles not easily defined, but generally they are broken down by the production time it takes to distill each fraction.

My personal preference of all the ylang ylang fractions gathered in the distillation process is the last fraction that is called ylang ylang III. It is less fluid, less intensely sweet, earthier and round, and has the most stabilizing effect on the nervous system.

YLANG YLANG OIL DISTILLATION CATEGORIES

Ylang ylang extra is the first fraction collected during the extraction process. It is usually the perfumers first choice and the most expensive distillation of the ylang ylang flower.

The next fractions collected are ylang ylang I, II and III, followed by ylang ylang complete, which is the complete distillation of the oil without interruption into fractions or parts.

(continued)

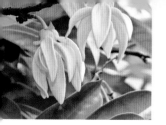

YLANG YLANG ESSENTIAL OIL

(CANANGA ODORATA): STEAM-DISTILLED FLOWERS—
BEAUTY OIL; NEUTRALIZES NEGATIVITY

Ylang ylang is high in sesquiterpenes. Sesquiterpenes are a class of chemical compounds commonly found in higher plants that give ylang ylang its powerfully sedative and antispasmodic properties.

Ylang ylang III, the last fraction collected during distillation, has a slightly thicker viscosity and an earthier and less intensely sweet scent. Ylang ylang III is composed almost entirely of sesquiterpene compounds.

Sesquiterpene compounds are known to stimulate the liver and endocrine glands. Ylang ylang essential oil also supports kidney and adrenal function and is good for weak knees and bladder control. Metaphysically, issues with the kidneys and bladder are related to excess emotion or fear that weakens the kidney and bladder function.

Inhalation of ylang ylang oil is useful for calming the nervous system and dispelling fear and anxiety. It is the first essential oil to consider when needing help to regulate and balance an over-stimulated nervous system. In my healing arts practice, it is common to see chronic lower back pain to result in those who experience ongoing anxiety, stress and fear.

Ylang ylang has the ability to help deepen cellular respiration and normalize breathing patterns which is helpful for treating panic attacks.

Research studies show that ylang ylang oil stimulates the central nervous system and helps alleviate depression.

A 2006 study performed in Thailand investigated the effects of ylang ylang oil on human physiology after transdermal absorption of ylang ylang oil. Forty healthy volunteers participated in the controlled experiments to assess skin temperature, pulse rate, breathing rate and blood pressure. The research showed that ylang ylang oil caused a significant decrease in blood pressure, as well as an increase in skin temperature. The participants using ylang yang oil reported feeling more calm and relaxed. The report concluded that these findings show some evidence that the usage of ylang ylang oil can cause relief of depression and stress in humans.

These results help explain why ylang ylang oil has been used successfully to soothe tachycardia and hypertension.

Ylang ylang oil's analgesic, anti-inflammatory, antispasmodic and sedative properties make it effective as a massage lubricant to relieve muscle aches and pains. It's also useful for relieving menopausal and PMS complaints like mood swings, nervousness, irritability and premenstrual cramps.

Ylang ylang oil is useful for calming the nervous system and dispelling fear and anxiety.

The concept of balancing the flow of yin and yang energies, as in Chinese medicine, is helpful for understanding ylang ylang oil's psycho-emotional effect on the nervous system and emotions. Ylang ylang's aroma is distinctly feminine, or yin. For this reason, when you are in an excessive masculine, or yang, state, inhalation of ylang ylang oil can serve to bring balance.

Ylang ylang oil stimulates the flow of emotion and enjoyment. It can be helpful for relieving any tendency to overexert yourself and helps you to relax your mind. When your mind is relaxed and open, you will naturally feel less anxious and more self-confident.

Often used in men's fragrances, ylang ylang oil is healing to the male psyche and supports the expression of emotional connection and intuition.

A cicatrizant, ylang ylang oil promotes wound healing and the formation of new skin cell tissues. It is often used in the beauty and skincare industry. Its regulating and balancing properties help balance sebum production, and it is suitable for all skin types. Its anti-infectious and antibacterial properties make it useful for preventing and controlling acne outbreaks. I use ylang ylang oil often in skincare formulations to harmonize the skin.

These same regenerative qualities make ylang ylang useful for stimulating new hair growth. I use it in hair care formulations to stop hair loss, as well as to address underlying issues of stress and to boost self-confidence. Simply add a drop of ylang ylang oil to your favorite shampoo or conditioner to experience benefits.

Ylang ylang oil blends well with many different oils or may be enjoyed as a single note on its own. For men's fragrances, blend with spice and wood oils like sandalwood, cedarwood, black spruce, thyme, cinnamon and cypress.

Dispense 1 to 3 drops of ylang ylang oil on a cotton ball or smell strip, close your eyes and inhale. Note in your journal the aroma qualities you can discern and the effects the oil has on your body, mind, spirit and emotions

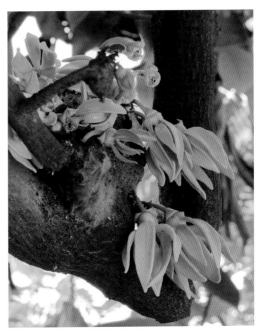

Often used in men's fragrances, ylang ylang oil is healing to the male psyche.

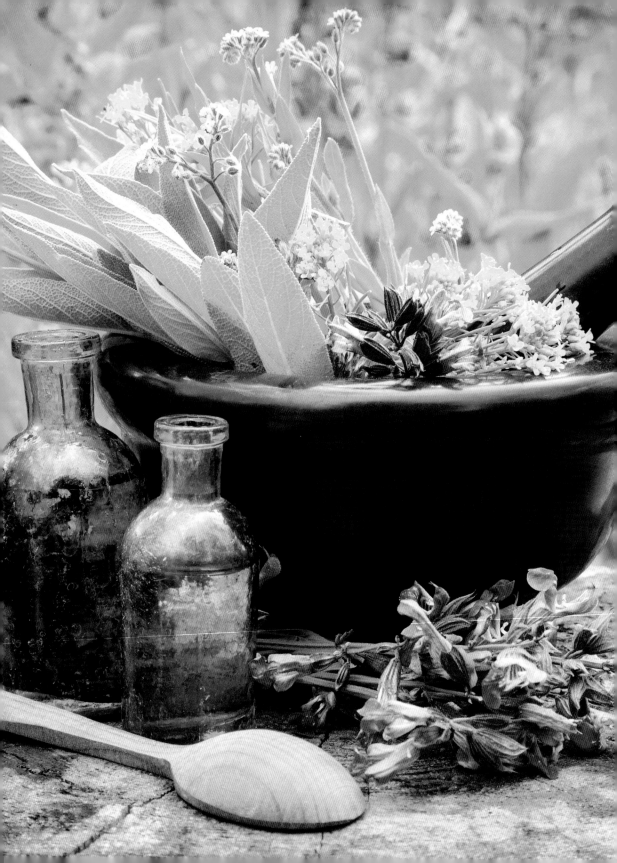

CHAPTER 7

Supplemental Oils

AMMI VISNAGA ESSENTIAL OIL (KHELLA PLANT SEEDS)

(AMMI VISNAGA): STEAM-DISTILLED HERB—NATURAL BRONCHODILATOR

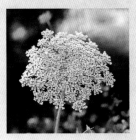 The best locations for growing and distilling *ammi visnaga* essential oil are Morocco and Egypt.

A native plant of North Africa, the ammi visnaga seed has been used in traditional herbal medicine for many years. The ammi visnaga seed has been used traditionally as an herbal remedy for treating kidney stones. It grows wild in the Middle East and Mediterranean regions and has been naturalized for growing in Australia and South America.

Ammi visnaga's slightly sweet, fresh, herbal and camphoraceous scent has subtle earthy and faintly dry, tea-like lower notes. Its antispasmodic, relaxant and bronchial dilating properties give ammi visnaga oil its potent ability to be useful for relieving asthma attacks.

Consider using ammi visnaga oil for relieving asthma symptoms, especially bronchial type, as well as allergies. Ammi visnaga may also be useful as a preventative for asthma attacks, as well as for relieving an attack by relaxing bronchial spasms.

Research shows ammi visnaga may decrease allergic reactions by stabilizing mast cell response to allergens and preventing histamine release.

Ammi visnaga's active chemical, khellin, is reported to be the botanical source for the pharmaceutical drugs Intal and Nasal Chromused, used for treating various respiratory conditions including asthma and emphysema.

(continued)

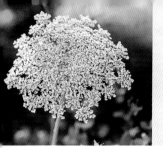

AMMI VISNAGA ESSENTIAL OIL (KHELLA PLANT SEEDS)

(*AMMI VISNAGA*): STEAM-DISTILLED HERB—NATURAL BRONCHODILATOR

In low doses, ammi visnaga is reported as being safe and has been used in traditional herbal medicine in the Middle East for years.

By relaxing coronary arteries, ammi visnaga may improve circulation within the heart, thereby easing the symptoms of angina.

Good for promoting healthy gums and teeth, ammi visnaga is a traditional remedy for treating kidney stones as it relaxes the ureter muscles to reduce the pain caused by a trapped stone, which aids release of the stone.

Research conducted in Egypt reported that ammi visnaga has a strong antispasmodic action on the small bronchial muscles, coronary arteries and urinary tubules. Ammi visnaga may be useful for lowering blood pressure and relieving angina symptoms.

Psycho-emotionally, ammi visnaga may be useful for calming feelings of anxiety and panic often associated with asthma.

Try 1 to 3 drops or more of ammi visnaga in your aroma diffuser or on a cotton ball or smell strip for direct inhalation. Inhaled, ammi visnaga's effects can last for up to six hours and shows practically no side effects. Ammi visnaga's odor is not especially pleasant, and for this reason, it's often blended with other bronchio-dilating essential oils to tone down its strongly herbal and medicinal scent. I recommend blending it with either blue tansy, rosemary or lemongrass oil.

CAUTION: Avoid during pregnancy and with babies and children. An extremely potent oil that is considered nontoxic in low doses, ammi visnaga is a photosensitizer. Avoid sunlight after application to the skin for up to twelve hours. Avoid with blood-thinning medications (coumarins). Avoid use on sensitive or damaged skin.

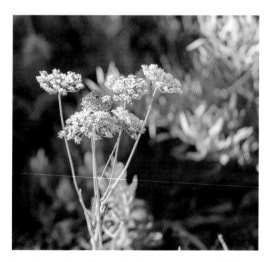

Psycho-emotionally, ammi visnaga may be useful for calming feelings of anxiety and panic often associated with asthma.

ATLAS CEDARWOOD ESSENTIAL OIL

(CEDRUS ATLANTICA): STEAM-DISTILLED WOOD—STRENGTHENS AND FORTIFIES MIND, BODY AND EMOTIONS

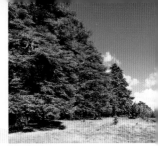

The best location for growing and distilling atlas cedarwood is Morocco.

A sweet, warm, rich, balsamic, woody aroma with fruity and honey undertones, atlas cedarwood oil has a fortifying effect on the mind and emotions and bolsters one's courage in times of great change and unsettled circumstances. In general, all cedarwood oils are very grounding and stabilizing to the nervous system.

The species is considered in danger of potential extinction from human use, due to the wood mafia and fires. In recent years, massive reforestation efforts have taken place in the Ifrane region of Morocco, and sustainable harvesting practices have begun. You can substitute Himalayan cedarwood oil in your blends that call for atlas cedarwood.

An aphrodisiac, cedarwood oil is used extensively in perfumery. Its fixative quality makes it useful for anchoring other oils in a blend. It blends especially well with other wood oils and citrus oils.

High sesquiterpene alcohol content gives atlas cedarwood its potent sedative action and makes it an excellent choice for soothing nervous tension, fear, anger, anxiety and depression. Use atlas cedarwood oil to promote meditative states of awareness. It is nourishing and balancing for the third chakra and supports a healthy ego.

Psycho-emotionally, atlas cedarwood oil may be especially helpful for boosting self-esteem, dispelling fear and giving you the strength and courage to face challenges.

Atlas cedarwood oil's regulating and tonic properties may be helpful for balancing the endocrine/glandular system and related symptoms.

Atlas cedarwood is often recommended for helping stop hair loss, especially related to stress. Its antiseborrheic properties are excellent for balancing too oily skin, hair and scalp conditions. Use it to control dandruff, as well as for skin conditions like acne, eczema, psoriasis and dermatitis.

An immune stimulant, atlas cedarwood oil promotes lymph circulation. This ability to stimulate the immune system, coupled with its mucolytic/expectorant properties, makes atlas cedarwood oil useful for relieving congestion and treating respiratory conditions like bronchitis, cough and excess phlegm.

Its antiseptic properties make atlas cedarwood oil useful in a diffuser to promote the killing of airborne bacteria. Blend with lemon oil to enhance this effect.

Its anti-infectious properties are useful for treating urinary tract infections, chronic urethritis, vaginitis, metritis and cystitis pain.

As a diuretic and tonic for the kidneys, try using atlas cedarwood for the relief of edema and simple water retention. Atlas cedarwood is also a popular beauty treatment. Its astringent, lipolytic and emollient properties make it effective for eliminating cellulite. Use it in a hot towel compress blended with pink grapefruit to enhance your results. (We have anti-cellulite blends for you to try in the "Spa and Beauty Treatments" section of this book on page 263.)

(continued)

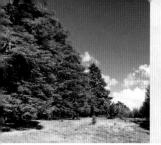

ATLAS CEDARWOOD ESSENTIAL OIL

(*CEDRUS ATLANTICA*): STEAM-DISTILLED WOOD—STRENGTHENS AND FORTIFIES MIND, BODY AND EMOTIONS

As a natural insect repellent, cedarwood oil has traditionally been used to prevent moths from infesting woolen clothing. It provides effective protection against mosquitoes and other insects, including fleas and ticks for your dog. Use a drop in your favorite dog shampoo. Be sure to check the "Animals and Pets" section on page 399 for recipes.

Atlas cedarwood oil blends well with many different oils, especially the wood and citrus oils including lemon, tea tree, lemongrass, patchouli, pink grapefruit, sweet orange, Himalayan cedarwood, black spruce, juniper berry, cypress, ylang ylang, bergamot, clary sage, geranium, spikenard and thyme.

Dispense 1 to 3 drops of atlas cedarwood oil on a cotton ball or smell strip, close your eyes and inhale. Note in your journal the aroma qualities you can discern and the effects the oil has on your body, mind, spirit and emotions.

CAUTION: Avoid in pregnancy as there is confusion among researchers about its abortive properties.

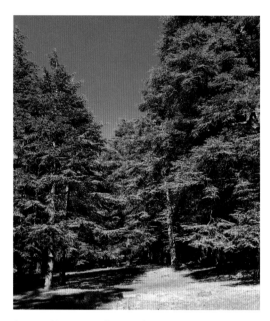

A natural insect repellant, cedarwood has traditionally been used to prevent moths from infesting woolen clothing.

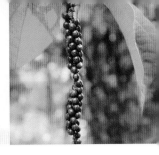

BLACK PEPPER ESSENTIAL OIL

(*PIPER NIGRUM*): STEAM-DISTILLED FRUIT—NEUTRALIZE NEGATIVITY
AND BREAK BAD HABITS

The best locations for growing and distilling black pepper are Madagascar and India.

Black pepper is distilled from the dried, whole, unripe fruit and has a soft, warm and spicy scent that's slightly woody with a dry top note that's similar to fresh cracked black peppercorns used in cooking.

As an analgesic, black pepper is especially good for muscular aches and pains. It may be helpful for relieving symptoms of arthritis, neuralgia, rheumatism, joint stiffness, sprains and strains, stiffness and poor muscle tone.

Its tonic action on the nervous, glandular and cardio-vascular systems makes black pepper useful for building strength and stamina for body, mind and emotions. It's excellent in a sports massage blend for warming and loosening the muscles before or after a sporting event.

Black pepper oil can be especially beneficial for relieving tired and achy muscles from overwork.

Psycho-emotionally, black pepper is often used to neutralize negativity and overcome addictions and bad habits like smoking or substance abuse. Its aphrodisiac properties have a reassuring and grounding effect and may help increase one's self-confidence and assertiveness to overcome challenges.

Black pepper's antiseptic and expectorant properties make it useful for relieving cold and flu symptoms like cough, sniffles, stuffy head, sore throat or nasal congestion.

A digestive stimulant, use black pepper to sooth symptoms associated with weak digestion and to stimulate digestive juices. Black pepper has been used to promote digestion of dairy foods in those who are lactose intolerant.

A rubefacient and stimulant, black pepper oil can increase your ability to pay attention and focus on important details and may be helpful for relieving mental lethargy and improving memory.

You can enjoy all the benefits of black pepper by using it as a food flavor.

Black pepper blends well with helichrysum, cypress, spikenard, basil, bergamot, fennel, frankincense, ginger, lavender, juniper, lemongrass, marjoram, myrrh, rosemary, sandalwood, ylang ylang and vetiver.

Dispense 1 to 3 drops of black pepper oil onto a cotton ball or smell strip, close your eyes and inhale. Note in your journal the aroma qualities you can discern and the effects the oil has on your body, mind, spirit and emotions.

CAUTION: Use in low dilutions of less than one percent as black pepper can be a skin irritant.

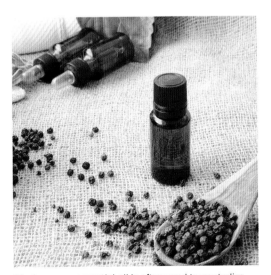

Black pepper essential oil is often used to neutralize negativity and overcome addictions like smoking or substance abuse.

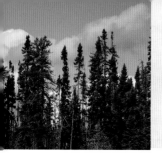

BLACK SPRUCE ESSENTIAL OIL

(*PICEA MARIANA*): STEAM-DISTILLED NEEDLES—REFRESHES, MENTAL CLARITY, PHYSICAL STAMINA

The best location for growing and distilling black spruce essential oil is Canada.

Inhaling the scent of black spruce has the power to restore your passion for life. If you love the great outdoors and enjoy the smell of high, pristine mountain tops, then you'll love the clear, crisp, clean aroma of black spruce oil. The scent of black spruce is vibrant, woody, balsamic, resinous and slightly sweet. Just like walking into a deep, green forest, black spruce oil can immediately free and uplift your senses.

Its high monoterpene content (65 percent) gives black spruce a wide spectrum of therapeutic actions similar to citrus oils. Essential oils high in monoterpenes are known to readily oxidize when left open to the light and air. Special care should be taken for proper storage to ensure potency for therapeutic results and to prevent oxidation.

Its high monoterpene content also gives black spruce its strongly anti-infectious, antifungal, antiviral, antiseptic (airborne) and expectorant properties. An effective immune stimulant, black spruce may be useful for treating a variety of respiratory conditions like bronchitis and asthma, as well as for preventing and treating cold and flu infections.

A regulating oil, black spruce has hormone- and cortisone-like properties that research has shown to stimulate the thymus gland and the hypothalamic–pituitary–adrenal axis (HPA). Through its regulating hormonal action, black spruce strengthens and stabilizes the entire nervous system and supports adrenal function. Its regulating action and its restorative and immune-stimulant properties make it helpful for regaining strength and building stamina after

illness. Those suffering from chronic fatigue syndrome (CFS) may benefit from black spruce's grounding, restorative and stabilizing effects.

Black spruce's warming and stimulating properties as well as its antispasmodic and anti-inflammatory action make it beneficial for relieving various muscle aches and pains, stiff joints, poor circulation, rheumatism, arthritis, strains, sprains, muscle cramps and spasms.

Psycho-emotionally, the hypnotic scent of black spruce can have a powerfully transformative effect on the human psyche. It can be useful for restoring your sense of purpose and the motivation to keep going. Black spruce promotes mental clarity and may be helpful for clearing mental confusion. Black spruce oil can give needed refreshment to the mind and emotions after one has endured much, or when needing to overcome a sense of defeat or failure. It may be useful for relieving extreme stress, anxiety and tension.

Black spruce oil blends well with many different oils including other conifer oils, citrus and spice oils, lavender, clary sage, ginger, bergamot, geranium, lemon, peppermint, sweet orange, spikenard, thyme and ylang ylang.

Dispense 1 to 3 drops of black spruce oil on a cotton ball or smell strip, close your eyes and inhale. Note in your journal the aroma qualities you can discern and the effects the oil has on your body, mind, spirit and emotions.

CAUTION: Black spruce oil becomes a skin irritant when the oil has oxidized. Due to its stimulating effect, avoid use during pregnancy and with young children and babies.

BLUE TANSY ESSENTIAL OIL (Moroccan Blue Chamomile)

(TANACETUM ANNUUM): STEAM-DISTILLED FLOWER TOPS—
ANTI-INFLAMMATORY, ALLERGY RELIEF, BREATHING AID

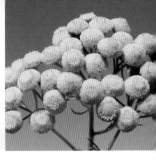

Blue tansy oil's high azulene content gives it a deep, vivid shade of blue (similar to German chamomile's color, though these two oils are not interchangeable).

Everyone loves the warm and friendly scent of blue tansy. Its aroma is delightfully fruity and slightly herbal with camphoraceous notes and a complex sweetness that's reminiscent of apples and spice.

Its naturally occurring antihistamine and anti-allergic properties make blue tansy especially effective for promoting allergy relief.

Blue tansy's bronchodilating effect makes it useful in blends for relieving symptoms of asthma and emphysema, and its anti-inflammatory properties help to reduce the swelling and itching often associated with allergies.

A long time sufferer of allergies and client of mine who used to get weekly shots and take daily medication to control symptoms reported that blue tansy had helped relieve both allergic reactions to environmental, as well as food, allergens. She had stopped taking allergy medication and no longer required shots.

As a regulating oil, blue tansy has a relaxing or invigorating effect depending upon the circumstances for which you are using it.

Blue tansy's powerful anti-inflammatory and antispasmodic action relieves stress and nervous tension and has an immediately calming effect on the nerves and nervous system. It is effective for relieving muscular aches and pains, sprains and strains, arthritis, rheumatism and sciatica.

Blue tansy's anti-inflammatory effect makes it an excellent first aid remedy for radiation burns from cancer treatment, as well as for inflamed or sun-damaged skin.

My friend Sylla used blue tansy oil as a spray-on mist, along with helichrysum, to relieve radiation burns from her breast cancer treatment. Customers who have used our radiation and other burn-care formulas made with blue tansy oil report how quickly they heal with little or no scarring.

Its anti-inflammatory effects make it useful for treating various skin conditions like bruises, itching, rash, irritation and dermatitis.

As an anthelmintic, blue tansy has been used to kill parasitic worms.

Blue tansy blends well with lemongrass, chamomile, ylang ylang, cypress, helichrysum and rosemary.

Dispense 1 to 3 drops of blue tansy oil onto a cotton ball or smell strip, close your eyes and inhale. Note in your journal the aroma qualities you can discern and the effects the oil has on your body, mind, spirit and emotions.

CAUTION: Avoid during pregnancy and with young children.

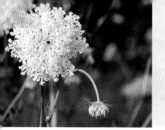

CARROT SEED ESSENTIAL OIL

(*DAUCUS CAROTA*): STEAM-DISTILLED SEED—SKIN REGENERATIVE

The best location for growing and distilling carrot seed oil is France.

Sweet and herbaceous, an artful distillation of carrot seed oil results in a lovely smelling oil. To me, it smells just like fresh pressed carrot juice. A carrot seed oil that is not artfully distilled has a bitter and unpleasant aroma that can ruin any blend. Small traces of carrot seed oil are often used by perfumers in oriental "fantasy" perfumes.

Primarily used for its holistic skincare effects, carrot seed's potent antioxidant and tonic properties promote elasticity and tone skin cell tissue through its ability to stimulate the formation of red blood cells.

Carrot seed oil is one of the very best essential oils (along with rose oil) for regenerating mature skin cell tissue and is often used in aromatherapy blends for natural skincare and for treating scars. Only a very small amount is needed to produce excellent results.

Additionally, carrot seed's cleansing and moisturizing properties make it an excellent choice for smoothing and softening mature skin, as well as fading deep facial lines, wrinkles and scars. Blend with rose and helichrysum oil to enhance this effect.

Harmonizing for all skin types, carrot seed oil's skin-nourishing and rejuvenating action makes it a useful addition to most facial and skincare formulas.

Its cooling effect is ideal for soothing sensitive or inflamed cell tissue. Carrot seed oil may be useful for treating acne, abscesses, boils and other skin disorders.

There is some evidence that carrot seed oil may improve liver and gallbladder function and may be especially helpful for treating hepatitis and colitis.

Carrot seed has been used to stimulate the production of milk in new mothers. As the scent is mild, it may be preferable to using the intensely sweet anise aroma of fennel oil (also recommended for this purpose), which can overpower the natural scent of the mother and interfere with important bonding.

Carrot seed oil blends well with citrus and spicy oils, geranium, rosemary, ylang ylang, cedarwood, cypress and lavender. For skin healing and tissue repair, blend carrot seed oil with other regenerative oils like rose, helichrysum, frankincense, myrrh, patchouli and spikenard.

Dispense 1 to 3 drops of carrot seed oil on a cotton ball or smell strip, close your eyes and inhale. Note in your journal the aroma qualities you can discern and the effects the oil has on your body, mind, spirit and emotions.

CAUTION: Some sources advise to avoid during pregnancy.

CINNAMON ESSENTIAL OIL

(*CINNAMOMUM ZEYLANICUM*): STEAM-DISTILLED LEAF—
POWERFUL ANTISEPTIC, WARMING TONIC, APHRODISIAC

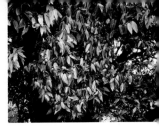

The best locations for growing and distilling cinnamon oil are Madagascar, Sri Lanka and India.

A sweet, spicy, warm, radiant and pungent oil, cinnamon's powerful antiseptic properties have been enjoyed and regaled for centuries. Cinnamon leaf oil and cinnamon bark oil are completely different. Cinnamon bark is distilled from the outer bark of the tree. Its color is deep reddish brown, and its aroma is much sweeter and more intense. It makes an excellent perfume-quality oil. Cinnamon leaf is distilled from the leaf, its aroma is less intense and sweet and its color is a light yellow to light reddish brown.

Cinnamon has a long history of traditional and esoteric uses as a plant aromatic. It was prized in ancient Egypt as a medicine, as a flavoring agent and for embalming. It is written about in the Bible.

Considered as precious as gold, cinnamon was widely traded as an aromatic plant, and its virtues are extolled in the Middle East and Orient for killing viruses and infectious diseases. Where cinnamon leaf oil was produced remained a mystery until 1270, when it was first reported being produced in Sri Lanka.

Modern research has revealed some of the mystery about cinnamon leaf's power to heal. It is high in phenols and other beneficial contents like eugenol, cinnamic aldehyde and linalool, which have all been reported to have potent effects as natural antimicrobial agents.

Cinnamon oil's properties are powerfully anti-infectious, antifungal, antiviral, antibacterial, antidiarrheal, antispasmodic and anti-parasitic as well as being strongly astringent, digestive and an immune stimulant.

Inhalation of cinnamon oil has proven effective for relieving respiratory infections.

Cinnamon leaf has been used for treating respiratory, musculoskeletal, digestive, cardiovascular, lymphatic, immune, urinary and reproductive conditions as well as nervous system complaints, among others.

Cinnamon is also anthelmintic, which means it expels parasitic worms (helminths) from the body by either stunning them as with vermifuges or killing them as a vermicide. Research into antimicrobial effects show that cinnamon oil inhibits and even completely destroys viruses, bacteria and fungi.

Cinnamon bark oil's antiseptic properties have been shown to be even more powerful for killing bacterial and fungal infections than cinnamon leaf.

(continued)

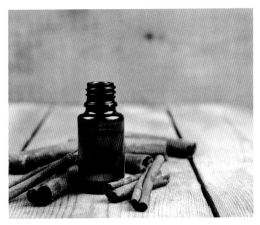

Cinnamon was prized in ancient Egypt as a medicine, a flavoring agent and for embalming.

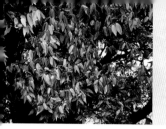

CINNAMON ESSENTIAL OIL

(*CINNAMOMUM ZEYLANICUM*): STEAM-DISTILLED LEAF—
POWERFUL ANTISEPTIC, WARMING TONIC, APHRODISIAC

Use cinnamon oil to keep the air fresh and free of "bugs" and to prevent the spread of infection. Everyone enjoys cinnamon oil's sweet, warm and spicy scent and its ability to prevent and relieve cold and flu symptoms.

Its antispasmodic, stimulant and astringent properties make cinnamon leaf oil helpful for relieving painful muscles and stiff joints.

Cinnamon leaf also has powerful aphrodisiac properties that are helpful for recovery after physical exhaustion and help build strength and stamina. Its warming and stimulating properties may be helpful for overcoming sexual impotence and relieving symptoms of frigidity.

Psycho-emotionally, cinnamon leaf oil arouses your emotional and psychic forces and stimulates creativity. It may relieve feelings of weakness, depression, emotional coldness, physical tension and any tendency to isolation.

Use cinnamon oil to relieve brain fog and lethargic states of energy. Cinnamon leaf oil warms your mind and emotions and may be helpful for dispelling feelings of loneliness.

During the winter months, cinnamon leaf oil is excellent to use when you feel chilled to your bones and can't get warm. It is helpful for relieving chilblains.

Enjoy the uplifting and warming scent of cinnamon leaf oil in your aroma lamp, or add a drop of it in a teaspoon (5 ml) of honey and stir into your favorite hot drink.

Cinnamon leaf oil also makes an excellent mouthwash and breath freshener and is often used as a first aid treatment for relieving toothache.

According to Ayurvedic medicine, cinnamon oil's warm and sweet scent is used to balance conditions of Vata imbalance such as flatulence, irritable bowel syndrome, constipation, anxiety and nervousness, premenstrual syndrome and insomnia. Cinnamon oil's warming action improves circulation and has a warming and grounding effect on excess Vata conditions.

Cinnamon leaf oil blends well with other spice oils and citrus oils including bergamot, clove, lemon, sweet orange, mandarin, thyme, rosemary, eucalyptus and tea tree.

Dispense 1 to 3 drops of cinnamon leaf oil on a cotton ball or smell strip, close your eyes and inhale. Note in your journal the aroma qualities you can discern and the effects the oil has on your body, mind, spirit and emotions.

CAUTION: Cinnamon leaf may be a skin irritant. It is suitable for skin application in weak dilutions of less than one percent. You may use it in a bath to warm you or in massage oil blends and hot compresses to relieve achy muscles and stiff joints. Due to its stimulating properties, avoid in pregnancy and with babies and children.

CLARY SAGE ESSENTIAL OIL

(*SALVIA SCLAREA*): STEAM-DISTILLED OR HYDRODIFFUSED FLOWERS—
RELIEVES DEEP TENSION

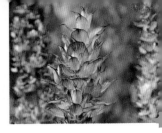

The best locations for growing and distilling are France and the United States.

Sweet, warm, exotic and sensuous with a slight herbal note, clary sage is an especially inviting aroma. Its intense floral scent has a deeply soothing effect on nervous tension for both men and women.

Clary sage comes from the Latin root, *clarus*, which means "clear." During the Middle Ages it was referred to as "clear eyes." The oil offers benefits for the eyes and for the nervous, hormonal and digestive systems.

Its strong yang character makes clary sage helpful for balancing excessive yin states which may occur during the normal menses cycle or in menopause.

As an aphrodisiac, clary sage was developed exclusively for the perfumery trade. When tested, clary sage was found to have more than 250 constituents giving it a broad spectrum of application for potential therapeutic use. Its high concentration of esters (70 percent or more), such as linalyl acetate, give clary sage its powerful antispasmodic and sedative action. This high concentration of esters may be responsible for clary sage's popular use to relieve premenstrual tension in women. It may also be helpful for reducing epileptic attacks.

Clary sage does have some reported use in the UK for easing painful contractions during labor and birth. Often blended with geranium oil, clary sage may help regulate and relieve female complaints associated with hormonal imbalance, such as irregular menses, menopausal symptoms, headache, nausea and depression.

Clary sage oil may be useful in a hot towel compress to relieve deep tension often associated with menstrual and intestinal cramps, as well as stomach, liver and gallbladder conditions.

According to aromatherapist Robert Tisserand, clary sage does have interesting anticancer activity. One study showed in vitro action against human breast cancer MCF-7 cells (Dimas et al 2006). An isomer, 13-epi-sclareol, also present in clary sage oil, also inhibited the growth of breast and uterine cancers in vitro. The study showed clary sage to be slightly more potent than Tamoxifen in its effect, but with no toxicity (Sashidhara et al 2007). This study suggests that the sclareol content in clary sage once thought to produce estrogen-like effects may in fact actually inhibit estrogen. Tisserand stated, "What we do know is that sclareol will not give you breast cancer."

A tonic, regenerative and revitalizing oil, clary sage may be excellent for treating nervousness, weakness, fear and depression.

(continued)

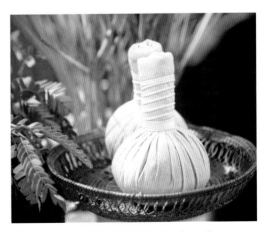

A hot compress with clary sage can relieve deep tension associated with menstrual cramps.

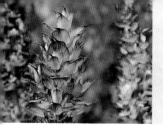

CLARY SAGE ESSENTIAL OIL

(*SALVIA SCLAREA*): STEAM-DISTILLED OR HYDRODIFFUSED FLOWERS—
RELIEVES DEEP TENSION

For some, clary sage's sedative action can be hypnotic on the mind and emotions, producing very tranquil and peaceful states. Used to stimulate lucid dreaming, clary sage can promote clear insight through your intuition.

Psycho-emotionally, clary sage oil nourishes your heart energies and can dispel negative thoughts and relax your mind to help you get through challenging or difficult circumstances. Clary sage may be useful for treating fatigue, stress, fear, anxiety, paranoia and mid-life crisis and for stimulating creativity, imagination and dreams.

Clary sage may be especially helpful for relieving stressful or tense physical and emotional states and conditions like migraine headaches.

Excellent in a sensual massage blend, clary sage promotes healthy circulation and is reported to be helpful for balancing circulatory problems like high blood pressure, varicose veins and hemorrhoids. It may also lower high cholesterol.

A research study on the use of clary sage and lavender conducted at Harris Methodist Hospital in Fort Worth, Texas showed that both oils calmed stress and relieved anxiety in over 57 percent of the ICU nurses involved in the study. It was noted that, "ICU nurses are called to participate in end-of-life decisions and patient resuscitations, and support families through a patient's journey. It is important for nurses to have outlets and options for stress relief."

Clary sage's calming, antiseptic and skin healing properties make it useful in beauty and skincare conditions that may be related to stress such as acne, boils and hair loss. It may also be a wrinkle reducer.

Its deodorant and astringent action make clary sage excellent for controlling body odor and excessive perspiration.

In Ayurvedic medicine, sweet aromas like clary sage are used to regulate and pacify both Vata and Pitta imbalances. Symptoms of Vata imbalance are premenstrual syndrome, insomnia, nervousness and anxiety or worry. Symptoms of Pitta imbalance include feelings of frustration and anger, a tendency to emotional upset and overreaction, high blood pressure and an inability to relax and go with the flow.

Clary sage oil blends well with geranium oils, bergamot, frankincense, lemongrass, lavender, ylang ylang, cedarwood and sweet marjoram.

Dispense 1 to 3 drops of clary sage oil on a cotton ball or smell strip, close your eyes and inhale. Note in your journal the aroma qualities you can discern and the effects the oil has on your body, mind, spirit and emotions.

CAUTION: As clary sage can stimulate a narcotic-like effect for some people, causing them to feel dizzy or light-headed, please avoid use when driving or needing to focus. Avoid during pregnancy.

CLOVE ESSENTIAL OIL

(*EUGENIA CARYOPHYLLATA*): STEAM-DISTILLED CLOVE BUD—
PAIN RELIEVER, ANTIFUNGAL

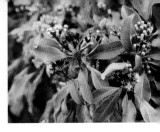

One of the best locations for growing and distilling clove oil is Madagascar.

Clove oil has a deep yellowish-brown color and a sweet, warm, radiant and penetrating peppery aroma. A valuable first aid oil for use alone or in a blend, clove oil is a powerful analgesic pain reliever and well known for having a numbing effect on the nerves. For this reason, clove oil has a reputation for being an effective emergency first aid remedy for toothaches.

For emergency care, add a drop of clove oil on a cotton swab and apply to the surrounding gum line of the affected tooth for immediate relief.

Research shows clove oil to be high in thymol, eugenol and cinnamaldehyde which have all been investigated on several microorganisms and parasites, including pathogenic bacteria, herpes simplex and hepatitis C viruses. In addition to its antimicrobial, antioxidant, antifungal and antiviral activity, clove oil was shown to have anti-inflammatory, cytotoxic, insect-repellent and anesthetic properties. Studies also demonstrate clove oil's antimicrobial activity against a large number of multi-resistant Staphylococcus epidermidis.

Since clove oil shares similar antiseptic and anti-infectious properties as cinnamon oil, it is powerful for treating a broad spectrum of viral, bacterial and fungal infections, including warts, herpes, athlete's foot and toenail fungus. Use clove oil for the prevention and treatment of infections.

Its stimulant properties make clove oil a helpful digestive aid, as well as useful for restoring loss of appetite due to illness. Clove bud oil's tonic and stimulating action make it useful for strengthening the mind and body.

Its anti-parasitic and anthelmintic properties make clove oil useful for dispelling intestinal worms and parasites.

A natural antihistamine and expectorant, clove is often recommended for various respiratory conditions such as asthma, sinus infections, bronchitis and other pulmonary conditions.

Its anti-inflammatory and anti-rheumatic properties make clove oil useful in blends for rheumatic-type pains. Clove oil may be helpful for relieving symptoms of arthritis, rheumatoid arthritis and various strains and sprains.

A stimulant and aphrodisiac, clove oil enhances memory retention and is good for relieving nervous exhaustion, fatigue, brain fog, lethargy and depressive states of mind.

Clove oil blends well with citrus and spice oils as well as other oils including bergamot, sweet basil, black pepper, cinnamon, ginger, lavender, lemon, sweet marjoram, peppermint, rosemary, thyme and tea tree.

Dispense 1 to 3 drops of clove oil on a cotton ball or smell strip, close your eyes and inhale. Note in your journal the aroma qualities you can discern and the effects the oil has on your body, mind, spirit and emotions.

CAUTION: Clove oil is known to irritate the skin and mucous membranes and is generally not for use in skincare, except in extremely weak dilutions of less than one percent. Please respect the power inherent in clove and use with extreme care.

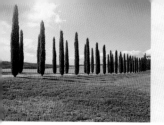

CYPRESS ESSENTIAL OIL

(*CUPRESSUS SEMPERVIRENS*): STEAM-DISTILLED LEAF—
POWERFUL ASTRINGENT, CLEANSER AND DETOXIFIER

Some of the best locations for growing and distilling cypress oil are Crete and France.

Cypress oil has a distinctly clean, fresh, sweet, herbaceous, woody and balsamic scent that's light and clear with a hint of spice. It is slightly reminiscent of pine and juniper berry. The oil is distilled from the leaves (needles) of the column-shaped evergreen cypress tree native to the Mediterranean region of Europe. Often planted close together to act as a screen from the elements, the cypress tree is a common appearance in many gardens and can be seen throughout southern Europe.

Frequently found in cemeteries, cypress has been considered a symbol of life after death and called "the tree of life and death." The ancient Greeks dedicated the cypress tree to the god Pluto, Lord of the Underworld, and, according to legend, the cross that Jesus was crucified on was made of cypress.

In the ancient temples of Egypt, cypress was burnt along with pine and juniper to cleanse the air. Cypress oil's medicinal uses were inscribed on papyri, and its wood was often used to fashion the sarcophagi of the Egyptian aristocracy.

Its antispasmodic properties make cypress oil a comforting fragrance, and it is often recommended during times of transition and uncertainty for both men and women. It may be especially helpful during times of recovery from grief and loss.

Cypress oil has a masculine, yang effect upon the human energy system. Its scent has the ability to stabilize and give direction and purpose during times of confusion. Its grounding effect helps curb excesses in body, mind and emotions. In perfumery, cypress is often used in men's colognes and aftershave lotions.

Psycho-emotionally, cypress oil acts to unify and give practical structure to the day-to-day matters of life. It provides support to the visionary and creative process, supporting you to bring your dreams into reality. Its antidepressant properties help to strengthen the heart energies, and it has the ability to comfort and soothe the emotions.

Cypress has been used for ritual cleansing and to promote health since ancient times. Cypress oil gives comfort, stimulates mental energy and supports one's capacity to concentrate and focus on priorities and develop new, healthy mental habits in the face of evolutionary change.

A hemostat and decongestant, cypress oil has the most powerful astringent action in aromatherapy. The ancient Chinese chewed the bark for gum issues and to control bleeding gums.

Cypress oil's properties act to tone and strengthen the circulatory and nervous systems and relieve circulatory and lymphatic congestion. Its powerful astringent properties make it useful for adding to shampoos to control excess oil and dandruff. Cypress oil can be useful for decongesting the prostate gland.

Cypress oil's regulating action may help balance hormonal action. It has been used as an effective treatment for female hormonal issues like irregular menstrual cycles, as well menstrual cramps and problems associated with menopause like hot flashes.

Cypress oil is often used for strengthening and supporting healthy functioning of the heart and circulatory system. It has been recommended for softening walls of hardened arteries and strengthening weak connective tissue. Its astringent action makes cypress effective for treating conditions associated with congestion of lymph or blood circulation such as muscle cramps, rheumatism and arthritis.

As a powerful vasoconstrictor and expectorant, cypress oil purifies the blood and is good for treating stagnant blood conditions and internal and external varicosities. Hippocrates is said to have recommended cypress for treating severely bleeding hemorrhoids, and it can be prepared as a topical salve to treat hemorrhoids.

As a diuretic, cypress oil may be helpful for relieving edema, swelling, fluid retention and bloating as well as good for controlling excess perspiration.

An immune stimulant, cypress oil supports a healthy immune system, and its antiseptic, antibacterial and antiviral properties inhibit and prevent infection. It may be useful for treating sore throat, sinusitis, laryngitis, asthma, bronchitis and cough.

According to Ayurvedic medicine—an ancient system of healing practiced in India—the spicy wood aroma and astringent and bitter qualities of cypress oil are ideal for pacifying imbalances of the Pitta and Kapha body-mind types. Symptoms of Pitta imbalance are high blood pressure, anger, frustration and emotional upsets. Symptoms of Kapha imbalance are high cholesterol, low metabolic forces, slow weight loss, fluid retention, stagnation and blockage, lethargy and depression.

Cypress oil blends well with many different oils including lavender, lemon, juniper berry, cinnamon leaf, sweet orange, peppermint, frankincense, myrrh, lemongrass, ylang ylang and sweet marjoram.

Dispense 1 to 3 drops of cypress oil on a cotton ball or smell strip, close your eyes and inhale. Note in your journal the aroma qualities you can discern and the effects the oil has on your body, mind, spirit and emotions.

CAUTION: Avoid in cases of pregnancy, high blood pressure and uterine and breast fibroids.

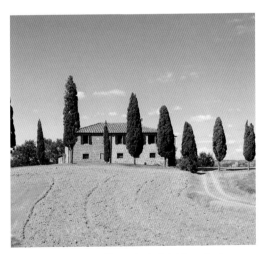

A diuretic, cyrpress oil may be helpful for relieving edema, swelling and fluid retention.

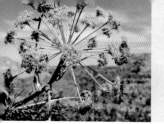

GALBANUM ESSENTIAL OIL

(*FERULA GALBANIFLUA*): STEAM-DISTILLED RESIN—SKIN HEALING, REGENERATIVE AND ANTI-INFLAMMATORY

The best locations for growing and distilling galbanum oil are Iran and Turkey.

Galbanum is a warm, balsamic, earthy and herbal scent with a hint of spice and a piney note. An aromatic gum resin produced from the umbelliferous Persian plant species of the genus ferula, galbanum oil is an "intensely green" aroma. To me, galbanum has a rich, earthy scent that's reminiscent of a freshly tilled garden. Garden gnomes busy at work always come to mind when I inhale the scent of galbanum.

Unlike any other oil in aromatherapy, galbanum has a musky and exotic presence and a strongly bitter taste. Its subtle balsamic, piney notes are said to be due to the presence of pinenes in its chemical makeup.

An ancient aromatic plant used for making incense, galbanum is mentioned being used for this purpose in the Book of Exodus. The galbanum plant belongs to the ferula family of plants originating in Iran, Turkey and Syria. Distilling galbanum is a complicated two-step process. The resin from galbanum roots is first converted to a resinoid compound then extracted by steam distillation.

The ancient Egyptians highly favored galbanum as a holy plant aromatic, and the reputed "green" incense of ancient Egypt is thought to be galbanum.

Its musty, green, exotic scent is greatly appreciated by modern-day perfumers. It has been used for making fine perfumes in the "green" family of scents.

One of the oldest plant medicines, Hippocrates used it, as did Pliny the Elder, an author and naturalist during the early Roman Empire who ascribed "extraordinary curative powers" to galbanum. Some of the mythology associated with galbanum has referred to it as the sacred "mother resin."

A rubefacient, galbanum's warming and tonic action and comforting scent may be enjoyed in a massage blend for relaxation and for releasing deep tension, muscle aches, arthritis and rheumatic pain.

Topically, galbanum oil's regenerative and anti-inflammatory properties have been used successfully for treating skin disorders and chronic inflammation. It may be useful for treating scars, boils, abscesses, ulcers, wounds, edema and swelling, skin rash and acne. As a skin tonic, galbanum may be useful in a blend for smoothing mature skin, lines and wrinkles.

Galbanum is said to help relieve pre-menstrual tension, cramps and menopausal symptoms and to strengthen female organs.

Psycho-emotionally, galbanum has a calming, balancing and grounding effect on the mind and emotions. It is useful for balancing extreme emotional states such as anger, frustration, nervous tension, erratic moods, emotional coldness, hysteria or paranoia. Galbanum is said to be helpful for removing psychic blocks and resolving old problems, especially of an emotional nature.

Galbanum oil blends well with many different oils including conifers, pines and other evergreens, as well as citrus oils, geranium, ylang ylang, lavender, patchouli, sandalwood and cedarwood. A trace of this oil is all that's needed for a truly remarkable blend.

Dispense 1 to 3 drops of galbanum oil on a cotton ball or smell strip, close your eyes and inhale. Note in your journal the aroma qualities you can discern and the effects the oil has on your body, mind, spirit and emotions.

CAUTION: Galbanum may be a skin irritant. Avoid during pregnancy.

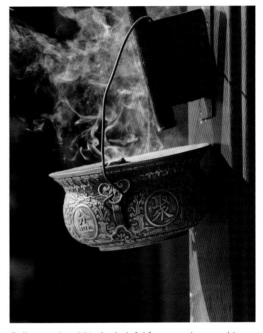

Galbanum is said to be helpful for removing psychic blocks and resolving old problems, especially of an emotional nature.

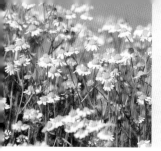

GERMAN CHAMOMILE ESSENTIAL OIL

(*MATRICARIA CHAMOMILLA*, SYNONYM: *MATRICARIA RECUTITA*):
STEAM-DISTILLED FLOWERS—CALMING PAIN RELIEVER

The best locations for growing and distilling German chamomile are Bulgaria and England.

The scent of chamomile is pleasantly sweet, fresh and fruity with delightful herbal after notes. In common use for more than 3,000 years, German chamomile has an established reputation as one of the most powerful anti-inflammatory and fever reducing oils in aromatherapy. It's thought to have been used for digestive complaints since at least the first century CE and is considered gentle enough for children.

The chamomile plant was revered by the Egyptians and used in cosmetic applications for at least 2,000 years. It's said that the Egyptians dedicated the chamomile plant to the sun and worshipped it above all other medicinal herbs for its healing properties. In her book, *Herb Garden*, Frances Bardswell calls chamomile the "plant's physician" as it has a remarkable healing effect on other plants.

Its high chamazulene content gives it a gorgeous, deep, vivid blue color. To maintain its intense shade of blue, chamomile needs to be refrigerated. Of course, studies on the psychology of color have shown that the color blue itself has a cooling effect on the psyche. Nature shows us the use of an oil by its inherent characteristics.

Studies have shown that German chamomile reduces inflammation, speeds wound healing, reduces muscle spasms and serves as a mild sedative to help with sleep.

It is excellent for treating red, inflamed and sensitive skin conditions. It has a long history of use in helping to relieve hot, irritated skin conditions like dermatitis, acne, cysts, boils, skin rash, eczema and psoriasis.

A regulating oil, German chamomile helps balance the body's natural sebum production and can be used for both oily and dry skin, hair and scalp conditions.

It's also excellent for treating all types of burns, as well as cuts, scrapes and abrasions. German Chamomile is reported to be useful for treating shingles outbreaks.

As a tranquilizer, German chamomile's sedative action can be helpful for relieving insomnia as it is calming to the nervous system, the mind and emotions.

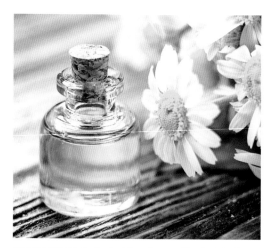

The Egyptians dedicated the chamomile plant to the sun and worshipped it above all other medicinal herbs.

As well as a sleep aid, German chamomile oil may also be useful for treating sleep disturbances and night fears. Inhale the scent of German chamomile just before sleep to encourage deep and restful sleep. (See caution.)

Its action to sooth and calm can be especially beneficial for relieving stress-related complaints like headache or indigestion.

Under the direction of a qualified aromatherapist and properly diluted, German chamomile is wonderful for anxious, pregnant moms. They can rely on its comforting scent as often as needed to help them relax and get rest.

German chamomile is the remedy of choice for fussy babies and wonderful for relieving colic, intestinal cramps and gas in newborns, as well as helpful for easing teething pain. Properly diluted in a carrier oil, German chamomile's gentle nature makes it perfect for soothing diaper rash.

German chamomile oil is lovely on its own. In a blend, use the more gently soothing and emotionally supportive oils like helichrysum, lavender, bergamot, rose, neroli, melissa, sandalwood, frankincense, geranium, roman chamomile, red mandarin, spikenard, vetiver and ylang ylang.

Dispense 1 to 3 drops of German chamomile oil on a cotton ball or smell strip, close your eyes and inhale. Note in your journal the aroma qualities you can discern and the effects the oil has on your body, mind, spirit and emotions.

CAUTION: German chamomile may make asthma and some allergies worse, so people with known sensitivities should not use it. If you're unsure if you have a sensitivity, do a skin patch test. Never use German chamomile oil during pregnancy as it may induce menstruation and/or premature labor due to its emmenagogue and uterotonic side effects.

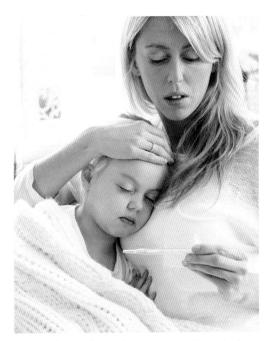

German chamomile's action to cool, soothe and calm can be especially beneficial for relieving a fever and is safe to use with children.

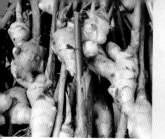

GINGER ESSENTIAL OIL

(*ZINGIBER OFFICINALE*): HYDRODIFFUSED (PREFERRED) OR STEAM-DISTILLED FRESH ROOT—NAUSEA REMEDY, DIGESTIVE AID, ENERGY TONIC AND APHRODISIAC

The best locations for growing and distilling are Sri Lanka and Madagascar.

The scent of fresh ginger root oil is sweet, warm, radiant and spicy. Its dry, hot, stimulating properties are well documented for relieving pain.

If you are feeling energetically low, inhale the scent of fresh ginger root oil. It will boost and give support to your life force energies, restoring their internal flow.

Ginger oil that is hydrodiffused has a more intense, golden color. The hydrodiffusion top-down method of distillation extracts more of the characteristic ginger notes, and the oil has a more intense full-bodied ginger aroma. This means less oil is usually needed in a blend, and the scent is more tenacious.

For immune system support, ginger root oil's tonic action serves to energize, ground and strengthen you after an illness. Its antiseptic properties make it effective as a preventative for infectious disease.

According to Chinese medicine, ginger root is a fever reducer with warming action. Its strongly yang nature regulates excess moisture, making it useful for elevating body temperature and relieving chills and fevers.

As a stimulant, ginger root oil helps improve circulation, increases body temperature and cellular respiration and may be useful for combating jet lag. Its antiemetic properties make it a helpful treatment for nausea, hangover and motion sickness. It's also used for lowering high cholesterol.

Its expectorant properties and its ability to boost the immune system makes it useful for treating illnesses caused by cold and dampness like the cold and flu, chills, fever, bronchitis, congestion, cough and sinusitis. Fresh ginger root may be helpful for treating ear, nose and throat conditions (ENT) like sore throat, tonsillitis and swollen lymph glands.

A powerful anti-inflammatory, analgesic and antispasmodic, ginger root oil improves blood circulation and is excellent for relieving muscle and joint aches and pains, sprains and strains and joint stiffness. It may also be helpful for relieving symptoms of headache, angina, arthritis and rheumatism.

Research was conducted using ginger and sweet orange aromatic essential oil for massage among elderly patients with moderate to severe knee pain. There was marked change reported for knee pain intensity, stiffness and physical function among all those receiving massage with aromatic oils.

A popular digestive aid, ginger root oil may be helpful for relieving toothache, cramps, loss of appetite, indigestion, constipation, heartburn, stomachache, anorexia and flatulence.

Psycho-emotionally, ginger root oil's restorative properties can help you to recover when you're feeling physically and emotionally burnt out, depleted or exhausted. Try fresh ginger root oil for relieving debility, nervous exhaustion and oversensitivity and to help ground and sharpen the senses.

In skincare, ginger root oil's rubefacient and moisture-regulating properties are useful for treating bruises, sores and carbuncles.

As an aphrodisiac, ginger may be helpful for treating male impotence and female frigidity.

Ginger root oil blends well with many different oils including cinnamon leaf, lemongrass, fennel, eucalyptus, black pepper, carrot seed and helichrysum.

Dispense 1 to 3 drops of fresh ginger root oil on a cotton ball or smell strip, close your eyes and inhale. Note in your journal the aroma qualities you can discern and the effects the oil has on your body, mind, spirit and emotions.

CAUTION: Exercise special care and respect when using fresh ginger root oil as it is a known skin irritant. For skin applications, use in a weak dilution of less than one percent.

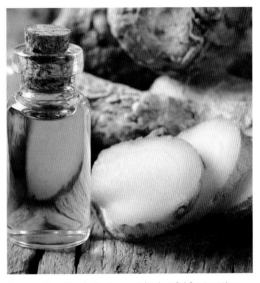

As an aphrodisiac, ginger may be hepful for treating male impotence and female frigidity.

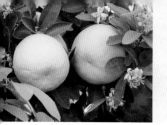

GRAPEFRUIT ESSENTIAL OIL

(CITRUS PARADISI): COLD-PRESSED (EXPRESSED) FRESH PEEL—
BODY CLEANSER, FAT BURNER, NATURAL WEIGHT LOSS AID

One of the best locations for growing and distilling grapefruit oil is the United States.

The aroma of grapefruit oil is fresh, citrusy and fruity. It is produced by cold-pressing the skin of the fruit. The bright, crisp and fruity scent of grapefruit oil energizes and uplifts the senses. The vapors of grapefruit oil stimulate the brain's neurotransmitters and can produce feelings of euphoria.

An immune stimulant and diuretic, grapefruit oil promotes body cleansing and the removal of toxins and excess fluids. It also increases your metabolism and helps to burn fat. Using grapefruit oil can help boost lymph gland activity. It can also help prevent and treat sluggish circulation and metabolism, which can lead to various health problems including allergies.

Grapefruit oil is rich in antioxidants. Its primary chemical constituent is limonene (up to 95 percent), which research has shown to have anti-cancer properties.

Its antiseptic and bactericidal properties kill bacteria (especially airborne bacteria). Studies have shown that grapefruit oil's antimicrobial properties are effective against many strains of bacteria like the dreaded Staphylococcus aureus (MRSA) and Candida albicans.

Grapefruit oil stimulates the liver and gallbladder function making it an excellent rejuvenating body tonic. Its action to increase circulation and tone the body makes it useful for regenerating skin cell tissues.

A key ingredient in many appetite suppressant formulas, grapefruit oil has been called the "dieter's friend." It is recommended in blends for regulating and treating eating disorders and for obesity issues.

An article in *Organic Style Magazine,* featuring twenty-five ways to lose weight naturally, listed inhalation of grapefruit oil at number twelve.

Research from the Institute of Aromatherapy in Toronto, Canada also reported that smelling grapefruit oil helps curb your "sweet" cravings.

Grapefruit can be used to regulate weight if used regularly. In my own practice, clients report success when using pink grapefruit to control their sweet cravings. Eliminating uncontrollable sweet cravings is an absolute must for many people suffering from Candida albicans. More and more research is linking over-consumption of sugar and high fructose corn syrup as a major contributor to obesity— now at an epidemic level in the United States— as well as cancer and other conditions.

To curb your food addictions, inhale the fresh, invigorating scent of grapefruit oil just before eating, going grocery shopping or whenever you feel tempted to grab something on impulse that you may later regret.

Grapefruit oil is an ingredient in many anti-cellulite blends. I've used pink grapefruit in appetite suppressant blends to successfully treat overweight clients who say it not only helps to diminish their appetite, but also improves their digestion and metabolism.

As a digestive aid, grapefruit oil has been reported to relieve a hangover from over-indulgence in food or drink.

Psycho-emotionally, grapefruit can enhance your feelings of self-esteem and definitely gives you an added sense of "I can do it!" Use grapefruit oil whenever you're feeling overwhelmed by life's challenges or when there's just too much going on. Grapefruit oil is also a great ally for when you're feeling drained by life circumstances. It can be a great friend to call upon to renew your optimism, as grapefruit oil can stimulate warm and happy feelings inside.

The effervescent quality of grapefruit's aroma makes it an ideal remedy for those grey, depressing mornings when you don't want to venture out from beneath your warm, safe covers. Keep a bottle of grapefruit oil by your bedside for a bit of morning zest to get you moving.

Add a drop of grapefruit oil to your favorite shampoo for a lustrous shine for dry, brittle hair. Grapefruit oil's astringent and tonic properties can also help eliminate oily hair, scalp and skin conditions like acne.

It is an excellent room freshener and deodorizer, as well as a disinfectant.

According to Ayurvedic medicine, the sour taste of grapefruit oil is used to regulate and balance conditions of Vata imbalance such as flatulence, constipation, anxiety, worry and restlessness, premenstrual syndrome and insomnia. The sour taste of grapefruit acts to improve the irregular digestive forces that are so characteristic of Vata body-mind types.

Grapefruit oil blends well with other citrus oils like lemon, sweet orange, mandarin and lime, as well as fennel, geranium, juniper berry and ylang ylang.

Dispense 1 to 3 drops of grapefruit oil on a cotton ball or smell strip, close your eyes and inhale. Note in your journal the aroma qualities you can discern and the effects the oil has on your body, mind, spirit and emotions.

CAUTION: As grapefruit oil is a phototoxin, please avoid exposure to direct sunlight or sunlamps for up twelve hours after application to the skin as pigmentation of the skin may result.

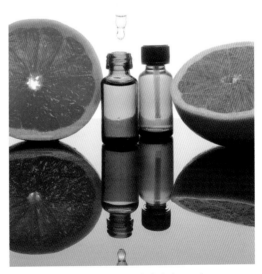

Research studies show grapefruit helps curb your "sweet" cravings.

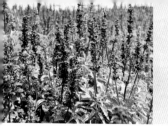

HYSSOP ESSENTIAL OIL

(*HYSSOPUS OFFICINALIS* AND *VAR. DECUMBENS*): STEAM-DISTILLED, FLOWERING PLANT—RESPIRATORY CONGESTION, COUGH SUPPRESSANT

The best locations for growing and distilling hyssop officinalis essential oil are France, Bulgaria and Italy. The best locations for var. decumbens are France and Spain.

A fairly rare oil, the scent of hyssop is warm, sweet, fresh, spicy and camphoraceous. Often used as an aromatic, medicinal plant, both varieties of hyssop oil may be useful as a cough reliever and suppressant. Hyssop oil has an established reputation for effectively treating respiratory conditions like asthma and allergies.

Hyssop is a very hardy, drought-resistant plant and thrives in the harshest climates where full sun and sandy soil are prevalent. The name hyssop is found in some translations of the Bible, and research suggests that some form of the hyssop plant was used in ancient times. According to biblical texts, hyssop was used for religious purification. A plant called hyssop was also used during the classical ages of the Greeks and Romans.

While many of their actions and effects are dissimilar, what both oils have in common is their anti-asthmatic and anti-inflammatory properties, making them suitable for alleviating swelling and inflammation and allergy and asthma symptoms. Both oils may also be useful for treating cough, bronchitis and cystitis. However, because *hyssop officinalis* is high in ketones (up to 58 percent), it is not recommended for prolonged use, whereas the *decumbens* variety is high in oxides (60 percent) and is considered less toxic and better suited for long-term use, in moderation.

Psycho-emotionally, both oils may be helpful for relieving anxiety, fatigue and nervous tension.

Hyssop oil blends well with citrus oils, especially lemon, lavender, rosemary, sage, ammi visnaga and clary sage.

Dispense 1 to 3 drops of hyssop oil on a cotton ball or smell strip, close your eyes and inhale. Note in your journal the aroma qualities you can discern and the effects the oil has on your body, mind, spirit and emotions.

CAUTION: Avoid both varieties of hyssop during pregnancy and with babies and children. Avoid the hyssop officinalis with the elderly and those with diagnosed seizure disorders or high blood pressure.

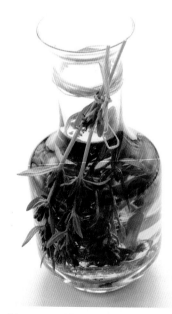

Hyssop oil has an established reputation for effectively treating respiratory conditions like asthma and allergies.

LEDUM ESSENTIAL OIL

(*LEDUM GROENLANDICUM*): STEAM-DISTILLED FLOWERING HERB—
THYROID AND IMMUNE SUPPORT

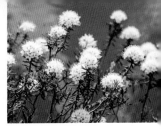

The best location for growing and distilling ledum essential oil is Canada.

A rare, herbal oil commonly referred to as Labrador tea or Greenland moss, ledum has a strongly medicinal aroma that is warm, spicy, herbaceous, radiant and penetrating. Traditionally, the ledum plant was used in herbal folk medicine and by Native Americans as a cure-all.

Ledum promotes the healthy function of respiratory and digestive systems. Its powerful action to detoxify, regulate, regenerate and decongest make ledum oil especially effective as a body cleanser and tonic. It may be useful for supporting healthy thyroid gland function, as well as decongesting the liver and treating hepatitis, Lyme disease, indigestion, flatulence and intestinal spasms.

An anecdotal study from Russia using ledum oil to treat Lyme disease, a tick borne bacterial infection, reported complete elimination of the bacterial pathogen involved in the disease.

Research in brain chemistry has discovered properties in many medicinal plants used by native cultures, such as ledum, to have sesquiterpenoid compounds. These compounds actively communicate within the human body to produce biological effects that are antitumoral, antimalarial, antimicrobial and anti-inflammatory, as well as tranquilizing to the nervous system.

Ledum oil may be effective for treating fever, flu and allergies. Kurt Schnaubelt PhD, of the Pacific Institute of Aromathery, recommends using ledum oil after acute illness. He considers it to be the number one choice for liver and kidney detoxification. He also recommends ledum for the treatment of nephritis and suggests using it to counteract the effects of insomnia and allergies.

Ledum oil's calming, antispasmodic and expectorant properties may be useful for relieving stomach upset and nervous indigestion. Ledum may also be beneficial for relieving bronchitis and cold and flu symptoms like nausea, aches and pains, congestion, sore throat and cough.

Its anti-inflammatory and regenerative healing properties make ledum oil useful for treating inflamed and irritated skin, cuts, wounds and allergic hypersensitivities.

According to Ayurvedic medicine, the warm and spicy aroma of ledum oil helps to regulate and pacify both Vata and Kapha doshas. Symptoms of Vata imbalance are premenstrual syndrome, constipation, insomnia, restlessness, nervousness, anxiety and worry. Symptoms of Kapha imbalance are high cholesterol, low metabolic forces, slow weight loss, fluid retention, stagnation and blockage, lethargy and depression.

Ledum oil blends well with lemon, pink grapefruit, fennel, carrot seed, sweet marjoram, thyme, oregano, cypress, lavender, blue tansy and spikenard.

Dispense 1 to 3 drops of ledum oil on a cotton ball or smell strip, close your eyes and inhale. Note in your journal the aroma qualities you can discern and the effects the oil has on your body, mind, spirit and emotions.

CAUTION: Though there is strong anecdotal evidence to support ledum's effectiveness, there is little research available. Generally, avoid use during pregnancy, with babies and children and with sensitive or damaged skin.

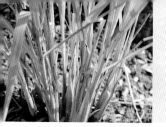

LEMONGRASS ESSENTIAL OIL

(*CYMBOPOGON CITRATUS* AND *FLEXUOSUS*): STEAM-DISTILLED OR HYDRODIFFUSED GRASS—RENEWS AND REFRESHES

The best locations for growing and distilling lemongrass are Haiti and India.

The scent of lemongrass is pleasant, fresh and lemony with an herbal note. Its effect is uplifting and refreshing to the mind, body and emotions. A regulating and tonic oil, lemongrass's action makes it an excellent oil to use for renewing your life force energy.

There are two varieties of lemongrass in common use today: *Cymbopogon citratus* and *Cymbopogon flexuosus*. While the effects are similar for both oils, C. citratus is more gentle in action and recommended for medicinal and culinary uses, while C. flexuosus is more of an industrial perfumer's oil.

Lemongrass oil has an affinity with the semiprecious stone citrine. Citrine is called the "merchant's stone." In China, the world's number one importer of citrine, merchants are said to place a chunk of citrine in the cash box to help the merchant attract income. It's thought that citrine will not only help you to attract wealth, but also help you to maintain a state of wealth.

Citrine is one of the few gemstone minerals in the world which does not hold or accumulate negative energy, but rather dissipates and transmutes it, releasing blockages on both physical and subtle levels. I use citrine, along with other select crystals and gemstones, to charge all of my essential oils and blends.

Lemongrass oil's natural astringent and diuretic properties promote lymph drainage. As I've mentioned before, the state of health of your lymph and immune system is directly related to your feelings of self-worth and self-esteem.

Psycho-emotionally, the digestive properties of lemongrass make it excellent for use in culinary dishes and may also have profound psychological and emotional effects. Using lemongrass oil helps you to digest and assimilate your life experiences. This digestive action stimulates and frees restricted conditions, helping you to move beyond self-imposed limitations. The renewing and refreshing properties of lemongrass help you to free negative mental patterns and allow them to flow.

As a regulating oil, lemongrass is helpful for stabilizing and promoting balance and harmony, especially the mood and emotions.

In traditional folk medicine, lemongrass has a long history of use. It was used to relieve muscle cramps, aches and pains and to lower blood pressure, relieve involuntary contractions like epilepsy, prevent vomiting, prevent and relieve cough, relieve rheumatic pain and inhibit and prevent infection. It is also a treatment for nervous and gastrointestinal disorders and fevers.

Recent research studies demonstrate lemongrass oil's sedative effect on the central nervous system. Its sedative properties are especially calming and soothing to your mind. Use lemongrass oil to promote relief of chronic mental states of anxiety, fear, worry and depression.

Lemongrass oil's powerful vasodilating (expansive), anti-inflammatory and sedative properties may be helpful for relieving muscle spasm as well as promoting regeneration and healing of soft tissue.

Other pharmacological studies show the remarkable capacity for therapeutic effects of the chemical constituents of Cymbopogon citratus. The effects of lemongrass include anti-amoebic, antibacterial, antidiarrheal, antifungal and anti-inflammatory properties. Other activities that have been studied include antimalarial, antimutagenicity (prevention of cell mutation and genetic alteration), antimycobacterial (prevention of bacteria like TB), antioxidant, hypoglycemic and neurobehavioral properties. The results of these studies "are very encouraging and indicate that this herb should be studied more extensively to confirm these results and reveal other potential therapeutic effects."

Historically, lemongrass has been used in traditional Indian Ayurvedic medicine for treating infections and reducing fever and inflammation. Its powerful vasodilating and regulating properties can provide fast and effective cooling relief for conditions of excess heat like hot flashes. Blend with blue tansy and peppermint oil to enhance this effect.

Lemongrass oil's regulating properties can be used to balance excess oily skin, hair and scalp conditions like seborrhea, dandruff and acne.

Its strong antiseptic and antifungal properties make lemongrass oil useful for treating fungal infections.

A natural insect repellent, lemongrass oil provides powerful protection from mosquitoes and insects and may be useful for preventing and eliminating fleas and ticks for your dogs.

Lemongrass oil blends well with peppermint, cedarwood, geranium, helichrysum, ylang ylang and conifers like spruce, fir and pine.

Dispense 1 to 3 drops of lemongrass oil on a cotton ball or smell strip, close your eyes and inhale. Note in your journal the aroma qualities you can discern and the effects the oil has on your body, mind, spirit and emotions.

CAUTION: Lemongrass oil is high in citral and may be a skin irritant.

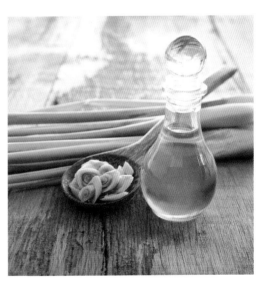

Lemongrass has been used in traditional Indian Ayurvedic medicine to relieve conditions of excess heat like hot flashes.

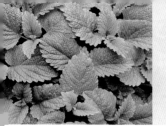

MELISSA ESSENTIAL OIL

(*MELISSA OFFICINALIS*): STEAM-DISTILLED FLOWERS AND LEAVES—
HEART PROTECTOR

The best locations for growing and distilling melissa oil are England, France and Bulgaria.

Also called lemon balm and "Balm of the Heart's Delight," the scent of melissa is sublime in character. The aroma is softly sweet and lemony with a clean, fresh, earthy coolness. Melissa oil may likely be the most adulterated oil in the perfume industry.

The aroma is characteristically fresh and clean, not at all murky, medicinal or citronella-like. As the yield of melissa oil from steam distillations is very low, the cost of pure melissa is extremely high. It takes approximately three tons (2,720 kg) of plant material to yield one pound (½ kg) of the pure essential oil. In fact, very little true melissa oil is distilled and available on the world market. Most of the melissa oil available commercially has been adulterated with lemongrass and citronella.

As a regulator, melissa oil can have both calming and uplifting effects depending on the circumstances for which it's used, and it can balance excess anxiety conditions.

Melissa oil has powerful anti-inflammatory and antiviral properties. It has been used effectively for treating herpes lesions. It may be useful for treating various infectious diseases such as the flu virus, smallpox and mumps.

Founder of the Tisserand Institute, Robert Tisserand's research indicates that melissa blended with rose otto is an effective treatment against shingles and cold sores. He recommends this blend neat for adults to treat cold sores. As it is a strong skin irritant, a dilution is advised.

Another study reported that "lemon balm oil is capable of exerting a direct antiviral effect on herpes viruses and concluded that melissa officinalis oil might be suitable for topical treatment of herpetic infections."

A heart protector, melissa oil has been used for treating tachycardia to slow the heartbeat and to relieve palpitations. Its hypotensive properties may also be useful for lowering blood pressure.

A nervine and mild sedative, in small doses melissa oil may be helpful for calming fear and anxiety and has been used for calming dementia agitation.

A study cited in the *Journal of Complimentary Medicine* reported melissa oil to be a safe and effective treatment for the management of agitation in severe dementia. The study indicated that pure melissa oil significantly reduced agitation and enhanced quality of life.

Laboratory studies on melissa oil showed that it inhibited GABA transaminase, which explains its anxiolytic (anxiety-reducing) effects.

As a digestive, melissa oil is often recommended for relieving nausea and indigestion, especially when associated with nervous tension.

Research was conducted on patients with mild to moderate symptoms of Attention Deficit Disorder (ADD). The study showed that those using melissa herbal essential oil experienced significant benefits in cognition after sixteen weeks of treatment.

Its antiallergic and antihistamine properties may make melissa oil useful for relieving allergy symptoms.

Psycho-emotionally, melissa oil's delightfully fresh scent may help ameliorate anger and restore the heart's natural rhythm of giving and receiving, allowing and accepting.

Melissa oil may also be helpful for integrating overwhelming feelings like shock, grief, terror and rage.

Blend melissa oil with frankincense oil to enhance its effectiveness for letting go, acceptance and greater depth of understanding.

As with helichrysum oil, melissa oil may help resolve past emotional trauma associated with early childhood memories or unconscious ancestral patterns.

Melissa oil blends well with rose, helichrysum, geranium, frankincense, bergamot, clary sage, clove, lemon, peppermint, sweet orange, mandarin, spikenard, thyme and ylang ylang.

Dispense 1 to 3 drops of melissa oil on a cotton ball or smell strip, close your eyes and inhale. Note in your journal the aroma qualities you can discern and the effects the oil has on your body, mind, spirit and emotions.

CAUTION: Use melissa oil in very low dilutions of 1 to 2 percent or less as its high aldehyde content makes it a strong skin irritant.

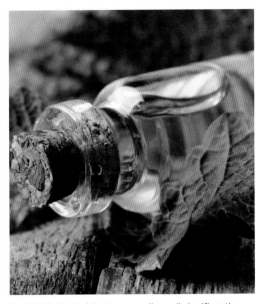

A study indicated that pure melissa oil significantly reduced agitation and enhanced quality of life in a group of patients with severe dementia.

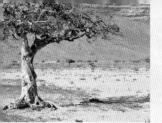

MYRRH ESSENTIAL OIL

(COMMIPHORA MYRRHA): STEAM-DISTILLED GUM RESIN TEARS—
RESTORATIVE TO THE BODY AND MIND

The best locations for growing and distilling myrrh oil are Ethiopia and Somalia.

Myrrh is sweet, warm, resinous, balsamic, smoky and woody with a hint of spice. Myrrh oil is an enduring aroma and maintains its character in any blend. You may use it to anchor other oils in a synergy blend.

Myrrh oil has a light to deep reddish-brown amber color. Its aroma is rich, deep, full-bodied and mellow. Ethiopian myrrh oil is generally considered a finer distillation from better tears. Myrrh comes from the Arabic word *murr*, which means "bitter" and probably refers to the myrrh resin's bitter taste.

An ancient and sacred oil, myrrh has been a popular healing oil since ancient times. It was valued by the Chinese as medicine, and the Egyptians used it for embalming their pharaohs, as well as for sun-worshipping practices. Greek soldiers used its resin to heal wounds and restore their strength after battle.

Traditionally, myrrh oil has been used for enhancing spiritual and emotional well-being. Thought to promote healthy functioning of the limbic (emotional) center of your brain, myrrh oil has a special beneficial effect on the endocrine (hormonal) glands and associated chakra energy centers.

Its tonic, restorative and stimulant properties make myrrh oil useful for promoting circulation of blood, lymph and nerve supply. Myrrh oil is also useful for stimulating cell tissues and restoring the physical energy of the body. Its vibrant tonic effect on cell tissues makes myrrh oil a wonderful tonic to help your body and mind recover after a long illness or physical and nervous exhaustion from overwork.

Research has shown myrrh oil to have many beneficial health constituents such as terpenoids, which are known to have anti-inflammatory and antioxidant properties. Myrrh oil can contain up to 75 percent sesquiterpenes. Sesquiterpenes are known to affect your hypothalamus, pituitary and amygdala glands, which control your emotions and hormonal response in the body.

Myrrh oil is excellent for restoring dry, cracked and mature skin cells. Its soothing, restorative and astringent action make it useful for relieving a wide variety of skin conditions including acne and sensitive, mature, oily, dry, wrinkled, chapped or cracked skin. Blended with helichrysum oil, myrrh oil is excellent for softening lines, scars and other adhesions.

Myrrh oil promotes healthy immune function and is good for treating respiratory conditions as its antiseptic and expectorant properties have a decongesting and drying effect on excess mucous as well as wet conditions like asthma, bronchitis, phlegm and respiratory congestion. Use myrrh oil for relieving coughs, colds and sore throat.

This same expectorant and decongestant action may be helpful for dispelling congestion and promoting healthy function of the thyroid, prostate and pituitary glands.

A study published in the *Journal of Medicinal Plant Research* by Chinese researchers reported myrrh resin extracts to be "effective against human gynecologic cancer."

Its strong antifungal properties make myrrh oil effective for eliminating athlete's foot, toenail fungus and ringworm. A client of mine reported he had suffered with a toenail fungus on his big toe for more than 20 years. It was a very severe case of toenail fungus that no topical or internal treatment had ever been able to eradicate. I recommended that he try myrrh oil neat directly on the toenail, once or twice a day. Within a month the toenail fungus was completely gone and has not returned.

As a natural digestive aid, myrrh oil promotes healthy digestive forces and may be helpful for treating stomachache, diarrhea, indigestion, flatulence and hemorrhoids.

Myrrh oil has been used to heal cold sores, canker sores, gingivitis, mouth ulcers and gum disease and to relieve toothache. It may be useful as a breath freshener as well as for mouthwash or toothpaste.

Myrrh oil is wonderful alone or can be blended with frankincense, helichrysum, bergamot, sweet orange, cinnamon, clove and rosemary to enhance its effects.

Dispense 1 to 3 drops of myrrh oil on a cotton ball or smell strip, close your eyes and inhale. Note in your journal the aroma qualities you can discern and the effects the oil has on your body, mind, spirit and emotions.

CAUTION: Due to its stimulating properties, please avoid myrrh oil during pregnancy.

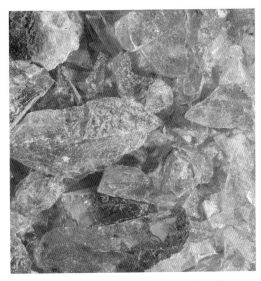

A study reported myrrh resin extracts to be "effective against human gynecologic cancer."

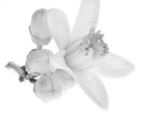

NEROLI ESSENTIAL OIL

(CITRUS AURANTIUM L, SSP. AMARA): STEAM-DISTILLED FLOWER—
INSPIRES PEACE AND HAPPINESS

The best locations to grow and distill neroli essential oil are Tunisia, France and Italy.

A divinely sweet, warm, honeyed, floral, orange aroma that's exotic and sensual, neroli is an exquisitely lovely oil from the blossoms of the bitter orange tree. I prefer the subspecies *amara* to the *bigaradia*. True neroli oil has a peaceful presence that lingers, wooing you to be still and enjoy life.

Neroli is also sometimes referred to as orange flower oil. Though derived from the same plant, the two extracts are distinctly different. Neroli oil is extracted by steam distillation, and orange flower is obtained by a method of extraction called enfleurage. Enfleurage is a cold-fat extraction process, in little use today, in which the oil's scent is absorbed into the fat (must have a low rancidity rate). The more common method of steam distillation injects steam into a still at slightly higher pressures and temperature to extract oils.

One of the most highly prized floral oils in perfumery, neroli was developed primarily for the fragrance trade. Its popularity began in the seventeenth century when the Duchess of Bracciano and princess of Nerola, Anne Marie Orsini, used the essence of the bitter orange tree flower to scent her bath and gloves. It's been called "neroli" ever since.

Various factors contribute to neroli being an extremely expensive oil. First, gathering the blossoms is labor-intensive as the neroli blossoms must be hand-picked. It takes vast quantities of the tender neroli blossom to distill even small amounts of the oil. Approximately one ton (900 kg) of neroli blossoms must be

gathered to make even a single quart (950 ml) of the pure essential oil, significantly adding to the cost of distilling the pure oil.

Ideally, the oil is best distilled immediately after harvesting and so must be very near the point of harvest. Finally, neroli oil does not keep as well as other floral oils and has a comparatively short shelf life.

The country of origin plays a key role in the quality of an aromatic scent, as does the distillation method and procedures for handling the oil.

A powerful aphrodisiac, neroli oil nourishes your feelings of self-love and acceptance. Neroli has an affinity with the precious diamond and is thought to strengthen the light and beauty within the human soul. A light winged messenger, neroli oil lightens the spirit and promotes inner peace and happiness. Even a fraction of a drop of pure neroli oil can have a profound effect on the human psyche.

A mild sedative, neroli's anxiolytic and anti-depressant effects are soothing and balancing to the mind and emotions and helpful for relieving anxiety and depression. Neroli oil may be beneficial for treating trauma and shock, as well as psychosomatic illnesses. A study conducted at a medical research center in Taiwan on the anxiolytic effects of neroli essential oil showed major decreases in levels of anxiety.

As a cardiotonic, neroli supports healthy cardio-vascular function. Neroli oil's hypotensive properties help lower high blood pressure and may be useful for treating varicosities and hemorrhoids. Energetically, neroli oil resonates with the open nature of the heart energy and serves to uplift and inspire. Its subtle vibration can produce immediate results in any stressful situation.

Psycho-emotionally, neroli oil promotes connection with your higher self and promotes self-confidence and your ability to relax and take action.

As a digestive aid, neroli oil has a calming effect on the intestines, liver and pancreas and may be useful as a compress for treating chronic diarrhea, colitis, flatulence and intestinal spasms.

Due to its high price, neroli, unlike other essential oils, has developed very little use in the food industry. It's thought that neroli oil may be one of the closely guarded secret ingredients in the Coca-Cola soft drink recipe.

As a neurotonic regulator, neroli improves elasticity of the skin. Its anti-inflammatory and anti-infectious properties make it especially useful for treating skin conditions like spider veins, scars, stretch marks, dry or oily skin, mature and sensitive skin and acne.

For chakra care, neroli is beneficial for balancing the higher chakras and helps open your heart and connect with your feeling, intuitive nature.

Neroli oil blends well with rose, helichrysum and melissa oils.

Dispense 1 to 3 drops of neroli oil on a cotton ball or smell strip, close your eyes and inhale. Note in your journal the aroma qualities you can discern and the effects the oil has on your body, mind, spirit and emotions.

CAUTION: Though a very gentle nontoxic, non-sensitizing, nonirritating oil, there are reports of phototoxicity when applied neat and directly on the skin.

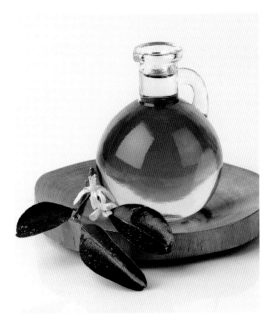

Neroli oil promotes connection with your higher self and enhances self confidence.

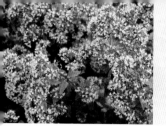

OREGANO ESSENTIAL OIL

(*ORIGANUM VULGARE*): STEAM-DISTILLED HERB—POWERFUL ANTIMICROBIAL

One of the best locations for growing and distilling oregano is Turkey.

The scent of oregano is intensely spicy, pungent, warm and radiant with herbal notes. Oregano oil is one of the most effective antibacterial oils in aromatherapy.

Its powerful antiseptic and antimicrobial action make oregano useful for treating a broad spectrum of infections. Distillations of oregano oil, especially high in carvacrol, are the most potent germ killers, along with the presence of thymol. Both carvacrol and thymol are present in thyme oil which is also known for its potent germ-killing ability.

A 1973 study by Hildebert Wagner demonstrated that a blend of essential oils had a broader spectrum of effectiveness against treating bacteria than a broad spectrum antibiotic, especially when treating upper respiratory bacterial infections. Effectiveness of essential oils for treating Candida albicans was also demonstrated.

Carvacrol has been shown to inhibit the growth of several strains of bacteria, and its low toxicity, pleasant taste and flavor make it especially useful as a food flavor to prevent and inhibit bacterial growth. The antimicrobial properties of oregano are believed to work by disrupting the bacteria membrane, causing it to die.

Numerous studies have shown the antimicrobial effects of thymol, ranging from "inducing antibiotic susceptibility in drug-resistant pathogens to powerful antioxidant properties." Research has also shown that naturally occurring biocides such as thymol and carvacrol "reduce bacterial resistance to antibiotics through a synergistic effect." Studies also showed thymol to be an effective fungicide.

These findings are especially relevant for the treatment of Candida albicans fungal infections that can cause severe systemic infections. Current treatments are not only highly toxic, but often result in drug-resistant Candida strains with low success rate.

Essential oils with the broadest spectrum of antibacterial and antifungal properties and the widest application include oregano, thyme, clove, cinnamon and tea tree.

Its antispasmodic action coupled with its powerful antiseptic action makes oregano oil helpful for soothing coughing fits and for treating bronchial infections.

Topically, oregano oil is also useful for relieving a wide variety of skin conditions, including eczema and psoriasis.

CAUTION: Oregano oil is a potent, "hot" antimicrobial and should be used with extreme caution. As it is a strong irritant to the skin and mucous membranes, use a less than 1-percent dilution for safe skin application. Avoid during pregnancy and with young children and pets.

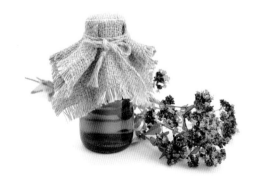

Oregano oil is one of the most effective antimicrobial oils in aromatherapy.

PALMAROSA ESSENTIAL OIL

(*CYMBOPOGON MARTINII*): STEAM-DISTILLED GRASS HERB—SKIN
AND WOUND HEALING

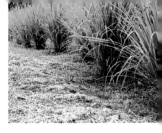

The best locations for growing and distilling palmarosa essential oil are Nepal, India and Indonesia.

One of the most popular oils in aromatherapy for treating skin problems like dry skin, rosacea, eczema and psoriasis, palmarosa has a sweet, herbal, rose-like, floral scent and is related to the lemongrass genus. Common names for palmarosa are Indian geranium and rosha grass. The oil is also widely used in the perfume industry because of its sweet-smelling floral rose aroma.

High in alcohols—specifically linalool and geraniol content (up to 95 percent)—palmarosa's powerful bactericidal properties may be useful for eradicating a wide spectrum of germs including thrush (*Candida albicans*) and E. coli.

The compound geraniol has also been shown to help stimulate cell growth, which can in turn repair damaged DNA.

A research study of essential oils extracted from the flower petals of palmarosa (*Cymbopogon martinii*), evening primrose (*Primula rosea*), lavender (*Lavandula angustifolia*) and tuberose (*Polianthes tuberosa*) reported that, "the essential oil extracted from Cymbopogon martinii showed the highest activity against both gram positive (Escherichia coli) and gram negative (Staphylococcus aureus) bacteria among the tested essential oils."

Research has also shown alcohol geraniol to be effective for treating autonomic nervous system imbalances. The autonomic nervous system is known to stimulate your hormonal production and response (refer to section on Geranium Oil on page 76). Palmarosa may be effective for treating genitourinary and reproductive issues like cystitis, vaginitis, cervicitis, urethritis and salpingitis. A uterine tonic, palmarosa may be a helpful aid for labor.

Palmarosa's regulating properties have also been reported to be helpful for normalizing thyroid function.

Research has also shown geraniol to be an effective plant-based mosquito repellent, and the rosy scent it imparts can be used to attract bees for pollination.

Palmarosa has been used for treating various respiratory conditions, including sinusitis, bronchitis, sore throat and inflammation of the ears and nasal mucous membranes.

Suitable for all skin types, palmarosa's regulating properties make it useful for balancing overly oily, dry or combination skin types. Its skin-healing, regenerative and antiseptic properties may be useful for treating numerous skin conditions including acne, dermatitis, eczema, rash, boils, abscesses, cuts, bruises, scars and wrinkles.

(continued)

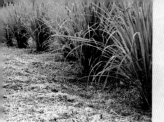

PALMAROSA ESSENTIAL OIL

(CYMBOPOGON MARTINII): STEAM-DISTILLED GRASS HERB—
SKIN AND WOUND HEALING

Psycho-emotionally, palmarosa's regulating effect may also be helpful for treating nervous exhaustion and stress-related symptoms such as fatigue and irritability. Palmarosa may be helpful for healing emotional wounds from betrayal and loss. It promotes feminine strength and courage, the capacity for endurance, stamina and stability.

Palmarosa oil blends well with geranium oils, floral oils, lavender, cedarwood, lemongrass, ylang ylang and patchouli.

Dispense 1 to 3 drops of palmarosa oil on a cotton ball or smell strip, close your eyes and inhale. Note in your journal the aroma qualities you can discern and the effects the oil has on your body, mind, spirit and emotions.

CAUTION: As a general rule, avoid during pregnancy, with young children and babies and without supervision of a qualified aromatherapist.

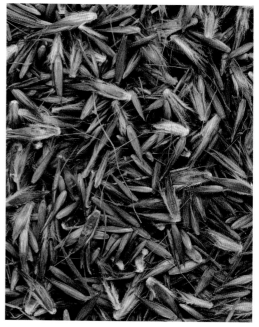

Shown here as seeds, and one of the most popular oils in aromatherapy for treating skin problems, palmarosa has a sweet, herbal and rose-like floral scent.

PATCHOULI ESSENTIAL OIL

(*POGOSTEMON CABLIN* AND *PATCHOULI*): STEAM-DISTILLED GRASS—
SENSUAL AND EARTHY, APHRODISIAC

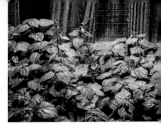

The best location for growing and distilling the cablin species of essential oil is Indonesia, and India is best for patchouli.

Patchouli cablin oil from Indonesia has a lighter color than the patchouli from India, but is just as heady with subtle differences in aroma. The Indonesian cablin is sweet and more full-bodied in character than the Indian patchouli and makes an excellent single-note perfume oil. The primary constituents of patchouli oil are sesquiterpenes (45 percent) and alcohols (as much as 33 percent), which gives patchouli its anti-influenza, anti-inflammatory and neuroprotective effects.

The heady scent of patchouli is earthy, sweet, resinous, warm, radiant, exotic and sensual. Its aroma became associated with the hippie culture of the 1960s and '70s, but the aromatic patchouli plant dates back to the days of the Egyptian pharaohs. Legend has it that King Tut had a large quantity of patchouli buried with him in his tomb.

Patchouli's aroma sings a warm, hypnotic hum to your senses with remarkable results. As an aphrodisiac and a mild sedative (in low doses), patchouli oil, with its high sesquiterpene and alcohol content, is one of the most relaxing, grounding and earthy scents in aromatherapy.

A powerful attraction oil, the strong, sensuous and throaty scent of patchouli has been highly prized in the perfume industry for centuries. In recent times, it has gained popularity as an alternative medicine, as well as for its use as incense and as an insect repellent.

A sedative in low doses and a stimulant in higher doses, inhalation of patchouli oil can leave you feeling breathless and overstimulate your senses, so take care. Use it sparingly as a little goes a long way.

An excellent skin tonic, patchouli oil's wound-healing and astringent properties make it useful for treating a broad range of skin conditions, including wrinkles and enlarged pores. Its regulating and regenerative properties act to strengthen skin cell tissue, as well as balance oily and combination skin conditions. Patchouli may be effective for controlling dandruff.

Similar in action to sandalwood and myrrh, patchouli oil is excellent for rejuvenating chapped, cracked, mature and sensitive skin. Its antiseptic properties make it useful for controlling acne outbreaks, wounds, eczema and psoriasis. Use along with pink grapefruit as an appetite suppressant and in treating cellulite.

Patchouli's tonic action may be helpful for stimulating digestion and increasing metabolism. It may also be useful for preventing flatulence and treating colitis.

Possibly an effective mosquito and insect repellent, blend patchouli oil with lemon tea tree to enhance this effect. Use in an outdoor aroma lamp, or put a few drops in a pool of melted candle wax on the patio.

Patchouli oil makes an excellent base note for anchoring a blend. It blends well with citrus and spice oils, floral oils, galbanum, ylang ylang, vetiver, myrrh, frankincense and sandalwood.

Dispense 1 to 3 drops of patchouli oil on a cotton ball or smell strip, close your eyes and inhale. Note in your journal the aroma qualities you can discern and the effects the oil has on your body, mind, spirit and emotions.

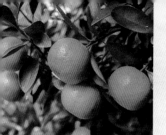

RED MANDARIN ESSENTIAL OIL

(*CITRUS DELICIOSA*): COLD-PRESSED PEEL—GENTLY CALMS AND SOOTHES

Mandarins grown and distilled in Italy are considered superior in the industry.

Red mandarin first began being widely cultivated in the early 1800s throughout the Mediterranean region where it thrives. It is one of the most commercially exported of all the citrus oils.

If you delight in the smell of fresh citrus, then you will love red mandarin. Its color is a deep orange to red, and the scent is sweet, fresh, warm, fruity and faintly floral like orange blossoms.

Many consider mandarin oil to be the same as tangerine and recommend using it interchangeably in blends; however, its aroma is distinctly different. While there are similarities in its analytical components, there are differences that make for a completely different quality and character.

Red mandarin's aroma has much more complexity and depth than tangerine oil. Though both have similar actions, mandarin oil is the more gentle and calming of the two, while tangerine oil is decidedly uplifting and great for when you're feeling grumpy.

A very comforting and soothing oil, red mandarin is gentle enough to use with children and during pregnancy, and frequently used in the birthing room by midwives.

Red mandarin is being used widely in medical centers by nurses as a comfort care measure for calming nervousness and agitation in patients, as well as a sleep aid. It can be effective for relieving nausea, similar in effect to ginger and peppermint. Red mandarin has also been used in nursing homes to calm agitation and promote sleep.

Psycho-emotionally, red mandarin has a natural affinity with the blood circulatory system and the heart. It acts to soothe and balance the heart energy center.

As with most citrus oils, red mandarin's antiseptic action makes it useful as a room spray to prevent and inhibit the spread of infection. It is excellent to use in children's playrooms.

Red mandarin oil blends well with other citrus oils like bergamot, tangerine, lemon and sweet orange as well as spice oils like cinnamon, clove and thyme. It also blends well with clary sage, geranium, lavender, sandalwood, vetiver and ylang ylang.

Dispense 1 to 3 drops of red mandarin oil onto a cotton ball or smell strip, close your eyes and inhale. Note in your journal the aroma qualities you can discern and the effects the oil has on your body, mind, spirit and emotions.

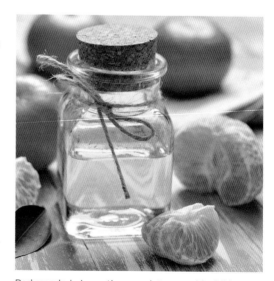

Red mandarin is gentle enough to use with children and during pregnancy.

ROSEMARY ESSENTIAL OIL

(*ROSMARINUS OFFICINALIS CT. VERBENONE* AND *CT. CINEOLE*):
STEAM-DISTILLED HERB AND FLOWERING TOPS—
RESTORATIVE, UNIVERSAL FIRST AID

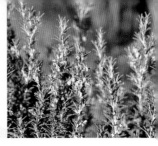

The best locations for growing and distilling rosemary verbenone are Corsica, Italy and France. Morocco is the best location for rosemary cineole.

An aromatic plant prized since ancient times, the powerful and pungent scent of rosemary is fresh, camphoraceous, warm and radiant like the sun. The woody and herbal aroma of the *verbenone* type is much less sharp than the *cineole* variety, which has a bitter bite to it.

Myth has it that the rosemary plant was draped about the goddess Aphrodite as she rose from the sea, born from the semen of the god Uranus. Legend also has it that the Virgin Mary transformed the color of the rosemary flower from white to blue when covering it with her blue cloak. It has since been called the "Rose of Mary."

A regulating oil with both stimulant and relaxant properties—depending upon the circumstances and the amount of oil used—the lovely verbenone chemotype is generally more relaxing in its effect than cineole.

Rosemary verbenone smells like the fresh-picked herb. Its soft fragrance is refreshing, lasting and pleasant. Either rosemary oil can take over a blend, so remember a single drop goes a long way.

Rosemary is an excellent first-aid oil to have on hand as its versatile nature gives it a multitude of uses. Use it alone or in synergy blended with other oils to enhance its effects. Rosemary oil has the highest hydrogen content of all the essential oils, which makes it a powerfully stimulating and warming oil.

Rosemary oil's antispasmodic action, along with its ability to stimulate and warm, make it effective for relieving symptoms of chronic fatigue, multiple sclerosis, gout, rheumatism, joint stiffness and muscular aches and pain.

With its long history of use, rosemary is one of the most highly valued oils of all the essential oils. It has been used as a sacred plant aromatic since ancient times. There are many folk songs attributed to its deep mystery and healing powers. Rosemary's place as a sacred healing oil has been lost in more recent times. Remnants of the rosemary plant have been discovered in Egyptian tombs, and its incense was used by the Egyptians for purification and healing.

Both Greeks and Romans are said to have made wreaths of rosemary to pay homage and give thanks to the gods. A universal healing herb, rosemary was reported to have been a chief ingredient in medicines made by alchemists and early scientists like Paracelsus. It is said that philosopher-healers of the Renaissance period regarded rosemary highly and praised its curative benefits in treating liver, heart, brain and eye disorders. Through the ages, rosemary has been used to celebrate life and to attract benevolent outcomes. No feast was ever without rosemary.

Its supreme skin-regeneration and wound-healing properties make rosemary verbenone especially useful for treating chronic skin conditions like broken veins, dermatitis, eczema, seborrhea and psoriasis.

(continued)

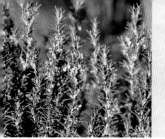

ROSEMARY ESSENTIAL OIL

(*ROSMARINUS OFFICINALIS CT. VERBENONE* AND *CT. CINEOLE*):
STEAM-DISTILLED HERB AND FLOWERING TOPS—
RESTORATIVE, UNIVERSAL FIRST AID

Excellent in skincare formulations for treating acne, wrinkles, scars and sun-damaged skin, its antiseptic and regulating action may be helpful for fighting infection and promoting glandular balance and function.

Its lipolytic properties make rosemary verbenone useful in an anti-cellulite formula. Blend with pink grapefruit, cypress or juniper to promote the breakdown of cellulite. Gentler and less stimulating than the more traditional cineole-rich rosemary, the verbenone chemotype is frequently recommended for its regenerative and nourishing properties.

Rosemary verbenone's skin-nourishing and regulating action make it excellent for treating mature skin and oily or dry hair, skin and scalp conditions. It may be useful for controlling dandruff. It is frequently used in hair treatment formulas to stop hair loss as well as stimulate new hair growth.

A male-patterned-baldness study compared Minoxidil (an over-the-counter hair loss treatment) to rosemary essential oil. Both were rubbed into the scalp daily. After six months, both groups experienced a significant increase in hair growth with rosemary users having less itchy scalps.

Rosemary verbenone may be helpful for regulating and balancing hormones. Try it in a hot compress for relieving numerous female complaints including irregular menstrual cycles, vaginitis, Bartholin cysts, menopausal symptoms and leukorrhea. Using rosemary oil is also said to remove causes which hinder conception.

Rosemary essential oil relieves blockage and stagnation and is known to fortify and protect the liver, gallbladder and heart and to enhance their function.

Its restorative properties make rosemary helpful for restoring, strengthening and balancing the nervous system and is said to provide protection against mood swings and glandular disorders.

Useful for restoring and balancing intestinal flora, rosemary verbenone may also be helpful for treating degenerative conditions of the bowel such as colitis, Crohn's disease and Irritable Bowel Syndrome (IBS).

Rosemary has been reported to strengthen and even restore sight. It is said to make the heart merry and to take away foolish imaginations.

Psycho-emotionally, rosemary oil's invigorating scent is reviving to the mind and emotions and is a wonderful aid for letting go of feelings of stress, frustration, inner resistance and a

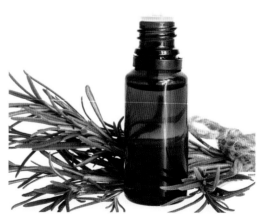

A study showed rosemary oil to significantly increase hair growth compared to over-the-counter hair treatments.

tendency to struggle. Rosemary oil enhances mental clarity and stimulates your taking creative action and is helpful in breaking free of negative habits. It may be especially good for clearing negative mental and emotional patterns, as well as negative situations. Combine with black pepper to enhance this effect.

A mental stimulant, rosemary essential oil stimulates the central nervous system and improves the intellect and left-brain recall of numbers and facts. It is a useful aid for meditation or in a study blend as it clears and stabilizes the mind. In ancient Greece and Rome, wreaths made of rosemary were said to be worn by students to improve mental focus and memory when studying or taking exams.

A 2013 study had two control groups in separate rooms. In one room there was a diffuser emitting the scent of rosemary. The other room had no diffuser. Both groups had memory exercises to complete. Subjects in the room with the scent of rosemary oil were shown to perform better. Blend rosemary with frankincense, sweet basil, orange or atlas cedarwood to enhance this memory-boosting effect.

Inhalation of rosemary oil has also been reported to be helpful for restoring the sensory abilities of smell, speech and sight!

Rosemary has been shown to be helpful for relieving mental fatigue, lethargy and physical exhaustion. A study of twenty healthy volunteers was conducted. Each subject inhaled the scent of rosemary. The study showed an increase in blood pressure, heart and respiratory rate. Along with this subjective experience of increased stimulation came reports of feeling refreshed. A great pick-me-up oil alone or in a blend, add rosemary oil to lemon, pink grapefruit or peppermint to enhance this effect.

Rosemary verbenone is recommended by many authorities for its cell-regenerating powers. It is excellent for the physical recovery of one's energy after an illness and may help to lower high blood sugar!

Its pronounced stimulating effect on the circulatory systems (lymph, nerve and blood) makes it especially helpful for increasing circulation, as well as for promoting cellular respiration and detoxification.

Rosemary's antiseptic and anti-infectious properties support a healthy functioning immune system. The chemotype of the cineole variety is most useful for stimulating immune function. Traditionally, rosemary plant aromatics were used to rid bad ghosts—like illness-causing bacteria.

(continued)

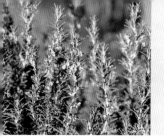

ROSEMARY ESSENTIAL OIL

(*ROSMARINUS OFFICINALIS CT. VERBENONE* AND *CT. CINEOLE*):
STEAM-DISTILLED HERB AND FLOWERING TOPS—
RESTORATIVE, UNIVERSAL FIRST AID OIL

Rosemary was one of the ingredients in the "Vinegar of the Four Thieves" recipe which hung in the Museum of Paris. It is said to be the original copy of the recipe posted on the walls of Marseilles during an outbreak of the Black Death which prevented the catching of the disease. Such herbal vinegars have been used as medicine since the time of Hippocrates.

The Four Thieves Legend

The story goes that during a great plague epidemic that swept through Europe there were four robbers who became well-known for robbing houses of plague victims. When they were finally caught and sentenced to death, they were promised their freedom if they gave their secret for how they escaped from catching the deadly pestilence sweeping the country. The recipe they gave included the plant infusion rosemary. After giving their recipe, the robbers were subsequently still put to death.

An immune stimulant, rosemary may be useful for relieving respiratory conditions like strep, bronchitis and sinusitis, as well as symptoms of the cold and flu.

Its mucolytic, decongestant and expectorant properties give rosemary its outstanding ability to relieve excess mucous conditions that is unsurpassed by other oils. Use rosemary for swelling, fluid retention edema, lung congestion and cough.

Inhalation of rosemary verbenone in moderation will clear blocked sinuses and relieve stuffy noses and sinus congestion. Blend rosemary with fennel in a hot compress or bath for stimulating and promoting the flow of chi (life force energy).

Rosemary's beneficial effects on the circulation of blood, lymph and nerve supply make it an excellent choice in a massage blend. Use rosemary verbenone for relieving symptoms of chronic fatigue and multiple sclerosis, gout and rheumatism and to relieve stiff joints and muscular aches and pain.

Rosemary verbenone is a favorite culinary herb for food flavoring and makes an excellent marinade! Combine one drop with ¼ teaspoon of olive oil and add at the end of the cooking process to maximize rosemary's benefits and flavors.

Rosemary oil blends well with many different oils including atlas cedarwood, basil, bergamot, eucalyptus, clary sage, bitter fennel, frankincense, grapefruit, lemon, lemongrass, sweet marjoram, oregano, thyme and peppermint.

Dispense 1 to 3 drops of rosemary oil on a cotton ball or smell strip, close your eyes and inhale. Note in your journal the aroma qualities you can discern and the effects the oil has on your body, mind, spirit and emotions.

CAUTION: Due to its highly stimulating properties, avoid using rosemary during pregnancy, if you have high blood pressure or a diagnosed seizure disorder.

ROSE OTTO ESSENTIAL OIL

(*ROSA DAMASCENA*): STEAM-DISTILLED FLOWER PETALS—
EMOTIONAL FREEDOM

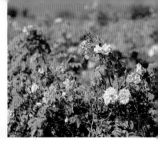

The best locations for growing and distilling rose oil are Bulgaria and Turkey.

An aphrodisiac, rose oil's fragrant nectar is sweet, floral, fresh, exotic and sensual. *Rosa damascena*, commonly known as Damask rose, is one of the most important species of the Rosaceae family and is primarily known for its perfuming effects.

Very gentle, rose oil can be used with babies and is one of the best oils to use for freeing the emotions. The scent of rose oil awakens you to new possibilities. Just a single drop can stimulate a transformative and lasting effect.

The rose plant species used to produce the pure essential oil is a large bushy plant with small- to medium-sized pink flowers. As with neroli, the petals must be harvested before sunrise when their oil content is at its peak. It takes about thirty roses to produce one single drop of rose oil, making it one of the most expense oils in aromatherapy.

Since ancient times, the rose has been a universal symbol of love. Its aroma has been celebrated for its power to touch and open the heart. Rose oil's power to awaken the human heart is unmatched by any other oil in aromatherapy.

Rose oil's ability to dissolve painful psychological and emotional blocks makes it your first choice when needing to calm your mind and emotions, whether you are male or female. Considered the fragrance of the goddess Aphrodite, the rose flower has been written about more than any other flower and is the most popular oil in perfumery.

Ancient legend has it that the Greek poet Sappho proclaimed the rose to be the "Queen of Flowers." Rose oil's feminine yin character makes it excellent for clearing and balancing the heart energies. It is often used in ceremonies for ritual cleansing of the auric field along with rose quartz crystal.

Its power to restore and elevate the emotions makes rose oil useful for healing emotional scars and letting go of old hurts and any bitterness. Blend rose oil with helichrysum oil to enhance this effect. Inhale the scent of rose oil to calm feelings of inner turmoil or jealousy. The scent of rose oil gently reduces your fears and reassures you that it is safe to let go and allow your heart to heal.

(continued)

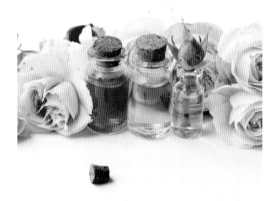

Rose oil is one of the best oils for freeing the emotions and is gentle enough to use with babies.

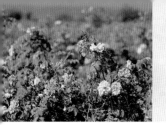

ROSE OTTO ESSENTIAL OIL

(*ROSA DAMASCENA*): STEAM-DISTILLED FLOWER PETALS—
EMOTIONAL FREEDOM

A beneficial remedy for depression, rose oil's powerful antidepressant properties are well documented. A study conducted on the relaxing effect of rose oil showed significant decreases in breathing rate, blood oxygen saturation and blood pressure, indicating a decrease in the stress response. Emotionally, subjects using rose oil were more calm, relaxed and less alert. This demonstrates that rose oil has a relaxing effect and is evidence that rose oil is effective for promoting relief of depression and stress.

Rose oil is excellent for smoothing major life transitions like puberty, marriage, birth, menopause and death. Its gentle scent gives comfort and support during times of sorrow. Rose oil is useful for relieving symptoms of hysteria, confusion and despair and allows for new growth. We are able to let possibilities flow in while gently letting go of the old ways and patterns in need of release.

An aphrodisiac, rose oil aids semen production in men and can be used for sexual difficulties. It may help alleviate impotence and frigidity for both men and women. Rose oil is a wonderful addition to any wealth attraction formula as it is said to allow the flow of prosperity, joy and happiness into one's life.

During the most decadent era of Rome (117–284 CE), historians report that rose petals were strewn in huge amounts at arenas, celebrations and marriage feasts. Still today, rose petals are strewn in celebration during marriage rituals, in wedding banquet halls and in honeymoon chambers.

As a tonic, regulator and nervine, rose oil has a deeply harmonizing and balancing effect upon the heart, the seat of the soul. It can bring you into balance and sync with life and helps strengthen your life force energies so that you are far less susceptible to illness. It may be helpful for relieving cardiac congestions and palpitations and to tone the liver, stomach and uterus.

Harmonizing for all skin types, rose oil's skin nourishing action makes it a useful addition to most facial and skincare formulas. Rose oil promotes cellular regeneration, and its cooling effect is ideal for soothing sensitive or inflamed skin cell tissue.

Beneficial for treating skin conditions like acne, eczema, psoriasis, shingles, herpes and dermatitis, rose oil's cleansing, moisturizing and tonic properties make it an excellent choice for smoothing and softening facial lines and wrinkles. It is especially nourishing and balancing for mature, sensitive and dry skin types. Use rose oil, along with helichrysum and carrot seed oil, to fade old scars and broken capillaries.

Rose oil has a long history of use in medicine. Since antiquity, physicians have praised its virtues to heal the lame and the sick. Its pharmacological effects have been studied, and most of the Central Nervous System (CNS) effects discovered are hypnotic, analgesic and anticonvulsant. The oil is reported to have respiratory, cardiovascular and laxative effects and is anti-diabetic, antimicrobial, anti-HIV, anti-inflammatory and antioxidant.

Rose oil's chemical structure is primarily made up of monoterpene alcohols. This biochemical combination is known as "the cold and flu synergy," as monoterpenes are known to stimulate expectorant action, as well as having antimicrobial properties.

Because rose oil's chemical structure is less drying than most expectorants, it is better tolerated by the kidneys and may be used more frequently. Its antiseptic properties make rose oil useful for treating pathogenic microorganisms as well as gingivitis, cold sores and gum problems.

Good for digestive complaints associated with emotional upset, rose oil's ability to reduce infection, as well as relieve cramps, makes it a useful remedy in a hot bath or compress for treating intestinal inflammation, IBS and Crohn's disease.

Rose oil is a wonderful women's oil because it is balancing for the genitourinary system and is known to have a balancing and regulating effect on female hormones and the menstrual cycle. Rose oil's astringent action promotes cleansing of the uterus and is helpful for relieving premenstrual tension and menopausal symptoms. It may be useful for treating urinary tract infections, cystitis and menstrual cramps, as well as regulating the menstrual cycle.

Rose oil may help relieve mood swings from hormonal fluctuations during pregnancy and is one of the most helpful oils to use for easing labor and delivery. Rose may also be useful for relieving postpartum depression.

According to Ayurvedic medicine, the softly sweet, floral, fresh aroma of rose oil is ideal for regulating and balancing all the doshas. Vata, Pitta and Kapha imbalances respond well to rose oil's regulating influence. Symptoms of Vata imbalance are premenstrual syndrome, constipation, insomnia, restlessness, nervousness, anxiety and worry. Symptoms of Pitta imbalance are high blood pressure, anger, frustration and emotional upsets. Symptoms of Kapha imbalance include high cholesterol, low metabolic forces, slow weight loss, fluid retention, stagnation and blockage, lethargy and depression.

Rose oil blends well with many different oils including helichrysum, Himalayan cedar wood (for male bereavement), geranium, clary sage, lavender, neroli, sandalwood, lavender and ylang ylang.

Dispense 1 to 3 drops of rose oil on a cotton ball or smell strip, close your eyes and inhale. Note in your journal the aroma qualities you can discern and the effects the oil has on your body, mind, spirit and emotions.

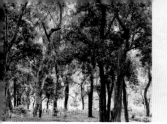

SANDALWOOD ESSENTIAL OIL

(*SANTALUM ALBUM*): STEAM-DISTILLED HEARTWOOD AND ROOTS—APHRODISIA
PROMOTES HARMONY

Some of the best locations for growing and distilling sandalwood are Mysore and Tamil Nadu in East India.

A sweet, warm, resinous, balsamic, earthy wood oil with a hint of spice, the scent of sandalwood oil is extremely tenacious. Sandalwood oil properly stored retains its fragrance for decades and is considered an inheritance-quality oil. Buy what you need to today, but you also invest for the coming decades. If you are a seller of essential oil, you can invest now for the future when you can resell the oil for a great return on your investment.

In the summer of 2006, the price of true Indian sandalwood essential oil escalated almost weekly. Scarcity of the raw material and Indian government restrictions on exportation made sourcing true sandalwood oil more and more difficult. Many vendors were no longer offering it. Since then, restrictions on exportation seem to be working as sandalwood oil is no longer on the endangered species list.

East Indian sandalwood oil containing a very high content of santalol usually indicates a strong aromatic scent, though this is not always the case. You should obtain a sample to check the quality of the oil before purchasing. Sandalwood oil distilled primarily from the very center of the heartwood or the roots of the tree usually has the purest and most intense aromatic scent.

After first distilling, the scent of sandalwood oil may be very gentle and lack the depth and fullness that it will mature into with age, but the characteristic aroma of that particular batch of sandalwood oil will be present.

As with all essential oils, the aromatic quality is greatly affected by many environmental factors, including the age of the tree being harvested (trees must be at least fifteen years of age) and the artistry of the distiller. Growing and distilling oils is often a time-honored profession, and the traditional practices for obtaining the finest quality oil from a plant are passed on through the family.

Sandalwood oil's character is very round and harmonizing. Its deep resonant nature is renowned for its regulating and grounding properties. Sandalwood's enduring fortifying properties will enhance any blend.

As a regulating oil, sandalwood has a balancing and harmonizing effect on the body, mind and emotions.

Sandalwood has been used extensively for centuries in Indian temples, as well as in churches around the world in religious ceremonies and for worshiping the Divine. Use sandalwood to enhance your meditation practice and to open and clear your solar plexus chakra, which connects you to the cosmic desire to manifest your divine soul's purpose and ensures a strong feeling of self-worth and empowerment.

A sedative and nervine, sandalwood oil is excellent for relieving nervous tension, insomnia, stress from a hectic life, grief, an agitated mind, feelings of isolation, compulsive and obsessive behavior, egocentricity, irritation, fear and control issues.

Its antidepressant properties make it useful for relieving negative mental and emotional states. Diffusing the scent of sandalwood oil readily clears negativity and restores harmony to the mind. Its life-sustaining, positive energies elevate your mind to higher ground where you can soar above life's worries to see things from a more balanced perspective. The big picture comes into view as sandalwood brings warmth and balance to your life.

Sandalwood's aphrodisiac properties are helpful for overcoming self-doubt, insecurity and hypersensitivity. If you're feeling overwhelmed by life, then inhale the fortifying scent of sandalwood oil. Its regulating and restorative action will slow your respiration and help calm your mind and emotions.

These same restorative effects make it a good tonic for the immune system. Its immune-stimulating properties act to increase white blood cell production.

Sandalwood diminishes overly egocentric drives and supports your ability to discern the needs and desires of others without feeling overwhelmed by them. Our connections with others is primarily a subconscious process guided by very subtle, nonverbal cues and signals. Sandalwood fosters your feelings of self-acceptance and your inner sense of connection so that your relationships with others can be strengthened and stabilized.

Research scientists have discovered the chemical substance responsible for sandalwood's erotic effect on your senses. A man's natural body scent is similar in chemical structure to the male hormone androsterone.

A pheramone, androsterone in light concentrations smells similar to sandalwood. It appears that sandalwood oil is similar to a man's natural body scent and, though barely perceptible, sends out a highly effective erotic signal to the opposite sex.

A cicatrizant, sandalwood oil has traditionally been used for skin regeneration and healing. Sandalwood is beneficial for mature skin and is known to balance both dry and oily skin conditions. Its natural antiseptic properties make sandalwood useful for relieving acne, skin rash, cracked or chapped skin, eczema and psoriasis. Blend with basil, helichrysum, chamomile or tea tree oils to enhance this effect.

(continued)

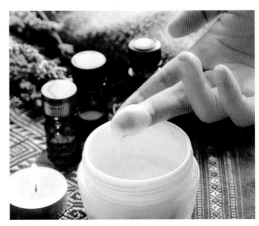

Its antidepressant properties make sandalwood oil useful, especially as a lotion, for relieving negative mental and emotional states.

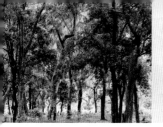

SANDALWOOD ESSENTIAL OIL

(*SANTALUM ALBUM*): STEAM-DISTILLED HEARTWOOD AND ROOTS— APHRODISIAC; PROMOTES HARMONY

Sandalwood's cardiotonic properties support the circulatory systems and enhance lymph, nerve and blood supply to all the organs and body systems.

According to Ayurvedic medicine, the sweet aroma of sandalwood oil is used to regulate and pacify both Vata and Pitta imbalances. Symptoms of Vata imbalance are premenstrual syndrome, constipation, insomnia, restlessness, nervousness and anxiety or worry. Symptoms of Pitta imbalance include feelings of frustration and anger, tendency to emotional upset and overreaction, high blood pressure and an inability to relax and go with the flow.

Sandalwood oil smooths and anchors any aromatic blend. True sandalwood oil matures with age and is considered an inheritance-quality essential oil. Sandalwood oil blends well with many different oils including rose, ylang ylang, melissa, neroli, sweet orange, mandarin, bergamot, lemon, frankincense, myrrh, galbanum and spikenard.

Dispense one drop of sandalwood oil on a cotton ball or smell strip, close your eyes and inhale. Note in your journal the aroma qualities you can discern and the effects the oil has on your body, mind, spirit and emotions.

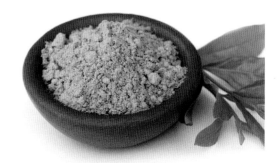

Sandalwood powder is excellent for treating a wide variety of skin conditions, and you may use it as an ingredient in your facial mask.

SWEET ORANGE ESSENTIAL OIL

(CITRUS SINENSIS): COLD-PRESSED (EXPRESSED) FRESH PEEL—LIGHT HEARTED, REJUVENATING TONIC, DISINFECTANT AND DEODORIZER

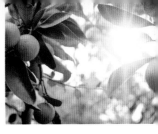

The best locations to grow and distill sweet orange oil are Italy, Portugal, France and the United States.

A gently rejuvenating and uplifting tonic, orange oil has a very sweet, fresh and citrusy aroma that's invigorating, warm and inviting.

As with other members of the citrus family, orange oil's natural astringency makes it an effective tonic for the circulatory and lymphatic systems.

Physically, sweet orange oil's stimulating and uplifting properties also makes it helpful for improving digestion, as well as relieving congested conditions. Use sweet orange oil to relieve muscle soreness after exercise, as it will help your body rest and recover.

Psycho-emotionally, sweet orange oil opens and lightens the heart energies, helping you to laugh and remember your sense of humor. When you need to lighten up, inhale the friendly scent of orange oil. Sweet orange oil has an affinity with the sun's light. It can inspire courage and help chase away any clouds of worry or self-doubt.

As an antidepressant, sweet orange oil is good for treating bouts of lethargy. Its harmonizing and tonic action promotes positive and happy feelings and pleasant emotions. Gentle enough to use with children, sweet orange is a wonderful oil to use in your child's playroom and may be useful for relieving nervousness and anxiety.

Research on sweet orange oil showed that it reduces anxiety. This may possibly be due to its high limonene content, an anxiolytic compound found in all citrus oils.

A study conducted in pediatric dental patients showed that sweet orange oil lowered cortisol and pulse rate, demonstrating its anti-anxiety effect. Similar reductions were also found in another control group of adult female patients.

Studies show that many essential oils have potential in dental hygiene. Sweet orange oil's natural antiseptic properties may be useful as a mouthwash for treating gingivitis and mouth sores.

A 2012 trial study found that a facial gel based on orange oil, sweet basil oil and acetic acid applied daily for eight weeks improved acne symptoms.

A natural diuretic, sweet orange is another citrus oil that's frequently used in anti-cellulite blends. Its astringent and lipolytic properties help break down fat cell deposits and cleanse and detoxify the tissues.

Around the house, sweet orange oil may be useful as an aromatherapy spray. Use it on countertops to disinfect surfaces and spray it into the air to eliminate odors. Sweet orange oil's antiseptic properties will immediately go to work to disinfect and freshen.

Sweet orange oil blends well with many different oils including citrus oils like bergamot, lemon, lime, mandarin and grapefruit and spice oils like clove, cinnamon, thyme, geranium, spikenard, patchouli, cypress, lavender and ylang ylang.

Dispense 1 to 3 drops of sweet orange oil on a cotton ball or smell strip, close your eyes and inhale. Note in your journal the aroma qualities you can discern and the effects the oil has on your body, mind, spirit and emotions.

CAUTION: Sweet orange oil may cause photosensitivity. Avoid exposure to direct sunlight after skin application.

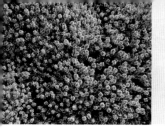

THYME ESSENTIAL OIL

(*THYMUS VULGARIS L.*): STEAM-DISTILLED FLOWERING TOPS AND
LEAVES OF THE HERB—POWERFUL ANTISEPTIC; IMMUNE SYSTEM

Some of the best locations for growing and distilling thyme oil are France, Germany, Morocco and Spain.

Dynamic, fresh and radiant, thyme oil's intensely spicy, pungent and herbaceous scent promotes a protective force field against a broad spectrum of viruses, bacteria and fungi.

Believed to bring courage to the one using it, the origin of the name thyme is related to both the Greek word *thymos*, "spirit" and the Egyptian word *tham*, a plant used for embalming in the mummification process. The Greeks used thyme for purification in their baths and as incense in their temples.

Of course, the thymus gland, which shares the same root word as thyme, plays a key role in the protective function of our immune system. One of the primary roles of the thymus gland is manufacturing T-cells which attack and kill foreign invaders like viruses and bacteria.

There are several varieties of thyme for distilling the oil with the most common being thymus vulgaris. A relative of oregano, thyme is a powerful immune stimulant and one of nature's most potent antimicrobial oils. Its fierce energy supports and protects the immune system and is unequaled by other aromatic plant oils.

A collaborative research study in Italy on the effects of thymol and carvacrol on Staphylococcus aureus and Staphylococcus epidermidis reported the "promising role of carvacrol and thymol as new lead structures in the search for novel antibacterial agents."

Thyme oil's powerful antiseptic, antibacterial and expectorant properties make it effective when diffused into the air for relieving

symptoms of asthma, bronchitis, pneumonia, sinusitis, cough, sore throat, colds and flu. It stimulates the formation of white blood cells and aids the oxygenation of cellular tissue for removal of toxic wastes during illness.

An effective natural agent against many bacterial strains, a study presented at the Society for General Microbiology's conference in Edinburgh pointed out that, "essential oils may be efficient and affordable alternatives to antibiotics in the battle against resistant bacteria."

Among the essential oils tested, cinnamon oil and thyme oil were reported to be most effective against the Staphylococcus species, including MRSA. Researchers pointed out that using natural agents like essential oils can help lower the use of antibiotics, thus minimizing the formation of new resistant strains of microorganisms.

Thyme is a natural decontaminant of food products. The journal *Food Microbiology* reported both basil and thyme oils to exhibit antimicrobial properties against the food contaminants Shigella sonnei and Shigella flexneri. Both the chemical contents thymol and carvacrol showed inhibitory benefits against these food contaminants.

Thyme oil, used as a preservative against spoilage in the food industry, also inhibits foodborne germs like salmonella, enterococcus, escherichia and the pseudomonas species.

Research on the antifungal activity of thyme essential oil (*Thymus vulgaris L.*) and thymol showed that thyme oil, "possesses a wide range spectrum of fungicidal activity."

Research on six essential oils published in the *Journal of Lipid Research* showed that thyme oil's anti-inflammatory properties had the same ability to suppress the inflammatory response as the popular antioxidant resveratrol. The study attributed this anti-inflammatory effect to the presence of the chemical carvacrol.

Thyme oil's powerful antispasmodic action improves circulation and is helpful for relieving sore muscles, aches, pains and various strains. Try it for relieving symptoms of arthritis, sciatica, rheumatism, gout, inflammation and swelling, sports injuries, painful joints and stiffness.

Pyscho-emotionally, thyme oil has been used traditionally since ancient times by the Egyptians and Greeks to promote physical and mental strength, to relieve fatigue, depression, anger and frustration, to improve the memory, to strengthen the nerves, to release mental blocks and trauma and to give courage. It is an excellent tonic for overcoming nervous exhaustion or to support physical recovery after a long illness.

Energetically, thyme oil's effect to boost your lymphatic system helps build self-esteem and confidence in your ability to heal. The lymph system is connected to one's sense of self-worth for being supported and protected in life.

Thyme oil may be an effective treatment as a gargle for thrush (candida albicans overgrowth in the mouth) and gingivitis. A research study on the antimicrobial efficacy of five essential oils against oral pathogens showed that peppermint, tea tree and thyme oil can act as an effective antiseptic solution against oral pathogens.

According to Ayurvedic medicine—an ancient system of healing practiced in India—the hot, spicy and herbal scent of thyme oil can be especially helpful for regulating and pacifying both Vata and Kapha doshas. Symptoms of Vata imbalance are premenstrual syndrome, constipation, insomnia, restlessness, nervousness, anxiety and worry. Symptoms of Kapha imbalance are high cholesterol, low metabolic forces, slow weight loss, fluid retention, stagnation and blockage, lethargy and depression.

Thyme oil blends well with many oils including eucalyptus, clove, cinnamon, cypress, lavender, lemon, peppermint and tea tree.

Dispense 1 to 3 drops of thyme oil on a cotton ball or smell strip, close your eyes and inhale. Note in your journal the aroma qualities you can discern and the effects the oil has on your body, mind, spirit and emotions.

CAUTION: As a skin irritant, avoid during pregnancy or in cases with a diagnosed seizure disorder, high blood pressure or hyperthyroidism.

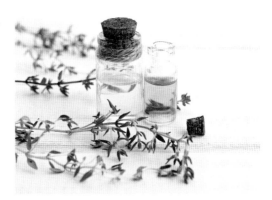

Thyme is believed to bring courage to the one using it.

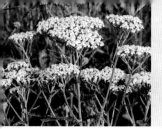

YARROW ESSENTIAL OIL

(*ACHILLEA MILLEFOLIUM L.*): STEAM-DISTILLED FLOWERS—
WOUND HEALING AND SMOOTHS TRANSITIONS

The best locations for growing and distilling blue yarrow oil are Bulgaria and Canada.

Rich in chamazulene content, yarrow has a sweet, warm, earthy, herbal and camphoraceous aroma. Its soft, full, herbal aroma is reminiscent of German chamomile and blue tansy, which also have a deep, vivid blue color from a high azulene content released during the heating process of distillation. Blue yarrow can stain, so take care.

Blue yarrow essential oil has been used since antiquity for its anti-inflammatory properties and to treat cold and flu symptoms. Blue yarrow is highly astringent and, historically, the fresh plant was used in folk medicine to stop nosebleeds, and one of its common names is nosebleed.

Another common name for blue yarrow is milfoil, which comes from its botanical name, *Achillea millefolium*, and alludes to the God Achilles' special fondness for the yarrow plant. Legend has it that Achilles used the sacred healing power of the yarrow plant to cure an injury to his Achilles tendon.

Its strongly antiseptic, astringent and anti-inflammatory properties make blue yarrow an exceptionally versatile oil. In bygone days, yarrow was commonly used to heal battle wounds. Its anti-inflammatory action is even more powerful than German chamomile or blue tansy oil. As a vascular tonic, blue yarrow may be helpful for treating varicose veins and hemorrhoids and promotes the healing of skin sores and open wounds.

A powerful restorative and analgesic pain reliever, yarrow strengthens and uplifts all of your organs and nervous and endocrine systems. Its antispasmodic action makes it excellent for treating various musculoskeletal complaints, from sports injuries and accidents to easing sore muscles and joints, strains and sprains. Blue yarrow may be an effective treatment for backache, arthritis and rheumatic pain.

Yarrow oil has a strongly cleansing and fortifying effect on the immune system and stimulates blood and lymph circulation. Its expectorant action may be helpful for relieving headaches related to sinus congestion, and its anti-allergic properties make it effective for relieving allergy symptoms.

Psycho-emotionally, blue yarrow has a stress-relieving and uplifting effect on the body and mind. It can help ease intense mental and emotional states that threaten to consume and overwhelm. Blue yarrow is a powerful ally when you're needing to allow the emergence of new vistas and fresh imaginations in your life.

It is said that the yarrow plant helps you to unite with life's paradoxical nature. Yarrow supports inner balance, stability, integration and wholeness. Its ancient cultural roots date back to a Chinese practice. Fifty wooden sticks made from the yarrow plant were used to cast the I Ching, which helped to determine correct actions for an individual to take when faced with a personal dilemma in the journey through life. The I Ching was always consulted when making an important decision.

Symbolically, the yarrow plant represents the opposites of heaven and earth being integrated harmoniously. For instance, the stem of the yarrow plant is strong and hard and has vertical and square markings, which represent yang or masculine qualities. While at the same time, the yarrow stem has characteristic yin or feminine qualities because it is round and hollow inside.

Yarrow is one of the best essential oils to use when faced with uncertainty during a challenging time. Use blue yarrow when you are at a crossroad in your life or during a great transition (such as puberty, change of location or home, marriage, menopause or life-threatening illness). It can help you unite and balance opposing forces within yourself and find your way.

To induce sleep, blend blue yarrow with German chamomile to promote calm and to soothe the mind and emotions.

Blue yarrow's regulating action may be helpful for balancing the menstrual cycle. Try it in a hot compress for relieving menstrual cramps, night sweats and hot flashes associated with menopause. It may also be useful for treating Pelvic Inflammatory Disease (PID). To treat vaginitis, use blue yarrow as a douche or in a sitz bath.

A digestive stimulant, blue yarrow may be helpful for treating constipation, cramps, gas, gout, indigestion and diarrhea, and promotes detoxification from overindulgence of drugs and alcohol.

Its regulating and stimulating action make yarrow oil useful for hair and skincare and for stimulating new hair growth. Add a drop of blue yarrow oil to your favorite shampoo to promote a healthy scalp and to strengthen your hair shaft. It is also an effective treatment for split ends.

Yarrow's astringent and regulating properties may be helpful for balancing overly oily skin, hair and scalp conditions, and its anti-inflammatory properties act to calm inflamed skin. Blend with sweet basil oil to treat acne or alone to relieve severe skin rashes and an assortment of skin irritations including eczema, psoriasis and seborrhea.

The antipyretic cooling action of all the blue oils (yarrow, blue tansy and German chamomile) make them helpful for relieving burns, including those associated with radiation treatment for cancer.

According to Ayurvedic medicine, the sweetly cooling and spicy aroma of blue yarrow is ideal for regulating and pacifying all the doshas or bodymind types. Vata, Pitta and Kapha imbalances respond well to blue yarrow's regulating influence.

Symptoms of Vata imbalance are premenstrual syndrome, constipation, insomnia, restlessness, nervousness, anxiety and worry. Symptoms of Pitta imbalance are high blood pressure, anger, frustration and emotional upsets. Symptoms of Kapha imbalance are high cholesterol, low metabolic forces, slow weight loss, fluid retention, stagnation and blockage, lethargy and depression.

(continued)

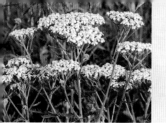

YARROW ESSENTIAL OIL

(ACHILLEA MILLEFOLIUM L.): STEAM-DISTILLED FLOWERS—
WOUND HEALING AND SMOOTHS TRANSITIONS

Blue yarrow oil blends well with many different oils including blue tansy, German chamomile, lemongrass, rosemary, helichrysum, cypress and ylang ylang.

Dispense 1 to 3 drops of blue yarrow oil on a cotton ball or smell strip, close your eyes and inhale. Note in your journal the aroma qualities you can discern and the effects the oil has on your body, mind, spirit and emotions.

CAUTION: Avoid during pregnancy. For children and babies you can safely substitute German chamomile. High ketone (thujone) content can cause headaches, so avoid prolonged use.

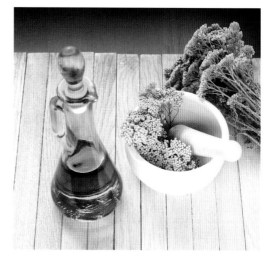

Yarrow is one of the best essential oils to use when faced with uncertainty and challenging times of transition.

ADDITIONAL OILS USED IN THIS BOOK

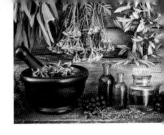

BASIL (*OCIMUM BASILICUM, CT LINALOOL*): STEAM-DISTILLED LEAF, EGYPT

AROMAS: Sweet, herbaceous, spicy, warm and radiant

USES: Focus support, to clear the mind, stay alert and aid memory

CAUTION: Avoid during pregnancy.

BIRCH (*BETULA LENTA*): STEAM-DISTILLED BARK, CANADA

AROMAS: Sweet, balsamic, warm, radiant, penetrating and woody

USES: Pain reliever, relieves muscle aches and pains

CAUTION: Its high methyl salicylate content (99%) makes birch oil harmful in high concentrations. Use in weak dilutions of less than 1%. Avoid in pregnancy, with babies and children. Avoid with sensitive or damaged skin.

JUNIPER BERRY (*JUNIPERUS COMMUNIS*): STEAM-DISTILLED BERRY, BOSNIA

AROMAS: Warm, fresh, radiant, spicy, balsamic, herbaceous, woody and piney

USES: Detoxifier, blood cleanser

CAUTION: Because of its stimulative effect on kidneys, avoid in pregnancy, in cases of acute chronic kidney or bladder infection, or with kidney disease.

MANUKA (*LEPTOSPERMUM SCOPARIUM*): STEAM-DISTILLED LEAF, NEW ZEALAND

AROMAS: Sweet, woody, earthy and balsamic

USES: Similar to tea tree in action, yet more gentle; the smell is sweet and mellow, not medicinal like tea tree

CAUTION: Neurotoxic. Short-term use of low dilutions of 1% or less is considered safe. Essential oils high in ketones need to be used with care in pregnancy.

SPIKENARD (*NARDOSTACHYS JATAMANSI*): STEAM-DISTILLED ROOT, NEPAL

AROMAS: Sweet, earthy, resinous, woody, exotic, sensual, warm and radiant

USES: Powerful sedative, spiritual healing and anointing oil

CAUTION: Avoid during pregnancy.

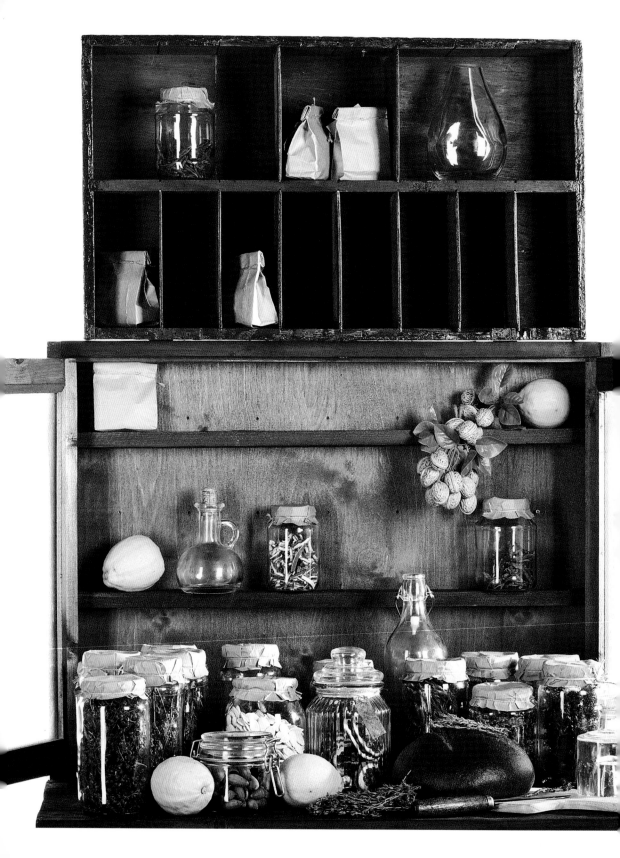

CHAPTER 8

Proper Storage of Essential Oils

As essential oils are highly volatile and quickly evaporate when exposed to the air, care must be taken to store them properly. This means keeping your essential oils tightly sealed in dark, colored-glass bottles. You want to store your oils in a cool, dark place, out of direct sunlight and out of the reach of children and animals. Artificial and fluorescent lighting can have a detrimental effect on essential oils and shorten their shelf life.

Pure essential oils will break down plastic and should never be stored undiluted in plastic bottles. Properly stored essential oils that have been sealed, unopened and kept in a cool, dark place will maintain their potency for many years.

The only exception to this may be the quicker evaporating citrus oils (such as grapefruit, orange, lime, mandarin and lemon) and conifers and firs (such as fir, pine and cypress). These oils have a shorter shelf life because high volatility leads to faster oxidation, causing them to lose any characteristic therapeutic properties, actions and effects.

Citrus oils are by far the most volatile of all the essential oils. Special care needs to be taken to keep them tightly sealed and stored in a darkened area that is both dry and cool. You can limit the amount of oxidation of your essential oils by keeping them in bottles that are filled to capacity in which there is no room inside the bottle for oxidation to occur.

You can consider refrigerating your citrus oils, blue oils, conifers and others to increase shelf life as long as the oils are kept in a dry condition and are stored for long-term use rather than being dispensed daily. Refrigerating your blue oils will help them retain their vibrant blue color. Never refrigerate rose oil, as it will thicken and congeal. Thicker, viscous oils have a low volatility rate and, as long as the bottle is filled to capacity, will have a very slow oxidation rate.

Shelf Life for Essential Oils

Many things can affect the shelf life of an essential oil. This is a general guide for a short list of essential oils. Proper storage can significantly increase the longevity of an oil's shelf life and its therapeutic quality. If stored in a dark, glass bottle that is filled to capacity and kept sealed, this guide will give you a general idea about shelf life.

NOTE: If an essential oil begins to appear cloudy, thicken or smell more acidic, it has likely begun to oxidize.

APPROXIMATELY 6 MONTHS– 2 OR 3 YEARS FROM DATE OF DISTILLATION:

Bay Laurel (*Laurus nobilis*)

Cypress (*Cupressus sempervirens*)

Eucalyptus* (*Eucalyptus globulus* and *radiata*)

Fir Needle (*Abies concolor*)

Frankincense (*Boswellia frereana*)

Grapefruit (*Citrus paradisi*)

Juniper Berry (*Juniperus communis*)

Lemon (*Citrus limonum*)

Lemongrass (West Indian) (*Cymbopogon citratus*)

Lime (*Citrus aurantifolia*)

Mandarin (*Citrus deliciosa*)

Nutmeg (*Myristica fragrans*)

Sweet Orange (*Citrus sinensis*)

Petitgrain (*Citrus aurantium*)

Pine (*Abies sibirica*)

Black Spruce (*Picea mariana*)

Tangerine (*Citrus reticulata*)

* If stored properly and/or refrigerated, eucalyptus can last up to 5 years.

APPROXIMATELY 3–4 YEARS FROM DATE OF DISTILLATION:

Ammi Visnaga (Khella Plant Seeds) (*Ammi Visnaga*)

Black Pepper (*Piper nigrum*)

Bergamot (*Citrus bergamia*)

Carrot Seed (*Daucus carota*)

Cinnamon Leaf (*Cinnamomum zeylanicum*)

Clove Bud (*Eugenia caryophyllata*)

Eucalyptus (*Eucalyptus globulus* and *radiata*)

Fennel, Bitter (*Foeniculum vulgare*)

Helichrysum (*Helichrysum italicum*)

Ledum (*Ledum groenlandicum*)

Myrtle (*Myrtus communis*)

Naiouli (*Melaleuca quinquenervia*)

Neroli (*Citrus aurantium var amara*)

APPROXIMATELY 4-5 YEARS FROM DATE OF DISTILLATION:

Basil (*Ocimum basilicum, ct linalool*)

Clary Sage (*Salvia sclarea*)

Eucalyptus (*Eucalyptus globulus* and *radiata*)

Geranium (*Pelargonium graveolens* and *roseum*)

German Chamomile (*Matricaria recutita*)

Ginger (*Zingiber officinale*)

Lavender (*Lavandula angustifolia*)

Palmarosa (*Cymbopogon martinii*)

Peppermint (*Mentha x piperita*)

Roman Chamomile (*Anthemis nobilis*)

Ylang Ylang (*Cananga odorata*)

APPROXIMATELY 6-8 YEARS FROM DATE OF DISTILLATION:

Cedarwood (*Cedrus atlantica* or *deodora*)

Myrrh (*Commiphora myrrha*)

Patchouli (*Pogostemon cablin*)

Sandalwood (*Santalum album*)

Vetiver (*Vetiveria zizanoides*)

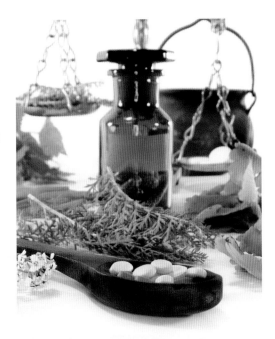

Stored properly, you can enjoy using your essential oils for many years.

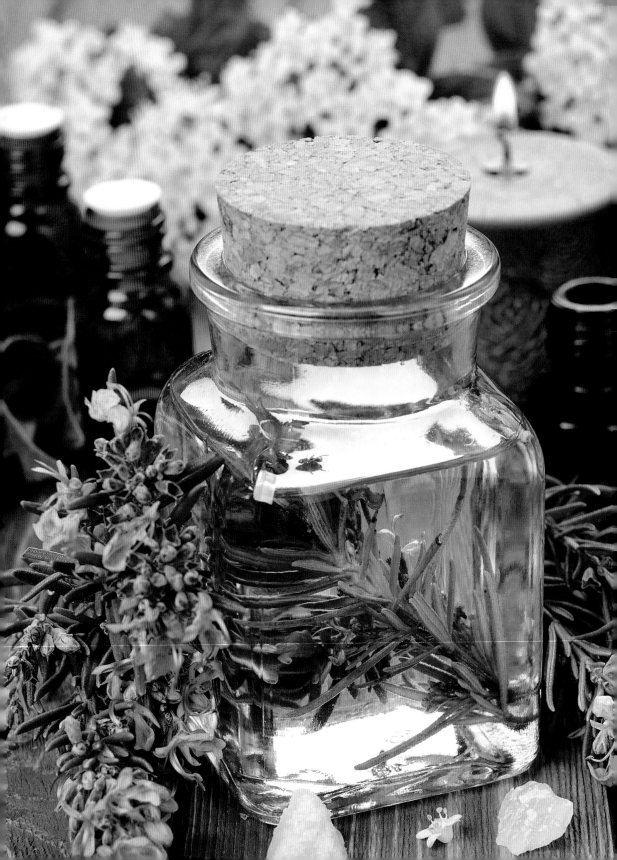

Aromatherapy Blending Guide (and Secrets)

I've always had a passion for music. There are a lot of analogies between aromatherapy blending and music. Formulating an essential oil blend is very much like making music. Like music, you can create essential oil blends that are very inspiring and uplifting to your senses, that help you to relax and unwind, relieve cold and flu symptoms and more.

Your taste in music is often reflected in the aromas you love most and the blends you feel inspired to create. If you like hot, spicy salsa music, you are probably attracted to hot and spicy oils. If you like music that's relaxing, you're probably drawn to calming oils. Maybe you like a combination of both relaxing and stimulating oils depending upon the circumstances and your desired results.

I love music everywhere except in my blending room. For me, blending is very much a meditative experience. I usually like to blend in silence with no distractions, so that I can completely focus on creating my blend.

I also use biodynamic blending methods that take into consideration phases of the moon, among other things. Just like how the best days for planting are noted in the farmer's almanac, there are best times to create your blends.

Music and blending have in common both craftsmanship and artistry. You have to learn how to touch and be touched by the oils. It's very much an intimate relationship that you develop with the oils. I've always had this intuitive, felt sense with essential oils. Some oils speak to me more loudly than others, but there is always a communion and partnership at the heart of my experience when blending oils.

Just like the finest culinary chefs with food ingredients or the most gifted musicians with their instruments, it's through developing an intimate relationship with the oils that you will learn how to create the greatest beauty and harmony when blending aromatic formulas. When you commune with your essential oils, you can produce incredible healing results in practice.

In aromatherapy, blending becomes craftsmanship when you learn how to use the tools of essential oils for healing. Craftsmanship is learning which essential oils to use for producing certain therapeutic results and discovering the method of application to use for the best outcomes and desired effects. When you learn the different techniques to use in practice, this is craftsmanship. Your craftsmanship allows the oils to achieve their greatest potential for promoting balance and healing.

Whereas artistry is when you're capturing the aromatic scents and creating harmony between ingredients and having those aromas enhance one another in a synergetic dance that is captivating to the senses.

Essential oils are not really tangible. They are aromatic vapors that quickly evaporate when they meet the elements of light, heat and air. Interestingly, it is the contact with the elements that releases the scent of essential oils. You actually feel aromatic scents. Your rational brain is not at all involved in your process of smell. Scent reaches the deepest part you!

Just as with music, there are top or high notes, middle notes and bottom or base notes. You want to create a blend of oils that can become like music, harmonious and pleasing to your senses, all while having the qualities needed to produce the desired therapeutic effects. When you make music with essential oils it moves beyond craftsmanship to artistry and becomes a visceral experience.

To keep your blends vibrant and consistent you have to use all your knowledge and the blending techniques you will learn. You will also need to connect with your blend exactly like a musician does to make music so that you and others can appreciate and benefit from using your essential oil blend.

My blending secrets will guide you step-by-step in exactly how to create the perfect blend. You will learn how to wed the artistry of blending with the craftsmanship needed to make each of your blends sing and achieve remarkable results.

After a little practice, you will know the aroma qualities and effects of many different essential oils and enjoy creating your very own aromatherapy blends to satisfy your personal needs!

To make a blend of essential oils for the first time, I recommend you start with a bottle that is larger than necessary so you have room to experiment and allow your blend to evolve. When I create a new blend, I usually start with a 1-ounce (30-ml), colored-glass bottle that can be tightly sealed with a screw cap.

You're experimenting with the oils to create your perfect blend, and it's best to have plenty of room to formulate your blend. Later you can transfer your blend to a smaller colored-glass, euro-dropper bottle for dispensing your oils. Right now you're in the blending creation mode.

Next you must decide for what purpose you want to use your essential oil blend. Is it a perfume or pain-relief oil, or is it for relaxation, beauty or skincare?

Essential Oil Blending Directions

1. Choose three essential oils (top, middle and base notes) you want to use in your blend.

2. Use an aromatherapy journal or a clean sheet of paper to write down the names of each essential oil you will be using to formulate your blend. You will record the number of drops of each oil you add to your blend. You will be writing down the recipe that you're creating.

3. Add 1-3 drops of your selected essential oil. Write down its aroma quality and characteristic effects and whether it is a top, middle or base note.

   I like to start with base notes as they are less volatile and will not have an immediate tendency to evaporate. The base note will also anchor the middle and high notes, so they're less susceptible to rapid evaporation. If you're going to walk away from your blend for any length of time, I recommend you cap the bottle tightly as a precaution to prevent evaporation. This also helps you develop your relationship with the oils. For me, aromatic blending is a sacred act of communion with the oils, and I'm always sending them my love and appreciation.

4. Add 1-3 drops of another of your selected essential oils. Write down its aroma quality and characteristic effects and whether it's a top, middle or base note.

5. Add 1-3 drops of your third essential oil, noting its aroma quality and characteristic effects, as well as if it is a top, middle or base note.

6. Cap the top of the bottle and shake vigorously, blending the oils.

Now it's time to sample your blend's aroma.

Dispense one drop onto a smell strip, tissue or cotton ball and inhale the aroma of your blend. When sampling the aroma, you will probably notice the scent of one of the essential oils more than the rest. This is usually the case. The lighter, higher, top notes are usually most discernible.

As your blend begins to synergize, the aroma qualities will change and take on a unique character. Allow space for this synergistic action to happen. You'll be glad you did. How you begin sets a firm foundation for your blend. You're gathering the information you need to create a truly mesmerizing blend. So take time for your blend to synergize.

Writing down your aroma experiences deepens your awareness of each essential oil and how it blends with other oils.

At a certain point, usually within 30 minutes, but sometimes longer, you'll notice the blend's aroma begins to stabilize. One of the reasons I use only 3-9 drops when first making a blend is that less time for synergy is required.

You will notice that the aroma of certain essential oils lingers longer in your memory.

Are you able to discern the individual oils? How have the oils changed or been enhanced by the other oils in the blend? Write down everything you notice about your experience of the three blended oils.

Now the next important question to answer is are you happy with the ratio of the oils? Does 1-3 drops of each oil in the blend seem the right ratio? Or, does your blend lack harmony?

The aromatic qualities and the language of aromas sing to your senses like muses inspiring you to formulate a balanced blend for harmonizing body, mind, spirit and emotions. Listen deeply as you experiment with your aromatic formulation. As you do this you will naturally get a feel for when to emphasize a particular aromatic note. You will begin to understand the language of aroma to achieve your desired results.

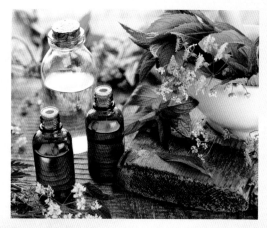

For me, aromatic blending is a sacred act of communion with the oils and I'm always sending them my love and appreciation.

Then add one additional drop of any one of the oils that especially called to you. You may feel that you want to experience more of that particular note in your blend. Be sure to record each drop you add to your blend in your journal or on your recipe sheet.

Mix the blend again and inhale. Follow the above guidelines for allowing your blend to synergize, and take time to fully experience it before moving forward. Take time to formulate your recipe slowly in gradual steps. Focus and pay close attention. Continue to notice and note your experience of the oils as you create your blend.

Continue to add one drop at a time of any of the oils that calls to you until you feel the blend is complete and pleases your senses.

Keeping track of the number of drops of each essential oil while blending ensures you won't forget the exact recipe of a blend should it be a memorable one for you.

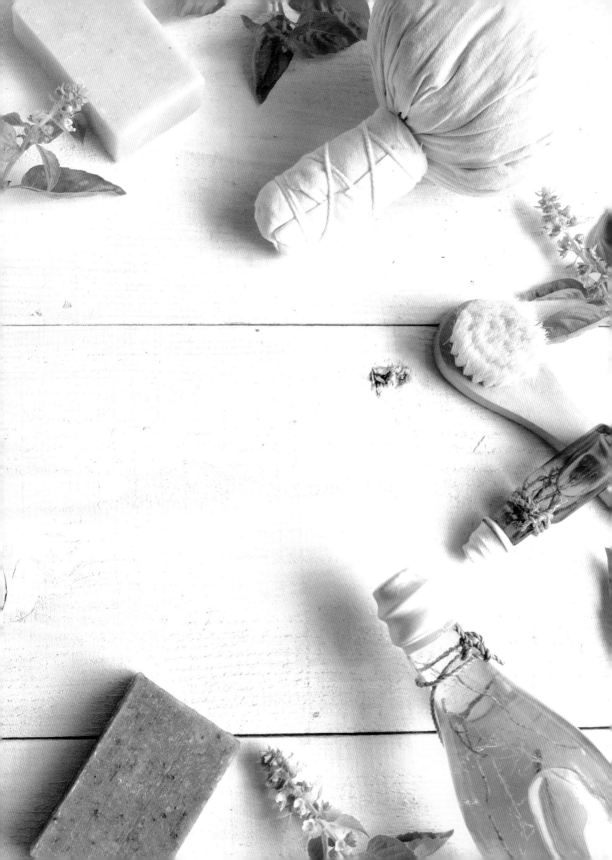

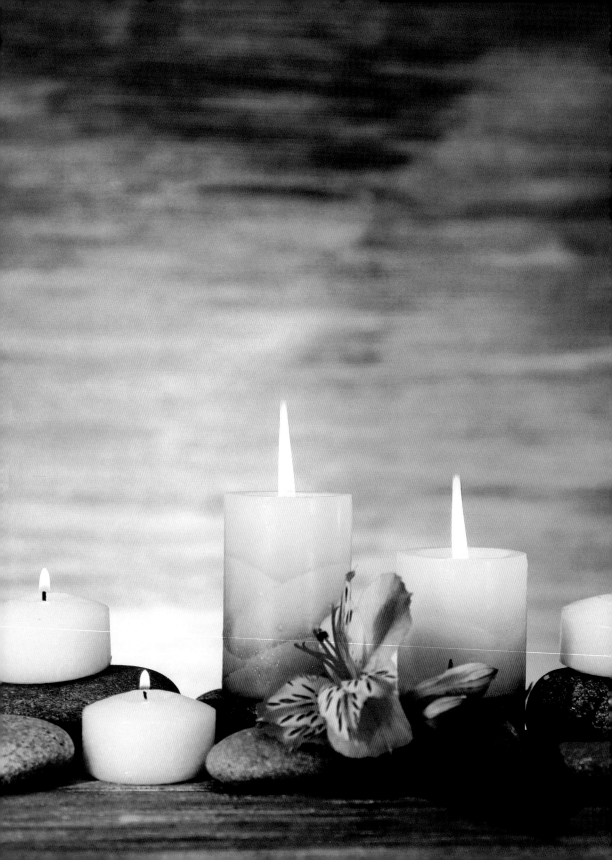

CHAPTER 10

Aromatherapy Formulas

After experimenting with creating your own essential oil blend, try these three types of starter aromatherapy blends. Allow your blend to synergize for at least 30 minutes, then pour your blend into a 1-ounce (30-ml) bottle of your favorite carrier oil in the recommended dilution amounts given for each blend.

1% DILUTION — HEADACHE RELIEF BLEND (9–15 DROPS TOTAL)

Eucalyptus, *Eucalyptus globulus*: 2 drops

Peppermint, *Mentha x piperita*: 3 drops

Lavender, *Lavandula augustifolia*: 4 drops

2% DILUTION — IMMUNE STIMULANT BLEND (15–18 DROPS TOTAL)

Lavender, *Lavandula angustifolia*: 5 drops

Manuka, *Leptospermum scoparium*: 5 drops

Eucalyptus, *Eucalyptus radiata*: 5 drops

5% DILUTION — SORE MUSCLE BLEND (30-45 DROPS TOTAL)

Marjoram, *Origanum majorana*: 10 drops

Peppermint, *Mentha x piperita*: 10 drops

Lavender, *Lavandula angustifolia*: 10 drops

Rub a little of your Headache Relief or Immune Stimulant essential oil blend diluted in carrier oil on your wrists, your temples or the sides of your neck or chest. Try the Sore Muscle Blend on a tense muscle or painful joint.

Use your blend several times at intervals over the next several days and notice what effect it has on you. Share your blend with family and friends, and ask them to report any effects they notice and how they enjoyed the oil. Make notes about all of your observations and how others who use the blend respond.

Also, notice if your essential oil blend changes over time. Does the scent of your blend smell the same on a smell strip as when applied to your skin? Or is it somehow different?

By trying out your essential blends with others and using different methods of application you are learning valuable information for creating essential oil blends that heal. Through exploring the uses and benefits of essential oils you will become confident about using them in your everyday life.

Next, try the following essential oil blends to test out your skills.

Massage Oil Blends

An aromatherapy massage has been shown to have therapeutic effects to calm your mind and emotions. It can also be used to promote muscle pain relief, speed healing of injuries and aid recovery from illness, physically demanding work and rigorous exercise.

An 8-month study was conducted on eight subjects who were given a weekly aromatherapy massage for 6 weeks. Each subject's level of anxiety and depression was measured using the Hospital Anxiety and Depression Scale (HADS) prior to their first massage and again after their final massage. Improvements were reported in six out of the eight test subjects.

Relaxation Formula

This formula is perfect as your go-to blend or for the beginner who is new to the world of aromatherapy massage. Always pleasing!

To a 5-ml euro-dropper bottle add:

Vetiver: 20 drops

Cypress: 20 drops

Lavender: 20 drops

Clary Sage: 10 drops

Bergamot: 30 drops

Close the cap tightly and shake the bottle vigorously to thoroughly blend the essential oils. Allow to synergize for 8 or more hours before using.

To make a ready-to-use relaxation blend, simply add 15–30 drops of your synergy blend to a 1-ounce (30-ml) bottle of your favorite carrier oil. Shake the bottle well to disperse the oils thoroughly. Use as a massage oil lubricant.

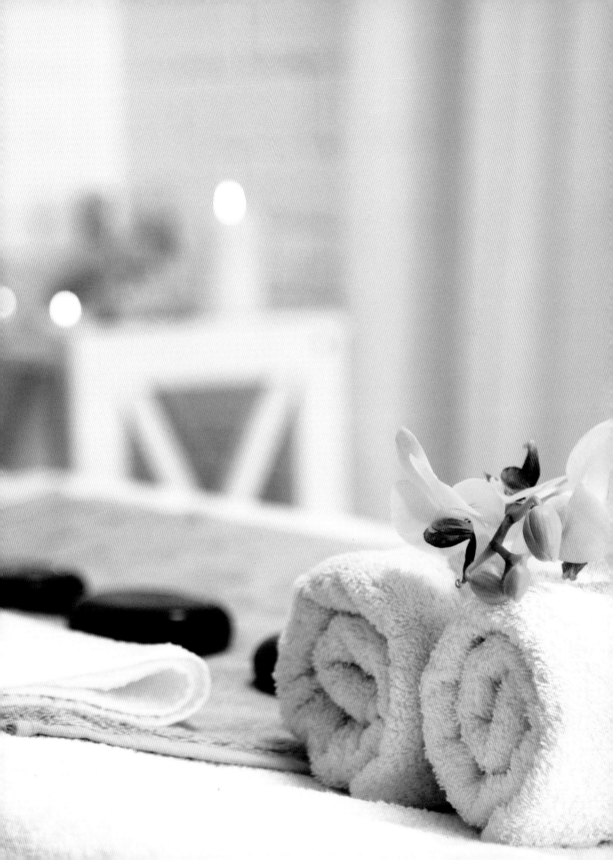

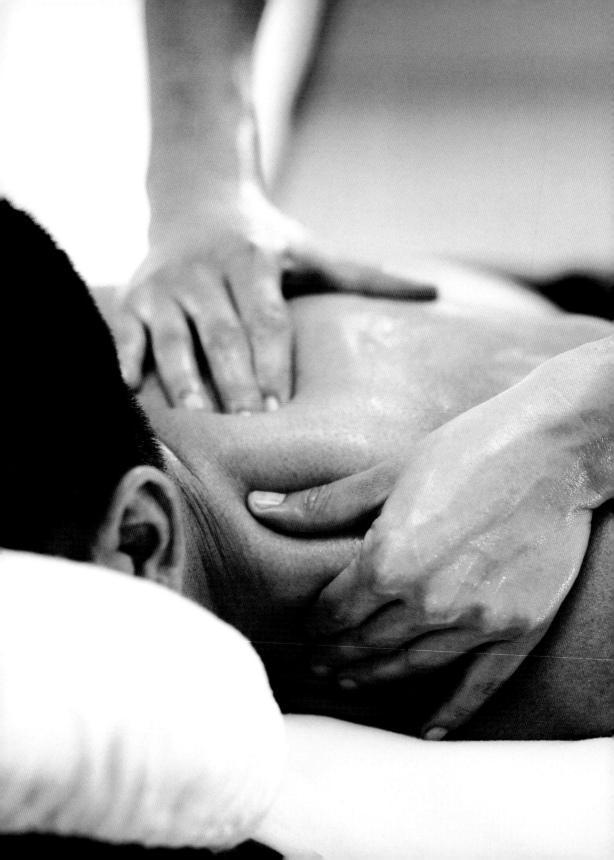

Sports Injury Formula

If you, a friend, a loved one or a client has an injury, especially one involving soft tissue, muscles, ligaments or tendons, this is a great blend you can rely on to speed healing and recovery.

To a 5-ml euro-dropper bottle add:

Sweet Marjoram: 40 drops

Helichrysum: 10 drops

Cypress: 40 drops

Peppermint: 10 drops

Close the cap tightly and shake the bottle vigorously to thoroughly blend the essential oils. Allow to synergize for 8 or more hours before using.

To make a ready-to-use sports injury blend, simply add 15–30 drops of your synergy blend to a 1-ounce (30-ml) bottle of your favorite carrier oil. Shake the bottle well to disperse the oils thoroughly. Use as a massage oil lubricant.

Calming Formula

When you need a blend that will help to ease and soothe an overly active or agitated mind and emotions, this is the blend to use.

~~~~~~

To a 5-ml euro-dropper bottle add:

Lavender: 20 drops

Sweet Marjoram: 20 drops

Ylang Ylang III: 20 drops

Roman Chamomile: 20 drops

Red Mandarin: 20 drops

Close the cap tightly and shake the bottle vigorously to thoroughly blend the essential oils. Allow to synergize for 8 or more hours before using.

To make a ready-to-use calming blend, simply add 15–30 drops of your synergy blend to a 1-ounce (30-ml) bottle of your favorite carrier oil. Shake the bottle well to disperse the oils thoroughly. Use as a massage oil lubricant.

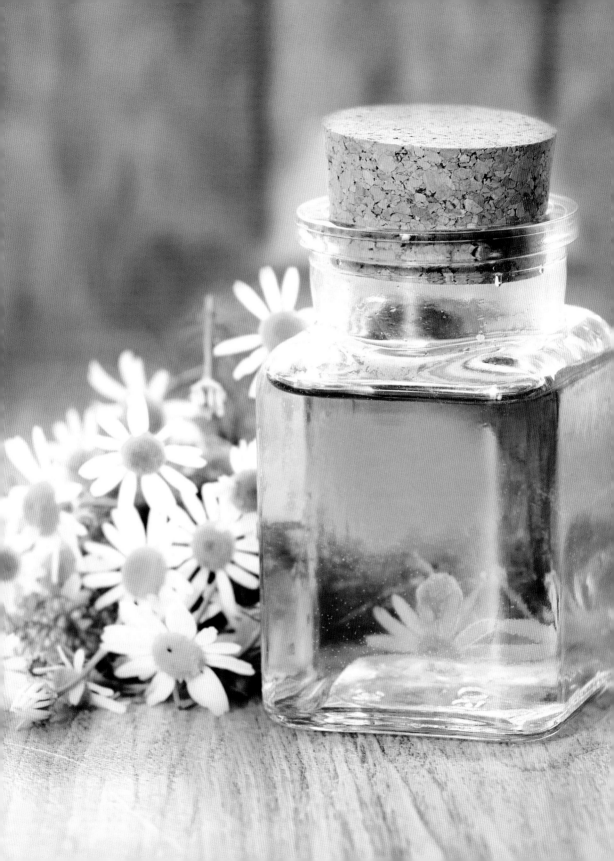

Restorative Formula

When your energy feels low, or you feel rundown or overly tired from not enough rest or sleep, or because you've been burning the candle at both ends, use this restorative formula. It will give your energy a boost, as well as freshen your thoughts and emotions and get you going in the right direction.

To a 5-ml euro-dropper bottle add:
Myrrh: 40 drops
Frankincense: 40 drops
Lemongrass: 10 drops
Galbanum: 1–2 drops
Black Spruce: 10 drops

Close the cap tightly and shake the bottle vigorously to thoroughly blend the essential oils. Allow to synergize for 8 or more hours before using.

To make a ready-to-use restorative blend, simply add 15–30 drops of your synergy blend to a 1-ounce (30-ml) bottle of your favorite carrier oil. Shake the bottle well to disperse the oils thoroughly. Use as a massage oil lubricant.

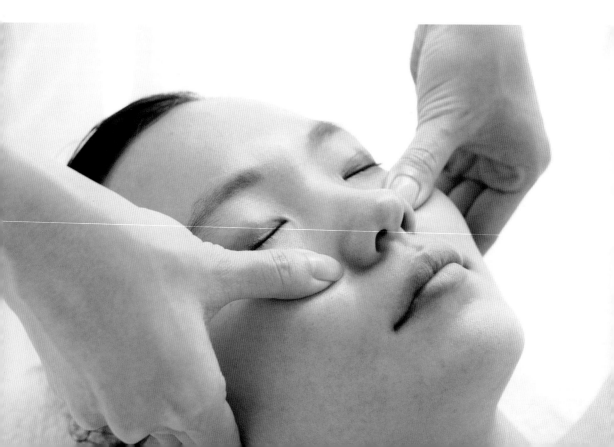

Muscle Pain Relief Formula

When your body feels sore and aches, this is a great oil you can rely on to ease your pain and give you the desired relief. It's also refreshing and restorative to your mind and emotions.

To 5-ml euro-dropper bottle add:

Sweet Marjoram: 80 drops

Ginger: 10 drops

Peppermint: 10 drops

Close the cap tightly and shake the bottle vigorously to thoroughly blend the essential oils. Allow to synergize for 8 or more hours before using.

To make a ready-to-use pain relief blend, simply add 15–30 drops of your synergy blend to a 1-ounce (30-ml) bottle of your favorite carrier oil. Shake the bottle well to disperse the oils thoroughly. Use as a massage oil lubricant.

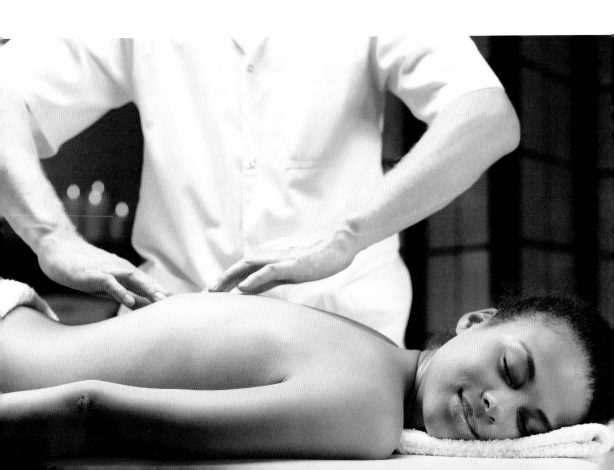

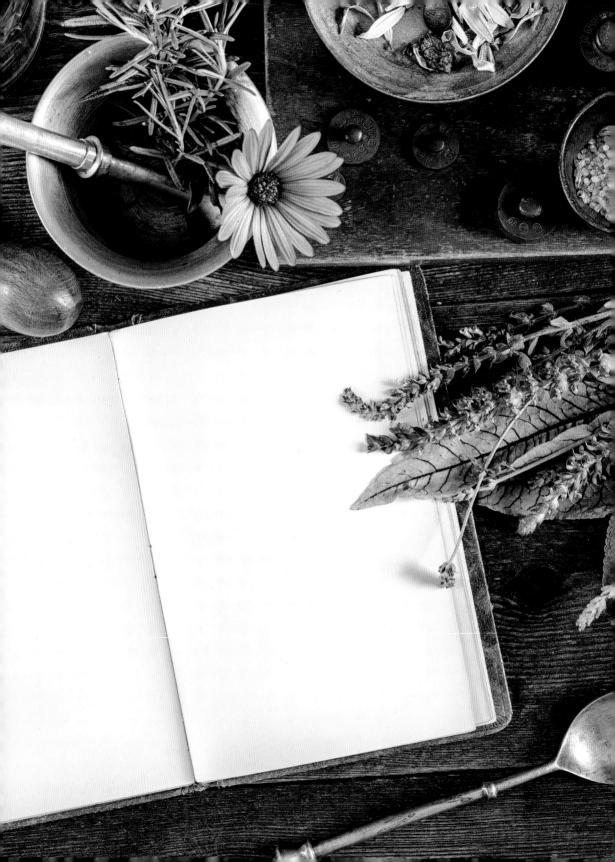

CHAPTER 11

Healing Blends

These blends will help you become more aware of how aromatherapy works as you continue to practice the art. Feel your confidence grow and bring relief to yourself and others with these Healing Blends.

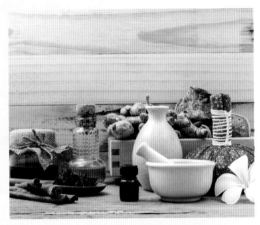

Create your own healing essential oil blends for alternative relief, relaxation and self-esteem.

Headache Relief Formula

Headache is the most common form of physical pain. More than 50 percent of adults in the U.S. will experience some kind of headache this year. Symptoms of a headache may include pain in the head and neck regions, loss of appetite, poor sleep, light headedness and dizziness. Headaches may be caused by many different conditions such as dehydration, toxicity in the body, cold and flu, head injury, structural deviations of the neck, dental and sinus issues, sleep deprivation, food allergies and intolerances, and medications, among others. There are three main types of headache experienced: migraines, tension headaches and cluster headaches. Commonly, the method of treatment used most often for headache is pain medication that can have unwanted side effects.

The essential oils in this Headache Relief Formula have been shown to be effective for relieving symptoms of tension and migraine headaches. The blend contains powerful analgesic pain relievers, vasoconstrictors and decongestants that promote circulation and shrink swollen membranes. The formula works best if used immediately at the first sign of a headache.

Tension and migraine headaches may be a sign of dehydration. Be sure to drink plenty of pure, fresh water daily. The guideline for sufficient water intake is generally half your body weight in ounces daily.

To a 5-ml, colored-glass, euro-dropper bottle add:
Peppermint: 20 drops
Marjoram: 20 drops
Eucalyptus: 20 drops
Lavender: 20 drops
Lemon: 10 drops
Juniper Berry: 5 drops
Basil: 5 drops

Cap the bottle tightly and shake vigorously to blend the essential oils. Allow to synergize for 8 hours or longer before using.

Dispense 1–3 drops on a cotton ball or smell strip and inhale the aromatic vapors of your headache relief blend for 10–15 seconds. You may repeat as needed. The formula is also effective when diffused into the air or used as a cool compress applied to the back of your neck.

To make a ready-to-use headache relief blend, simply add 15–30 drops of your synergy blend to a 1-ounce (30-ml) bottle of your favorite carrier oil. Shake the bottle well to disperse the oils thoroughly. Apply a few drops of your ready-to-use headache relief blend to sinus points around your nose and forehead, as well as on the back of your neck.

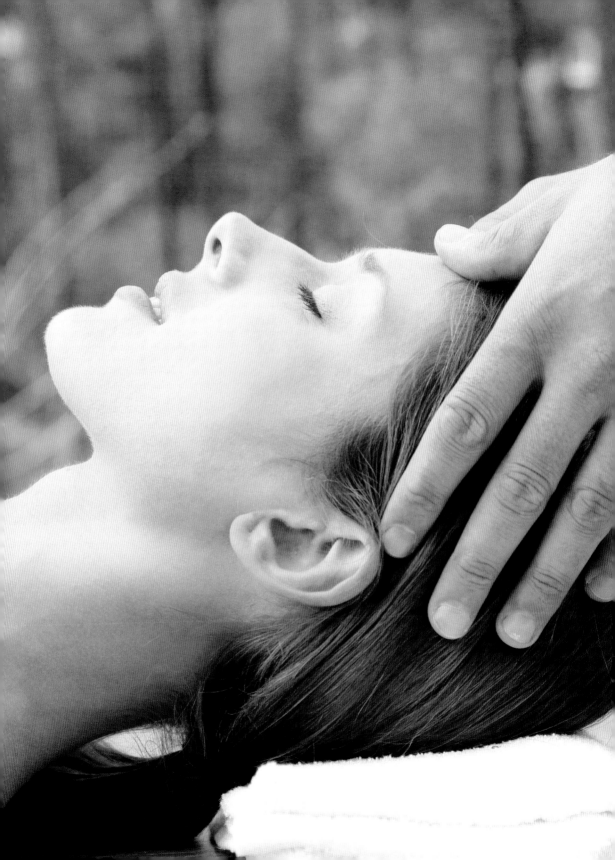

Headache Relief Formula 2

A second headache relief formula to try. It contains the same analgesics and vasoconstructors with more gentle feel when using. It promotes circulation and shrinking of swollen membranes. It's best if used at the first signs of headache.

To a 5-ml, colored-glass, euro-dropper bottle add:
Peppermint: 30 drops
Sweet Marjoram: 30 drops
Lavender: 10 drops
Eucalyptus: 30 drops

Close the cap tightly and shake the bottle vigorously to thoroughly blend the essential oils. Allow to synergize for 8 or more hours before using.

Dispense 1–3 drops on a cotton ball or smell strip and inhale the aromatic vapors of your headache relief blend for 10–15 seconds. You may repeat as needed. This formula may also be effective as a cool compress.

To make a ready-to-use headache relief blend, simply add 15–30 drops of your synergy blend to a 1-ounce (30-ml) bottle of your favorite carrier oil. Shake the bottle well to disperse the oils thoroughly. Apply a few drops of your ready-to-use headache relief blend to sinus points around your nose and forehead, as well as on the back of your neck. Best results are obtained when you use your headache relief blend at the first signs of a headache. Clients report with regular use their headaches diminish in severity, are less frequent or may stop altogether.

Migraine Relief Formula

About 15 percent of the world's population experiences migraines. A migraine is a recurring type of primary headache that affects half of the head with throbbing pain that lasts for up to 72 hours. Associated symptoms, which may be mild to intense, include nausea, vomiting and sensitivity to movement, light, heat, sound and smell. Most people report having an aura before a migraine episode, which is a visual cue that signals a migraine is about to occur.

Thought to be caused by a combination of both genetic and environmental influences, migraines may be inherited through one's family of origin. Changing hormone levels may also play a role as the fluctuation increases pressure on the blood vessels and nerves of the brain, resulting in a migraine.

The essential oils in this formula have been shown to be effective as a comfort care measure for relieving the painful symptoms associated with a migraine headache.

To a 5-ml, colored-glass, euro-dropper bottle add:
Peppermint: 40 drops
Lavender: 20 drops
Cypress: 20 drops
Frankincense: 20 drops

Close the cap tightly and shake the bottle vigorously to thoroughly blend the essential oils. Allow to synergize for 8 or more hours before using.

Dispense 1–3 drops on a cotton ball or smell strip and inhale the aromatic vapors of your migraine relief blend for 10–15 seconds. You may repeat as needed. This formula may also be effective as a cool compress.

To make a ready-to-use headache relief blend, simply add 15–30 drops of your synergy blend to a 1-ounce (30-ml) bottle of your favorite carrier oil. Shake the bottle well to disperse the oils thoroughly. Apply a few drops of your ready-to-use migraine relief blend to sinus points around your nose and forehead, as well as on the back of your neck. Best results are obtained when you use your migraine relief blend at the first signs of a migraine. Clients report that with regular use their migraines diminish in severity, are less frequent or may stop altogether.

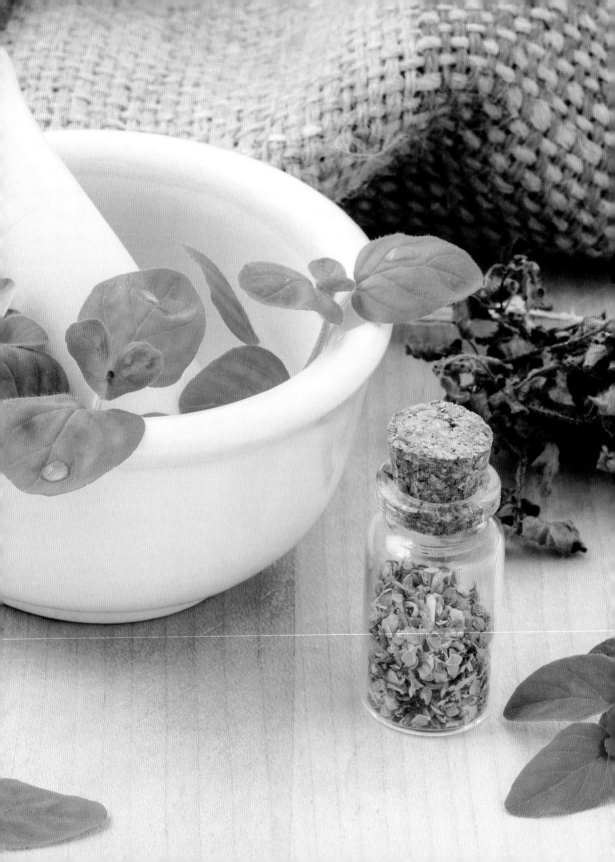

Pain Relief Formula

Research shows that pain, and the suffering it brings, is the number one driving force behind the alternative and complementary health care movement. As humans, we all seek to move toward pleasure and away from pain. These are the two forces that drive all human behavior.

Physical pain is an unpleasant sensation that may involve damage to tissues that is also experienced emotionally. No one likes to experience pain and will do whatever necessary to move away from it. Whether your pain is acute (short-term) or chronic (long-term), essential oils can help to provide symptomatic relief, as well as promote natural healing.

The essential oils in this comfort care formula may be effective for relieving symptoms of physical pain and the accompanying emotional discomfort.

To a 5-ml, colored-glass, euro-dropper bottle add:

Peppermint: 20 drops

Helichrysum: 20 drops

Sweet Marjoram: 20 drops

Ylang Ylang III: 10 drops

German Chamomile: 30 drops

Cap the bottle tightly and shake vigorously to blend the essential oils. Allow to synergize for 8 hours or longer before using.

Dispense 1–3 drops on a cotton ball or smell strip and inhale the aromatic vapors of your blend for 10–15 seconds. You may repeat as needed. This formula is also effective when diffused into the air.

To make a ready-to-use massage blend, simply add 15–30 drops of your synergy blend to a 1-ounce (30-ml) bottle of your favorite carrier oil. Shake the bottle well to disperse the oils thoroughly. Dispense 1–3 drops. Inhale the scent first and then gently apply a few drops of your ready-to-use blend to the area of pain and massage in thoroughly.

Muscle Pain Relief Formula

The medical term for muscle pain is myalgia. It is a common symptom in many disease processes, though commonly it's most often associated with chronic tension, overuse, over-stretching, injury, strain to a muscle or group of muscles and trauma. Muscle pain is also common to those who suffer with chronic fatigue syndrome.

To a 5-ml, colored-glass, euro-dropper bottle add:

Cypress: 30 drops

Sweet Marjoram: 35 drops

Ylang Ylang III: 10 drops

Lavender: 10 drops

Lemongrass: 5 drops

Peppermint: 5 drops

Helichrysum: 5 drops

Close the cap tightly and shake the bottle vigorously to thoroughly blend the essential oils. Allow to synergize for 8 or more hours before using.

Add 15–18 drops of your synergy blend to a 1-ounce (30-ml) bottle of your favorite carrier oil. Shake the bottle well to disperse the oils thoroughly. Apply a few drops and massage in to relieve strained or sore muscles, ligaments and tendons. Taking a hot shower or bath before applying will increase blood flow to enhance your results. Applying just before bed can be helpful for promoting deep and restful sleep, as well as supporting deep healing and recovery. It may also be effective as a hot compress.

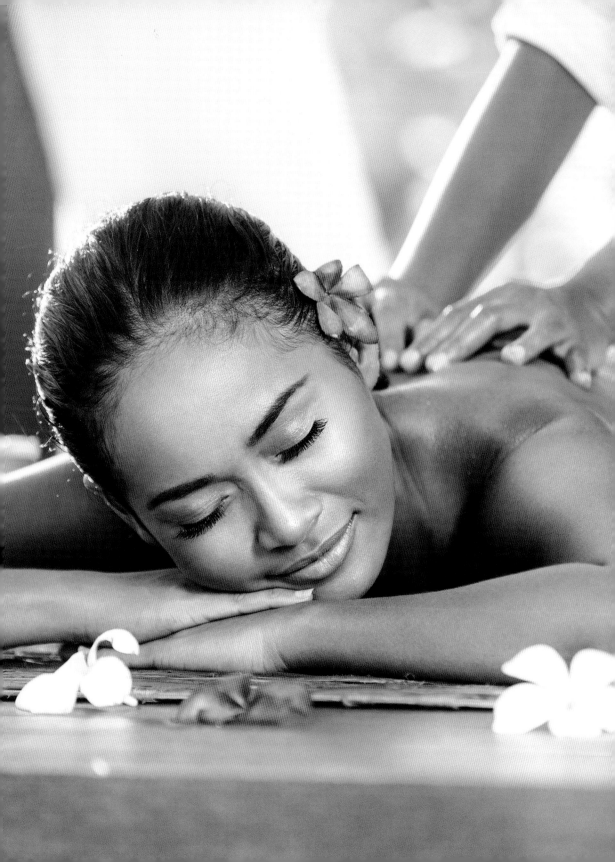

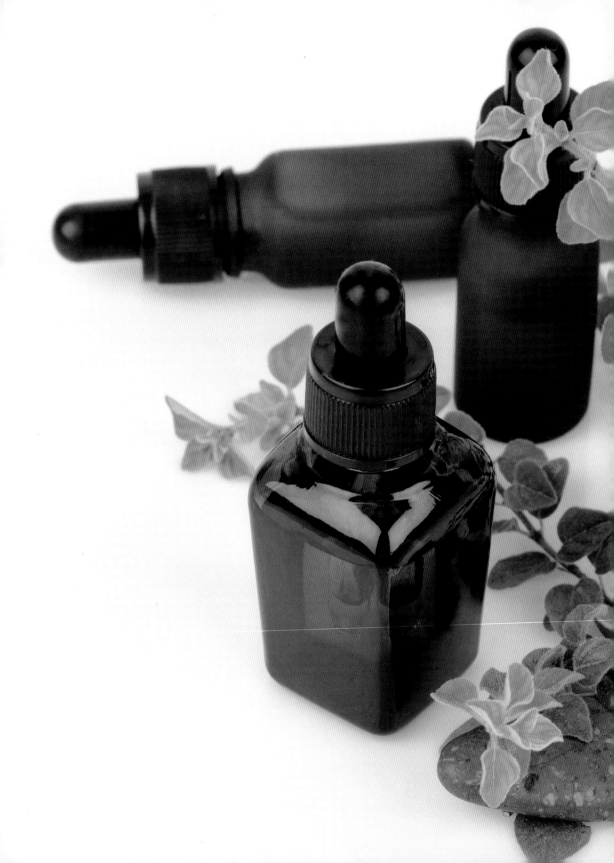

Sciatica Pain Relief Formula

The word sciatica dates back to 1451. It is a medical condition characterized by shooting pain that usually radiates down one leg from the lower back. There may also be associated weakness or numbness present in the leg and foot. It's estimated that up to 40 percent of all people will have sciatica at some time in their life.

To a 5-ml, colored-glass, euro-dropper bottle add:

Cypress: 10 drops

Sweet Marjoram: 20 drops

Ylang Ylang III: 20 drops

German Chamomile: 40 drops

Black Pepper: 10 drops

Close the cap tightly and shake the bottle vigorously to thoroughly blend the essential oils. Allow to synergize for 8 or more hours before using.

Add 15–18 drops of your synergy blend to a 1-ounce (30-ml) bottle of your favorite carrier oil. Shake the bottle well to disperse the oils thoroughly. Apply a few drops and massage in to relieve sciatica pain. Taking a hot shower or bath before applying will increase blood flow to enhance your results. Applying just before bed can be helpful for promoting deep and restful sleep, as well as supporting deep healing and recovery. It may also be effective as a hot compress.

Nerve Pain Relief Formula

The medical term for nerve pain is neuralgia. Neuralgia is a form of chronic pain that occurs when there is damage to a nerve. It is characterized by sharp, shooting pain that can be intermittent or ongoing. Nerve pain is often associated with symptoms of sciatica and herpes, among others.

To a 5-ml, colored-glass, euro-dropper bottle add:

Cypress: 20 drops

Sweet Marjoram: 20 drops

Lavender: 15 drops

Ylang Ylang III: 20 drops

German Chamomile: 20 drops

Black Pepper: 5 drops

Close the cap tightly and shake the bottle vigorously to thoroughly blend the essential oils. Allow to synergize for 8 or more hours before using.

Add 15–18 drops of your synergy blend to a 1-ounce (30-ml) bottle of your favorite carrier oil. Shake the bottle well to disperse the oils thoroughly. Apply a few drops and massage in to relieve nerve pain. Taking a hot shower or bath before applying will increase blood flow to enhance your results. Applying just before bed can be helpful for promoting deep and restful sleep, as well as supporting deep healing and recovery. It may also be effective as a hot compress.

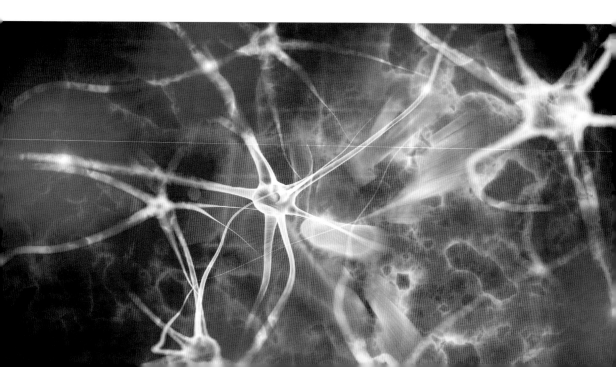

Fibromyalgia Pain Relief Formula

Recognized as a disorder by the U.S. National Institutes of Health and the American College of Rheumatology, fibromyalgia is a chronic, widespread and painful medical condition of the muscles and surrounding connective tissues characterized by an increased response to pressure from the outside environment. Fibromyalgia seems genetically inherited through the family of origin and is often associated with chronic fatigue. Other associated symptoms include anxiety and depression, poor digestion, bowel and bladder issues, post-traumatic stress disorder and sensitivity to light, sound and temperature.

Natural treatment of fibromyalgia includes getting plenty of rest, exercising regularly and eating a whole-foods diet. Essential oils can play an important role as a comfort care measure to alleviate the painful symptoms associated with fibromyalgia.

To a 5-ml, colored-glass, euro-dropper bottle add:

Cypress: 20 drops

Sweet Marjoram: 30 drops

Ylang Ylang III: 30 drops

Peppermint: 20 drops

Close the cap tightly and shake the bottle vigorously to thoroughly blend the essential oils. Allow to synergize for 8 or more hours before using.

Add 15–18 drops of your synergy blend to a 1-ounce (30-ml) bottle of your favorite carrier oil. Shake the bottle well to disperse the oils thoroughly. Apply a few drops and massage in to relieve fibromyalgia or rheumatic pain. Taking a hot shower or bath before applying will increase blood flow to enhance your results. Applying just before bed can be helpful for promoting deep and restful sleep, as well as supporting deep healing and recovery. It may also be effective as a hot compress.

Arthritis Pain Relief Formula

Arthritis is a joint disorder characterized by chronic pain, inflammation and swelling of one or more joints. There are many kinds of arthritis with the most common being osteoarthritis. Getting adequate rest and eating a healthy, whole-foods diet can be helpful. Studies show that regular exercise helps increase range of motion and flexibility and strengthens the joints and the entire physical body.

To a 5-ml, colored-glass, euro-dropper bottle add:

Cypress: 20 drops

Sweet Marjoram: 20 drops

Ylang Ylang III: 20 drops

Peppermint: 20 drops

Black Pepper: 10 drops

Ginger: 10 drops

Close the cap tightly and shake the bottle vigorously to thoroughly blend the essential oils. Allow to synergize for 8 or more hours before using.

Add 15–18 drops of your synergy blend to a 1-ounce (30-ml) bottle of your favorite carrier oil. Shake the bottle well to disperse the oils thoroughly. Apply a few drops and massage in to relieve arthritic-type pain. Taking a hot shower or bath before applying will increase blood flow to enhance your results. Applying just before bed can be helpful for promoting deep and restful sleep, as well as supporting deep healing and recovery. It may also be effective as a hot compress.

Tendinitis Relief Formula

Tendinitis is characterized by pain and inflammation of a tendon and is most commonly caused by excessive overuse or strain. Most commonly, tendinitis injuries occur in the upper shoulder girdle and rotator cuff attachments, as well as the elbow region; however, injury to the Achilles tendon is also quite common.

From years of treating tendinitis injuries, I've learned that the best methods of treatment include complete rest from using the injured tendon for a period of time—up to 6 weeks—along with hot and cold contrasting aromatherapy baths, ice packs and hot compresses. Otherwise, tendinitis can develop into its chronic cousin tendinosis, which is much more challenging to treat and requires a different treatment protocol.

To a 5-ml, colored-glass, euro-dropper bottle add:

Sweet Marjoram: 40 drops

German Chamomile: 20 drops

Helichrysum: 20 drops

Black Pepper: 10 drops

Ginger: 10 drops

Close the cap tightly and shake the bottle vigorously to thoroughly blend the essential oils. Allow to synergize for 8 or more hours before using.

If you're using a 10-percent dilution of any of the pure essential oils, add them directly to your bottle of carrier oil before application.

To make a topical, ready-to-use oil, simply add 18 drops of your formula to a plastic dispensing bottle filled with your chosen carrier oil. Shake well to disperse the oils in the carrier before applying 1–3 drops and massaging into the area. This formula may also be effective as a contrasting hot and cold aromatherapy bath or compress.

Leg Cramp Relief Formula

Leg cramps can be extremely painful and occur suddenly without notice as a usually voluntary leg muscle or muscle group suddenly goes into an excessive involuntarily contraction, causing extreme shortening of the leg muscle tissue. A leg cramp can last for several seconds, minutes or even hours. Though the associated cause is not completely understood, cramping of a skeletal muscle, such as leg cramps, may be from excessive exercise, dehydration, low levels of minerals (magnesium, potassium, calcium and sodium) or poor circulation.

It's reported that, "around 40% of people who experience skeletal cramps are likely to endure extreme muscle pain, and may be unable to use the entire limb that contains the 'locked-up' muscle group. It may take up to seven days for the muscle to return to a pain-free state."

Leg cramps may occur anytime, however a large number of them are nocturnal, which means they happen at night, disrupting your normal sleep.

To a 5-ml, colored-glass, euro-dropper bottle add:

Sweet Marjoram: 40 drops

Peppermint: 20 drops

Cypress: 20 drops

Lavender: 10 drops

Helichrysum: 10 drops

Close the cap tightly and shake the bottle vigorously to thoroughly blend the essential oils. Allow to synergize for 8 or more hours before using.

If you're using a 10-percent dilution of any of the pure essential oils, add them directly to your carrier oil.

Add 10–15 drops of your pure essential oil formula to a 1-ounce (30-ml), colored-glass misting bottle filled with light coconut oil. Light coconut oil is light enough that it will not clog the atomizer sprayer. Shake the bottle vigorously to disperse the formula in the carrier oil before using.

To make a ready-to-use oil, simply add 10–15 drops of your formula to a plastic dispensing bottle filled with your chosen carrier oil. Shake well to disperse the oils in the carrier before applying gently to the area of leg cramping. Clients report that applying the Leg Cramp Relief Formula after taking a warm shower or bath and just before bed helps them sleep more deeply and prevents nocturnal leg cramps.

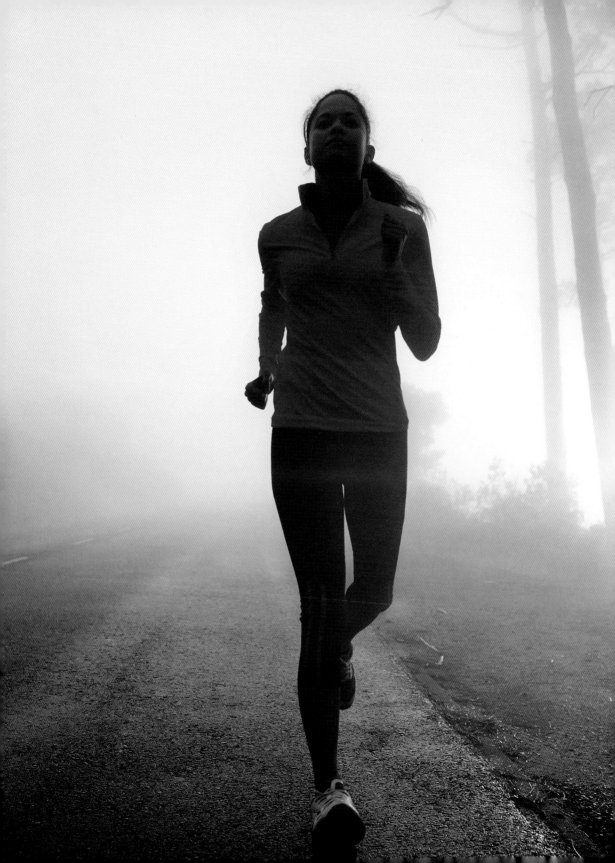

Constipation Relief Formula

Constipation has been linked to many illnesses and health risks, including vitamin and mineral deficiency, poor immune response, toxicity, poisoning and a variety of chronic pain syndromes and food allergies.

The Constipation Relief Formula has a distinctly rejuvenating and warming effect and contains essential oils with calming, astringent and restorative properties known to be effective for stimulating digestion and assimilation and for promoting healthy functioning of the stomach, pancreas and intestines.

To a 5-ml, colored-glass, euro-dropper bottle add:

Basil: 10 drops

Cypress: 20 drops

Sweet Orange: 20 drops

Sweet Marjoram: 20 drops

Black Pepper: 10 drops

Peppermint: 20 drops

Close the cap tightly and shake the bottle vigorously to thoroughly blend the essential oils. Allow to synergize for 8 or more hours before using.

Use 10–15 drops of your Constipation Relief Formula on a poultice as a hot compress over the lower abdomen or in a sitz bath (page 247) to promote relief of constipation symptoms. You may repeat as needed.

Nausea Relief Formula

Nausea is an unsettled sensation in your upper stomach that causes you to feel sick. Feelings of nausea can trigger an involuntary urge to vomit and hinder daily activity. Common causes associated with nausea include motion sickness, vertigo, dizziness, migraine, stomach flu, depression, anxiety, medications and food poisoning.

To a 5-ml, colored-glass, euro-dropper bottle add:

Peppermint: 60 drops

Ginger: 20 drops

Lemon: 20 drops

Cap the bottle tightly and shake vigorously to blend the essential oils. Allow to synergize for 8 hours or longer before using.

Dispense 1–3 drops on a cotton ball or smell strip and inhale the aromatic vapors of your Nausea Relief Formula for 10–15 seconds. You may repeat as needed. This formula is also effective when diffused into the air.

To make a ready-to-use nausea relief blend, simply add 15–30 drops of your synergy blend to a 1-ounce (30-ml) bottle of your favorite carrier oil. Shake the bottle well to disperse the oils thoroughly. Apply a few drops of your ready-to-use nausea relief blend to sinus points around your nose and forehead, as well as on the back of your neck.

CAUTION: Though research shows ginger and peppermint to be effective for nausea relief, pregnant women should not use without supervision of a qualified health professional or aromatherapist due to their stimulating effect.

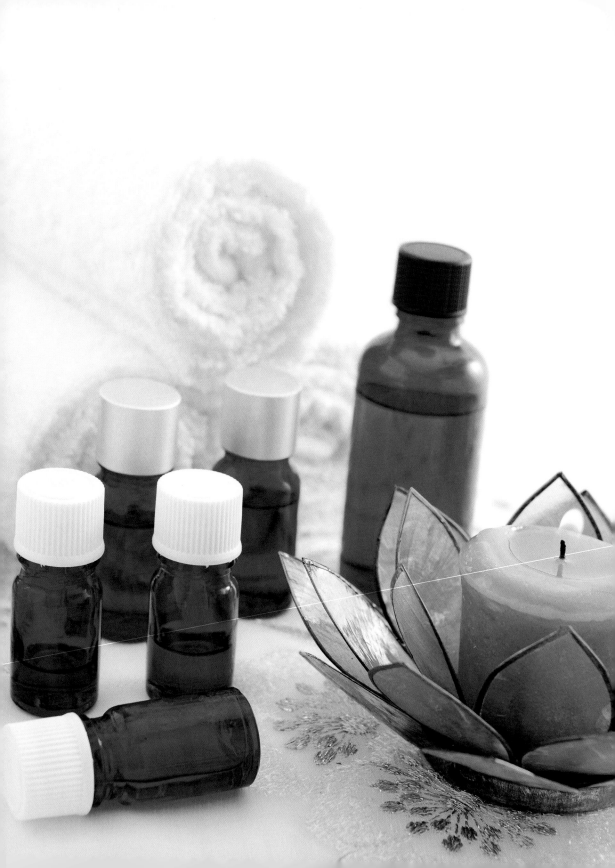

Burn Care Formula

Burns can be caused by heat, radiation, electricity or friction, though statistics show most result from fires and hot liquids. Substance abuse and smoking have also been linked to the probability of getting burns.

There are four kinds of burns. First-degree burns affect the superficial layers of the skin. These are red without blisters, result in minimal pain and last only a few days. Next, there are second-degree burns that cover a larger area of skin with blistering and more intense pain. These require more time to heal and may result in scarring. A third-degree burn covers an even larger area and often has no pain due to nerve damage, and the area is stiff. This type of burn requires special treatment for healing to occur, as the tissue is so injured the body's own natural healing ability needs assistance. A fourth-degree burn involves an even larger area of tissue and may include muscles, tendons or bones, which may be charred black. This can lead to the loss of the injured body part.

The essential oils in this formula have been shown to be effective as a comfort care measure for relieving painful symptoms associated with first and second degree burns, as well as for stimulating the body's own natural healing ability to promote rapid healing and prevent scarring.

To a 5-ml, colored-glass, euro-dropper bottle add:
German Chamomile: 20 drops
Lavender: 40 drops
Helichrysum: 20 drops
Geranium Roseum and Graveolens: 20 drops

Close the cap tightly and shake the bottle vigorously to thoroughly blend the essential oils. Allow to synergize for 8 or more hours before using.

If you're using a 10-percent dilution of any of the pure essential oils, add them directly to your carrier oil.

Add 10–15 drops of your pure essential oil Burn Care Formula to a 1-ounce (30-ml), colored-glass misting bottle. Shake the bottle well each time before using to disperse the oils in the water. Gently mist around the burn area to promote fast cooling relief and healing of the tissue.

To make a burn care gel or oil, simply add 10–15 drops of your formula to a plastic dispensing bottle filled with your chosen carrier of aloe vera gel or oil. Shake well to disperse the oils in the carrier before applying gently around the burn area. This formula may also be effective as a cool compress. Clients report it has prevented peeling and scarring of tissue.

Sunburn Relief Formula

Sunburn results from an overexposure to ultra violet light, most often from the sun. Symptoms of overexposure include reddening of skin tissue that feels hot and painful to the touch; light-headedness or low energy may also result. As the skin heals, it may peel as new skin tissue is formed and, in extreme cases, overexposure may result in permanent scarring of skin tissue. Excess exposure to the sun's ultra violet light is also the primary cause of non-malignant skin tumors.

As a preventative measure, sun protection such as hats and long sleeves are advised when in the sun for long periods or during the peak hours of midday sun. Sunscreen is another way to prevent sunburn. It has been shown that moderate exposure to the sun that results in sun tanning can actually prevent sunburn as it increases the melanin content in your skin, which is the skin's natural protection against overexposure to the sun.

The essential oils in this formula have been shown effective as a comfort care measure for relieving painful symptoms of sunburn, as well as stimulating your body's own natural healing response and may prevent peeling.

To a 5-ml, colored-glass, euro-dropper bottle add:
German Chamomile: 20 drops
Blue Tansy: 20 drops
Lavender: 30 drops
Helichrysum: 20 drops
Rose: 10 drops

Close the cap tightly and shake the bottle vigorously to thoroughly blend the essential oils. Allow to synergize for 8 or more hours before using.

If you're using a 10-percent dilution of any of the pure essential oils, add them directly to your carrier oil.

Add 10–15 drops of your Sunburn Relief Formula to a 1-ounce (30-ml), colored-glass misting bottle. Shake the bottle well each time before using to disperse the oils in the water. Gently mist around the burn area to promote fast cooling relief and healing of the tissue.

To make a burn care gel or oil, simply add 10–15 drops of your formula to a plastic dispensing bottle filled with your chosen carrier of aloe vera gel or oil. Shake well to disperse the oils in the carrier before applying gently around the burned area. This formula may also be effective as a cool compress. Clients report it has prevented peeling and scarring of tissue.

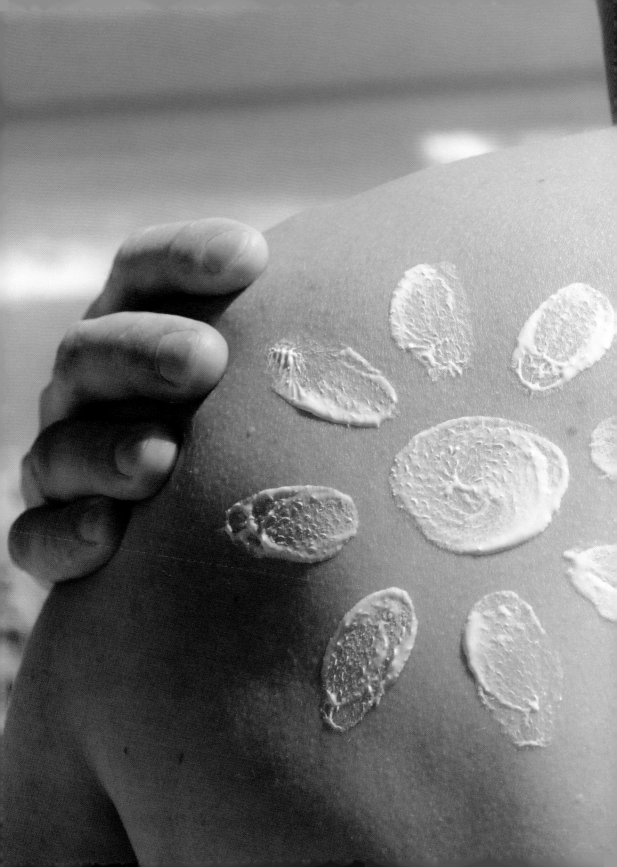

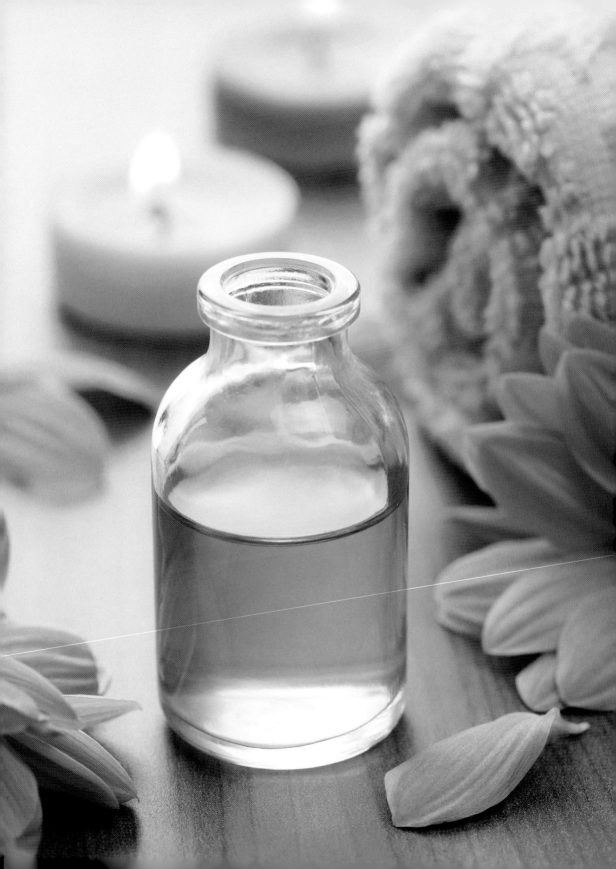

UV Radiation Burn Relief Formula

Damage to the skin may occur with excessive UV radiation that results in redness, inflammation and swelling to the damaged skin and surrounding area. The sun is the most common cause of high exposure to ultra violet light, but radiation therapy when undergoing cancer treatment is another cause of radiation burns. The oils in this formula have been shown to be effective for relieving the painful symptoms associated with radiation burns, as well as helpful for stimulating natural healing of tissue with little or no peeling of tissue or scarring afterward.

To a 5-ml, colored-glass, euro-dropper bottle add:

German Chamomile: 20 drops

Blue Tansy: 40 drops

Geranium Roseum and Graveolens: 20 drops

Lavender: 10 drops

Helichrysum: 10 drops

Close the cap tightly and shake the bottle vigorously to thoroughly blend the essential oils. Allow to synergize for 8 or more hours before using.

If you're using a 10-percent dilution of any of the pure essential oils, add them directly to your carrier oil.

Add 10–15 drops of your pure essential oil burn care formula to a 1-ounce (30-ml), colored-glass misting bottle. Shake the bottle well each time before using to disperse the oils in the water. Gently mist around the burn area to promote fast cooling relief and healing of the tissue.

To make a burn care gel or oil, simply add 10–15 drops of your formula to a plastic dispensing bottle filled with your chosen carrier of aloe vera gel or oil. Shake well to disperse the oils in the carrier before applying gently around the burn area. This formula may also be effective as a cool compress. Clients report it has prevented peeling and scarring of tissue.

Mosquito and Insect Protective Repellent Formula

Generally regarded as pests, both mosquitoes and insects are usually very small in size, but can be a huge nuisance or even dangerous to one's health. The mosquito itself feeds on the blood of its hosts, and its saliva can cause irritation to the skin with uncomfortable symptoms like burning and itching. Some mosquitoes are known to pass on very harmful and serious infections like malaria, West Nile virus and dengue fever.

All of the essential oils in this formula are known to protect against mosquito and insect bites, some of which can be quite serious. Research studies have actually shown that peppermint oil not only repels insects in general, but the dengue-fever carrying mosquito as well.

To a 5-ml, colored-glass, euro-dropper bottle add:

Palmarosa: 40 drops

Lemongrass: 20 drops

Lemon Tea Tree: 10 drops

Atlas Cedarwood: 10 drops

Patchouli: 10 drops

Peppermint: 10 drops

Close the cap tightly and shake the bottle vigorously to thoroughly blend the essential oils. Allow to synergize for 8 or more hours before using.

If you're using a 10-percent dilution of any of the pure essential oils, add them directly to your carrier oil.

Add 10–15 drops of your pure essential oil formula to a 1-ounce (30-ml), colored-glass misting bottle filled with either purified water or light coconut oil. Light coconut oil has a light enough consistency that it will not clog the atomizer spray. Shake the bottle well each time before using to disperse the oils. Gently mist onto clothing or around an area you wish to protect from mosquito and insect bites. You will only need to shake the bottle with carrier oil vigorously once to disperse the oils evenly before using. The oil will stay on longer and have a longer lasting effect. You can also dispense drops of pure essential oil formula on a pool of melted candle wax or in an aroma lamp to diffuse into the air.

Allergic Skin Reaction Relief Formula

Allergic skin reactions are a hypersensitive immune response to a substance that triggers abnormal symptoms like itching, burning, blisters, redness, rash, pain, hives, swelling and inflammation.

Allergies are common. Reports indicate that about 20 percent of people have experienced a skin reaction like eczema, which is common among young children.

There are many substances that can trigger an allergic skin reaction, including:

- Insect bites from bees, wasps and spiders

- Common foods (i.e. gluten, eggs, dairy, nuts and fruits)

- Chemicals or medications

- Metals (i.e. gold in jewelry)

The best way to avoid allergic skin reactions is to eliminate the allergens that cause them.

To a 5-ml, colored-glass, euro-dropper bottle add:
Blue Yarrow: 20 drops
Ylang Ylang III: 20 drops
Palmarosa: 30 drops
Geranium Roseum and Graveolens: 10 drops
German Chamomile: 10 drops
Helichrysum: 10 drops

Close the cap tightly and shake the bottle vigorously to thoroughly blend the essential oils. Allow to synergize for 8 or more hours before using.

If you're using a 10-percent dilution of any of the pure essential oils, add them directly to your carrier before application.

Dispense 1–3 drops on a cotton ball or smell strip and inhale the aromatic vapors of your blend for 10–15 seconds to promote calming of your immune system and allergic response. You may repeat as needed.

Add 10–15 drops of your pure essential oil Allergic Skin Reaction Relief Formula to a 1-ounce (30-ml), colored-glass misting bottle. Shake the bottle well each time before using to disperse the oils in the water. Mist gently around the area of the allergic skin reaction.

To make a topical gel or oil, simply add 10–15 drops of your formula to a plastic dispensing bottle filled with your chosen carrier of aloe vera gel or oil (light coconut oil recommended). Shake well to disperse the oils in the carrier before applying gently around the affected area. Avoid direct application onto the allergic skin reaction until the skin has begun to clear. This formula may also be effective as a cool compress.

Poison Ivy and Oak Irritation Relief Formula

More than 50 million people annually are affected by allergic reactions to poison ivy and poison oak. Only a small percentage of people, about 15–30 percent, have no allergic reaction.

Poison ivy and oak have similar symptoms for which essential oils can be used as a natural remedy to control symptoms and speed healing. Symptoms include burning, itching, reddish inflammation, swelling, irritating skin lesions, non-colored bumps, painful rash and oozing blisters.

Poison ivy and oak aren't spread by touching the blisters themselves, but rather by having direct contact with the oily fluid inside the blisters that can stay on your skin and clothes. That's why it's important for you to wash your hands and all clothing soon after exposure.

To a 5-ml, colored-glass, euro-dropper bottle add:
German Chamomile: 20 drops
Blue Tansy: 20 drops
Helichrysum: 20 drops
Palmarosa: 20 drops
Blue Yarrow: 10 drops
Cypress: 10 drops

Close the cap tightly and shake the bottle vigorously to thoroughly blend the essential oils. Allow to synergize for 8 or more hours before using.

If you're using a 10-percent dilution of any of the pure essential oils, add them directly to your carrier oil.

Add 10–15 drops of your pure essential oil Poison Ivy and Oak Irritation Relief Formula to a 1-ounce (30-ml), colored-glass misting bottle filled with purified water. Shake the bottle well each time before using to disperse the oils in the water. Mist around the affected area to promote fast relief of symptoms and speed healing.

To make a leave-on gel or oil, simply add 10–15 drops of your formula to a plastic dispensing bottle filled with your chosen carrier of aloe vera gel or oil. Shake well to disperse the oils in the carrier before applying gently around the area. This formula may also be effective as a cool compress or in a bath. Be sure to wash hands thoroughly with a sanitizing agent after direct contact with poison oak or ivy on the skin.

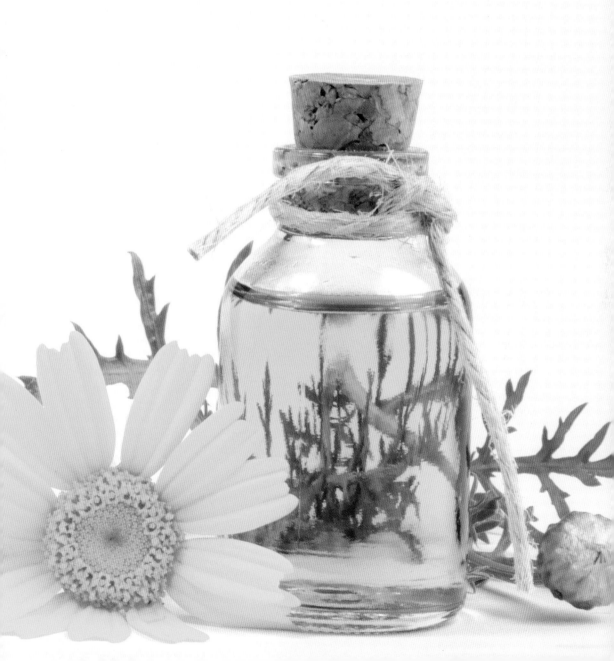

Warm Bath Treatment

A warm bath can bring relief when nothing else will. Especially good for soothing allergic skin reactions, baths may also be used to relieve poison ivy and oak irritations.

Allergic Skin Reaction Relief Formula (page 199)
4 cups (90 g) raw, uncooked oats

In a bowl, add 10–15 drops of your essential oil blend to 4 cups (90 g) of raw, uncooked oats. Mix the blend thoroughly into the oats, cover and set aside while you draw a warm bath. Add the oats with the essential oil blend to your bath water and stir into the water. Relax in the bath for 10–20 minutes. This method of treatment is especially good for soothing an outbreak of hives.

CAUTION: You may wish to do a skin allergy test for each of the essential oils in the formula before using.

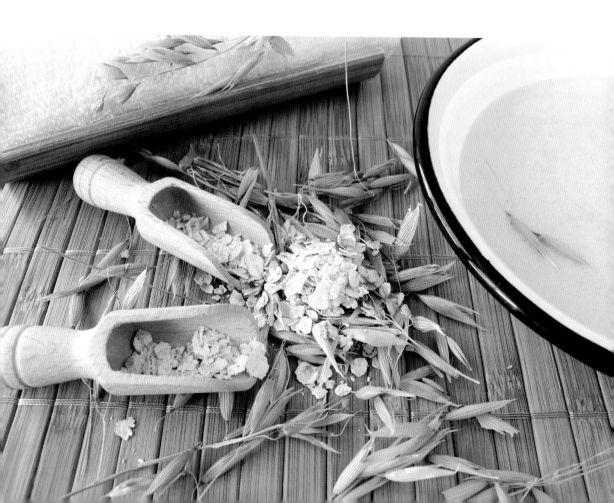

Scar Formula

Scars naturally occur on areas of the skin after there has been an injury. Scar tissue formation, which is made up of protein (collagen), is a normal function of tissue repair after an injury, and the appearance of scarring is common.

A scar treatment of essential oils is most effective when applied immediately after an injury to the skin, though even old scars can become noticeably less apparent or even disappear completely. This depends upon the severity of the injury to the skin, the age of the scar and other factors like diet and quality of skin tissue.

To a 5-ml, colored-glass, euro-dropper bottle add:

Helichrysum: 20 drops

German Chamomile: 20 drops

Rose: 20 drops

Palmarosa: 10 drops

Geranium Roseum and Graveolens: 10 drops

Ylang Ylang: 5 drops

Carrot Seed: 5 drops

Lavender: 5 drops

Myrrh: 5 drops

Close the cap tightly and shake the bottle vigorously to thoroughly blend the essential oils. Allow to synergize for 8 or more hours before using.

If you're using a 10-percent dilution of any of the pure essential oils, add them directly to your carrier oil and shake well to blend before application to the skin.

To make a ready-to-use dilution for direct application to the skin, add 10–15 drops of your pure essential oil Scar Formula to a 1-ounce (30-ml) plastic dispensing bottle. Or you can add 5–8 drops of formula to a 0.5-ounce (15-ml), colored-glass, euro-dropper bottle filled with your chosen carrier oil. Shake well to disperse the oils in the carrier before gently applying to the area of the scar. This may be applied first as a warm compress (to soften tissue) before applying the ready-to-use blend.

Foot Bath for Athlete's Foot or Toenail Fungus

A foot bath is a way to focus your essential oils to a specific area. The warm water increases circulation and action of oils.

1 cup (500 g) Epsom or sea salts

10–15 drops Athlete's Foot Formula (page 205) or Toenail Fungus Formula (page 207)

Foot bath

In small ceramic bowl, combine 1 cup (275 g) salts and 10–15 drops of the essential oils formula. Blend in thoroughly and set aside. Fill your foot bath with hot water (98°F–101°F [36°C–38°C]). Add the scented salts into the foot bath water and stir. Soak your foot/feet, being sure to submerge and cover the toenails completely in water. Soak for 10–20 minutes or until the water cools. Towel dry and allow the area to remain open to the air as much as possible. Wearing open-toed sandals can be helpful.

FOR USE IN BETWEEN FOOT BATHS

Add 10–15 drops of your pure essential oil formula to a 1-ounce (30-ml) colored-glass misting bottle filled with light coconut oil. Light coconut oil will not clog the atomizer sprayer. Shake the bottle vigorously to disperse the oils before applying to the affected area.

To make a toenail fungus gel or oil, simply add 10–15 drops of your formula to a plastic dispensing bottle filled with your chosen carrier of aloe vera gel or oil. Shake well to disperse the oils in the carrier before applying. Be sure to wash hands thoroughly with a sanitizing agent after direct contact with the area.

Athlete's Foot Formula

Athlete's foot is a common infection of the feet caused by a fungus. The medical term used for it is *tine pedis*. Some of the characteristic signs and symptoms associated with athlete's foot are redness, itching, burning, peeling and blisters. As fungal infections thrive in moist environments, between the toes of the feet are the most commonly infected areas because of poor air circulation to keep the area dry. Fungal infections may also occur on the hands, toenails, as well as the fingernails.

To a 5-ml, colored-glass, euro-dropper bottle add:

Clove: 40 drops

Tea Tree: 20 drops

Thyme: 20 drops

Lemon: 20 drops

¼ cup (130 g) Epsom or sea salts

Foot bath

Close the cap tightly and shake the bottle vigorously to thoroughly blend the essential oils. Allow to synergize for 8 or more hours before using.

Add 10–15 drops of your pure essential oil Athlete's Foot Formula to a carrier of ¼ cup (130 g) Epsom or sea salts and mix thoroughly. You can add more drops of the athlete's foot blend in subsequent foot baths if well tolerated.

Fill your foot bath with hot water (98°F–101°F [37°C–38°C]), add scented salts and stir into foot bath water completely. Soak your foot/feet for 15–20 minutes or until the water cools. Dry with a clean hand towel.

Next, apply a 10-percent, ready-to-use dilution of the athlete's foot fungus blend around the infection to be absorbed into your skin.

It's best to leave your feet open to the air and keep the area as dry as possible; wearing open sandals may be helpful. You may apply your ready-to-use blend as often as needed between foot soaks. Be sure to wash your hands thoroughly with a sanitizing cleanser after direct contact with the infected area.

Perform your athlete's foot bath at least once or twice daily for 3–6 weeks, or even longer in some cases, depending upon how severe your case of athlete's foot is.

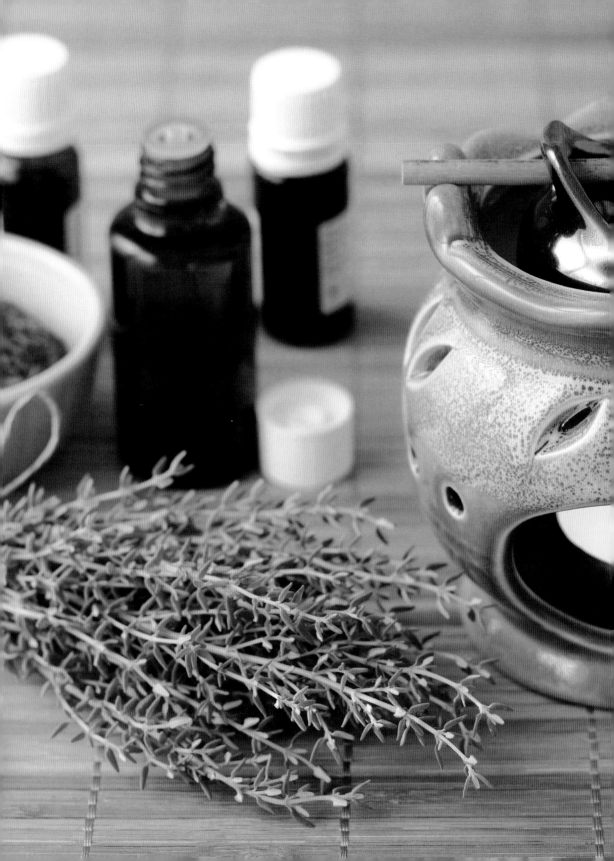

Toenail Fungus Formula

The medical term for toenail fungus is *tinea unguium*. Though it may also affect the fingernails, the most common malady of the nail is toenail fungus, which affects 10 percent of the population.

Toenail fungus appears as a thickened, brittle and discolored nail bed varying in colors from a black, reddish orange to yellow and green. As the infection worsens, the nail begins to break down and pieces of the nail detach from the nail bed, which becomes red, inflamed and painful. Advanced toenail fungus can also have quite an offensive smell.

The research shows that the most important factors for preventing a toenail fungal infection are good blood circulation and ventilation of the toes and feet. Also, toenail fungus seems to run in the family, so if your father had toenail fungus you're far more likely to have it yourself. Men are far more often affected by the disease than women.

Essential oils are effective for destroying a toenail fungal infection, promoting healing of the nail bed and stimulating growth of a new nail matrix.

To a 5-ml, colored-glass, euro-dropper bottle add:
Clove Bud: 30 drops
Myrrh: 30 drops
Lemon: 20 drops
Thyme: 10 drops
Lavender: 10 drops
¼ cup (130 g) Epsom or sea salts
Foot bath

Close the cap tightly and shake the bottle vigorously to thoroughly blend the essential oils. Allow to synergize for 8 or more hours before using.

Add 10–15 drops of your pure essential oil Toenail Fungus Formula to a carrier of ¼ cup (130 g) Epsom or sea salts and mix thoroughly. You can add more drops of the athlete's foot blend in subsequent foot baths if well tolerated.

Fill your foot bath with hot water (98°F–101°F [37°C–38°C]), add scented salts and stir into foot bath water completely. Soak your foot/feet for 15–20 minutes or until the water cools. Dry with a clean hand towel.

Next, apply a 10-percent, ready-to-use dilution of the toenail fungus blend around the infection to be absorbed into your skin.

It's best to leave your feet open to the air and keep the area as dry as possible; wearing open sandals may be helpful. You may apply your ready-to-use blend as often as needed between foot soaks. Be sure to wash your hands thoroughly with a sanitizing cleanser after direct contact with the infected area. Perform your toenail fungus footbath at least once or twice daily for 3–6 weeks, or even longer in some cases, depending upon how severe your case of toenail fungus is.

Warts Formula (non-genital)

Warts are usually small, rough patches of growth that look somewhat like a head of cauliflower. They are caused by a viral infection, and common areas of infection are the hands and feet. Though the common wart is considered benign, its appearance causes concern for many, especially children and young adults, with a 12–24 percent rate of occurrence. Warts are contagious and may spread through contact with open areas and broken skin.

To a 5-ml, colored-glass, euro-dropper bottle add:

Tea Tree: 10 drops

Cinnamon Leaf: 20 drops

Lemon: 20 drops

Thyme: 10 drops

Myrrh: 20 drops

Clove Bud: 20 drops

¼ cup (130 g) Epsom or sea salts

Foot bath

Close the cap tightly and shake the bottle vigorously to thoroughly blend the essential oils. Allow to synergize for 8 or more hours before using.

Add 10–15 drops of your pure essential oil Wart Formula to a carrier of ¼ cup (130 g) of Epsom or sea salts and mix thoroughly. You can add more drops of the wart blend in subsequent footbaths if well tolerated.

Fill your footbath with hot water (98°F–101°F [37°C–38°C]), add scented salts and stir into the foot bath water completely. Soak the area of your wart for 15–20 minutes or until the water cools. Dry with a clean hand towel.

Next, apply a 10-percent ready-to-use dilution of the wart blend directly on the wart, and let the oils be absorbed into the skin.

It's best to leave the wart open to the air and keep the area as dry as possible. You may apply your ready-to-use wart blend as often as needed between soaks. Be sure to wash your hands thoroughly with a sanitizing cleanser after direct contact with the infected area.

Perform your wart bath at least once or twice daily for 3–6 weeks or even longer in some cases.

Herpes Formula

There are two types of herpes simplex virus, type 1 (HSV-1) and type 2 (HSV-2). Herpes simplex-1 is more common, effects the mouth and is referred to as a cold sore. HSV-2 is what causes the genital type of herpes infections. Both are transmittable by direct contact with the body fluids and lesions of an infected individual. The communicable disease may still be transmitted even when asymptomatic. Genital herpes is considered a sexually transmitted disease (STD). Though condom use can decrease the risk of infection, the most effective prevention is to avoid any genital contact. At the start of this millennium, it was estimated that more than 536 million people (16 percent of the world's population) were infected with HSV-2. Most people with HSV-2 are asymptomatic and do not realize that they are infected.

This formula contains some of the most potent antimicrobial and antiviral essential oils known in aromatherapy and may be helpful for promoting relief and faster healing for symptoms of herpes outbreaks. Be careful to apply the herpes formula around the herpes lesion, not directly on an open lesion!

To a 5-ml, colored-glass, euro-dropper bottle add:
Bergamot: 20 drops
Palmarosa: 20 drops
Myrrh: 10 drops
Helichrysum: 10 drops
Rose: 10 drops
Cypress: 5 drops
Lavender: 5 drops
Lemon: 5 drops
Oregano: 1 drop
Thyme: 1 drop
Galbanum: 5 drops

Close the cap tightly and shake the bottle vigorously to thoroughly blend the essential oils. Allow to synergize for 8 or more hours before using.

If you're using a 10-percent dilution of any of the pure essential oils, add them directly to your carrier oil.

(continued)

Herpes Formula (Continued)

Add 10–15 drops of your pure essential oil formula to a 1-ounce (30-ml), colored-glass misting bottle of purified water or light coconut oil. Light coconut oil is light enough that it will not clog your atomizer sprayer. Shake the bottle well each time before using to disperse the oils in the water. Lightly mist around the area of the herpes outbreak to promote fast relief and healing of tissue. If using light coconut oil, you will only need to shake the bottle vigorously once to disperse the oils evenly in the carrier before using.

To make a herpes ready-to-use gel, simply add 10–15 drops of your formula to a plastic dispensing bottle filled with your chosen carrier of aloe vera gel. Shake well to disperse the oils in the carrier before applying gently around the infected area. This formula may also be effective as a cool or warm compress.

CAUTION: Oregano oil is a potent, "hot" antimicrobial and should be used with extreme caution. As it is a strong irritant to the skin and mucous membranes, use a less than 1-percent dilution for safe skin application. Avoid during pregnancy and with young children and pets.

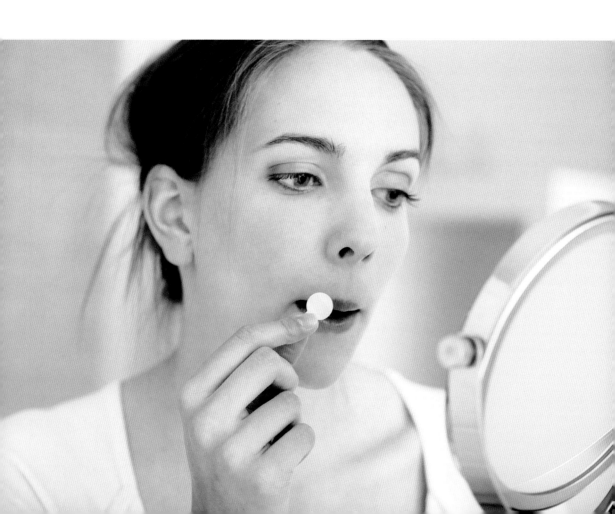

Ringworm Formula

Ringworm is caused by a fungal infection of the skin. The medical term for ringworm is *dermatophytosis*. As with all fungi, ringworm thrives in warm, moist environments where there is little or no air circulation. It's thought that 20 percent or more of the population is infected with ringworm, with athletes being the most commonly affected by this skin condition.

Ringworm appears as enlarged raised rings of the fungi on the skin and thus the name ringworm. An infection on the skin of the feet by dermatophytosis is called athlete's foot and in the groin it is called jock itch. Ringworm is contagious and spreads between humans. Animals, including dogs and cats, can also become infected by the disease.

Signs of ringworm infection include:

- Raised red, itchy patches on the skin that resemble a ring

- Red patches with blisters that drain and ooze

- Bald patches on the scalp or fur of an animal

- Discoloration and cracking in severe cases

Fungi like ringworm thrives in warm, moist environments and is often picked up in public shared facilities like gyms, saunas or swimming pools. Sharing exercise equipment that has not been disinfected properly and communal sharing of towels and other wearable gear is considered to be the primary cause of the disease. The number one prevention is to avoid sharing clothing and sports equipment and to always wear protective footwear like thongs when using public facilities.

To a 5-ml, colored-glass, euro-dropper bottle add:
German Chamomile: 20 drops
Blue Tansy: 20 drops
Palmarosa: 20 drops
Spikenard: 20 drops
Helichrysum: 10 drops
Lavender: 10 drops

Close the cap tightly and shake the bottle vigorously to thoroughly blend the essential oils. Allow to synergize for 8 or more hours before using.

If you're using a 10-percent dilution of any of the pure essential oils, add them directly to your carrier oil.

(continued)

Ringworm Formula (Continued)

Add 10-15 drops of your pure essential oil Ringworm Formula to a 1-ounce (30-ml), colored-glass misting bottle filled with purified water. Shake the bottle well each time before using to disperse the oils in the water. Lightly mist around the area to promote fast relief of itching and to promote healing.

To make a ringworm gel or oil, simply add 10-15 drops of your formula to a plastic dispensing bottle filled with your chosen carrier of aloe vera gel or oil. Shake well to disperse the oils in the carrier before applying gently around the area. This formula may also be effective as a cool compress. Always thoroughly wash your hands with a sanitizing soap after direct contact with the infection.

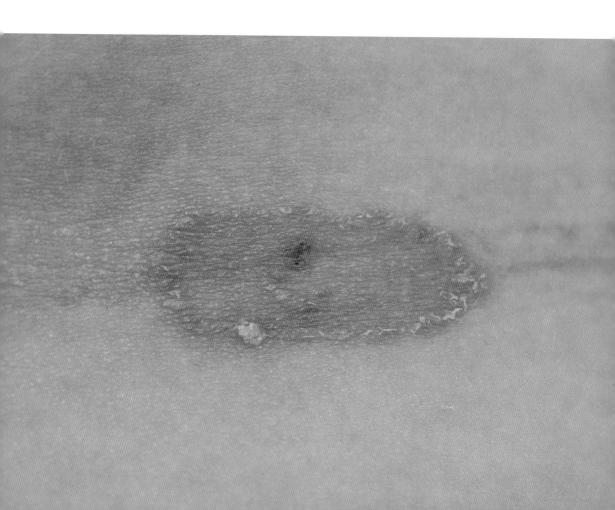

Ringing Ear Relief Formula

The medical term for ringing ear is *tinnitus* which comes from the Latin word *tinnīre* meaning "to ring." Tinnitus is often described as a ringing or buzzing sound, though sometimes clicking, roaring and hissing are other terms used to describe the sound. It can come from one or both ears and be either loud or soft and high or low pitched. Ringing ear can cause depression, nervousness and anxiety in 1–2 percent of people, while most tolerate it very well. Tinnitus is thought to be brought on from a number of causes such as ear infections, stress, certain medications, allergies, Ménière's disease, head injury, nerve damage, poor circulation or earwax buildup.

Preventative care includes avoiding listening to loud music, especially through headphones.

The Ringing Ear Relief Formula contains essential oils with calming, astringent and restorative properties known to be effective for relieving symptoms of tinnitus, especially when associated with congestion or poor nerve conduction and circulation.

To a 5-ml, colored-glass, euro-dropper bottle add:

Cypress: 20 drops

Lemon: 20 drops

Helichrysum: 40 drops

Birch: 10 drops

Juniper Berry: 10 drops

Close the cap tightly and shake the bottle vigorously to thoroughly blend the essential oils. Allow to synergize for 8 or more hours before using.

Use your Ringing Ear Relief Formula as a poultice to relieve congestion and symptoms related to poor congestion and nerve conduction. You may repeat as needed. To make a ready-to-use Ringing Ear Relief blend, simply add 15–30 drops of your synergy blend to a 1-ounce (30-ml) bottle of your favorite carrier oil. Shake the bottle well to disperse the oils thoroughly. Apply a few drops of your blend to the front and backside of your ear with tinnitus symptoms and massage in.

Sleep Formulas

Studies show that sleep deprivation causes one out of every six fatal car accidents. The research also shows that 17 continuous hours without sleep not only decreases your alertness and performance, but also increases your blood alcohol levels enough to be classified as a drunk driver. Disastrous events like the Valdez oil spill and Chernobyl have been linked to human errors due to sleep deprivation.

A modern malady, sleep deprivation was not experienced before the invention of electric lights. Before indoor lighting, people followed their natural sleep cycles and went to bed soon after sunset and rose again at sunrise, which resulted in more hours of sleep.

The research indicates that if it takes you more than 10–15 minutes to fall asleep, then you're sleep deprived. An excellent sign that you are not sleep deprived is when you're tired enough to immediately fall into a deep state of dreamless sleep and wake-up feeling refreshed and alert.

The essential oils in both of these sleep formulas promote deep and restful sleep and have been shown effective for relieving symptoms of sleep loss, insomnia and night terrors. They help calm anxiety and worry and are helpful for restoring the body's natural sleep cycles.

Sleep Formula 1

The essential oils in this formula help you relax more easily, so you fall asleep and stay asleep.

To a 5-ml, colored-glass, euro-dropper bottle add:
Lavender: 10 drops
Clary Sage: 10 drops
Ylang Ylang III: 20 drops
German Chamomile: 20 drops
Spikenard: 20 drops
Red Mandarin: 20 drops

Cap the bottle tightly and shake vigorously to blend the essential oils. Allow to synergize for 8 hours or longer before using. If you're using a 10 percent dilution of any of the pure essential oils, add them directly to your bottle of carrier oil before application.

Dispense 1–3 drops on a cotton ball or smell strip and inhale the aromatic vapors of your sleep blend for 10–15 seconds. You may repeat as needed. This formula is also effective when diffused into the air or used as an aromatic spray.

To make a ready-to-use blend, simply add 15–30 drops of your synergy blend to a 1-ounce (30-ml) bottle of your favorite carrier oil. Shake the bottle well to disperse the oils thoroughly. Apply a few drops of your ready-to-use blend to sinus points around your nose and forehead, as well as on the back of your neck. This is also excellent in your bath as a nighttime relaxation soak just before bed.

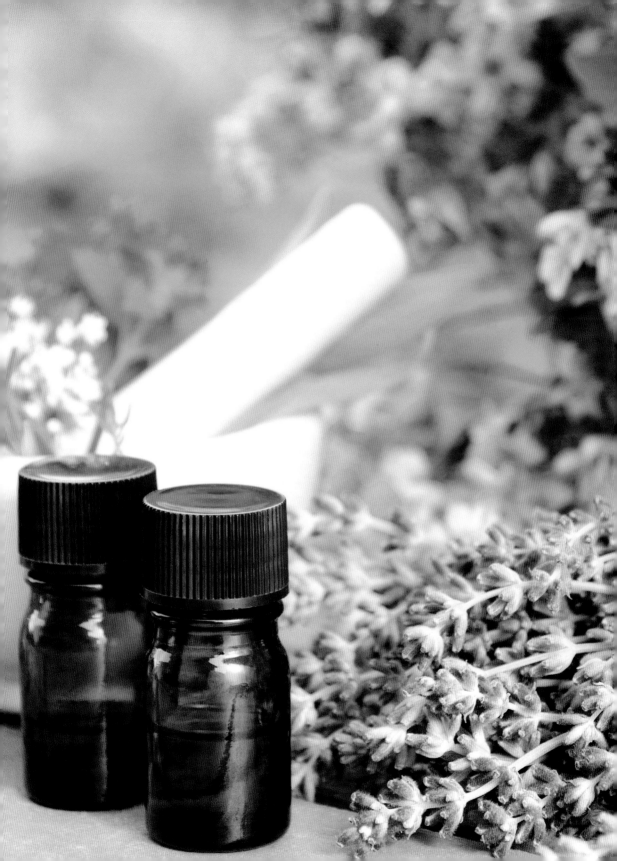

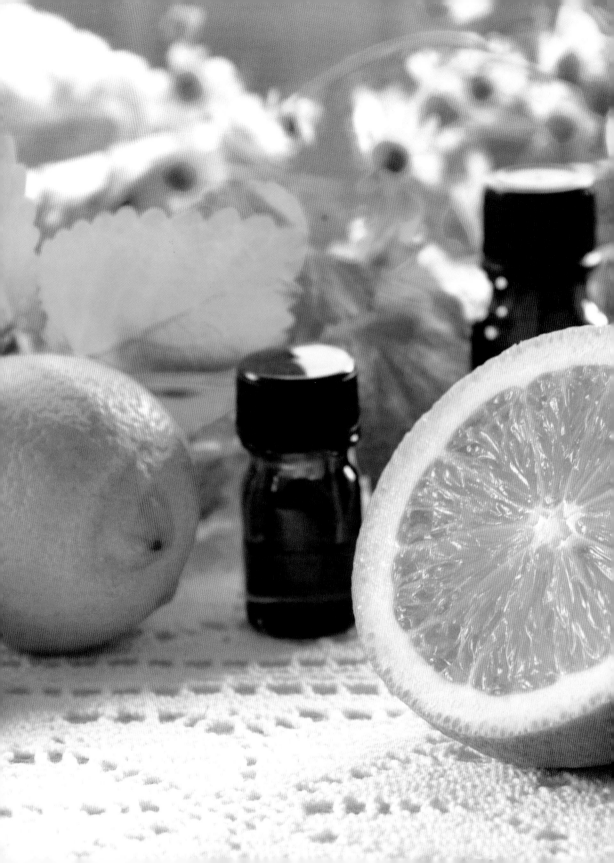

Sleep Formula 2

This second sleep formula is for those of you who want an alternative sleep formula to try or who wish to avoid the use of clary sage. Some women prefer not to use clary sage and previously it was thought to have mild phyto (plant) estrogen-like properties. (Read the latest research about clary sage on page 107.)

To a 5-ml, colored-glass, euro-dropper bottle add:

Red mandarin: 40 drops

Ylang ylang III: 20 drops

German Chamomile: 20 drops

Spikenard: 10 drops

Vetiver: 10 drops

Cap the bottle tightly and shake vigorously to blend the essential oils. Allow to synergize for 8 hours or longer before using. If you're using a 10 percent dilution of any of the pure essential oils, add them directly to your bottle of carrier oil before application.

Dispense 1–3 drops on a cotton ball or smell strip and inhale the aromatic vapors of your sleep blend for 10–15 seconds. You may repeat as needed. This formula is also effective when diffused into the air or used as an aromatic spray.

To make a ready-to-use blend, simply add 15–30 drops of your synergy blend to a 1-ounce (30-ml) bottle of your favorite carrier oil. Shake the bottle well to disperse the oils thoroughly. Apply a few drops of your ready-to-use blend to sinus points around your nose and forehead, as well as on the back of your neck. This is also excellent in your bath as a nighttime relaxation soak just before bed.

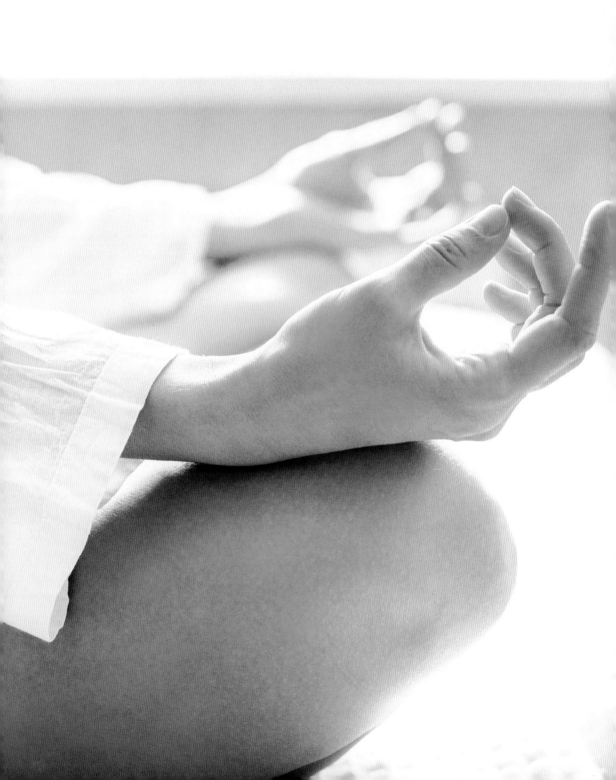

CHAPTER 12

Healthy Lifestyle

Cleansing and Detoxification Formula

The body naturally cleanses and detoxifies itself perfectly. Using essential oils for cleansing and detoxification in this context simply means gently stimulating the body's own natural healing processes to enhance cleansing and detoxification. Part of a cleansing and detoxification program might include removing any processed foods and eating only natural whole foods that the body uses more efficiently for cellular regeneration and healing.

A nerve and blood tonic, the detoxification formula contains essential oils with powerful astringent, circulatory and immune stimulant properties. The properties are known to be effective for stimulating lymph drainage and may also be effective for internal cleansing of the liver and gallbladder when abstaining from toxic substances like drugs and alcohol. This blend may also promote heavy metal detoxification (HMD).

To a 5-ml, colored-glass, euro-dropper bottle add:
Juniper Berry: 40 drops
Cypress: 20 drops
Lemon: 20 drops
Myrrh: 10 drops
Rosemary: 10 drops

Close the cap tightly and shake the bottle vigorously to thoroughly blend the essential oils. Allow to synergize for 8 or more hours before using.

Use the Cleansing and Detoxification Formula as a poultice over the liver and gallbladder area or in a bath to promote cleansing and detoxification. You may experiment with other methods of application (refer to the "How to Use Essential Oils" section on page 29) for even more suggestions about how to use the Cleansing and Detoxification Formula to find out what works best for you.

Weight Loss Program

Most people know that dieting doesn't work, and the research shows that the very process of dieting itself increases your body's natural tendency to gain weight. Researchers call this "diet-induced weight gain," and it is considered a factor in the increasing obesity epidemic.

A study of more than 2,000 sets of twins from Finland, from sixteen to twenty-five years of age, showed that after embarking on just one dieting weight loss plan, the dieting twin was two to three times more likely to become overweight compared to the non-dieting twin. Furthermore, with each subsequent restricted plan to lose weight, their risk increased for becoming overweight.

In conclusion, researchers agree, "It is now well established that the more people engage in dieting, the more they gain weight in the long-term."

Restricted food intake or dieting is also associated with food binging, overeating and eating disorders.

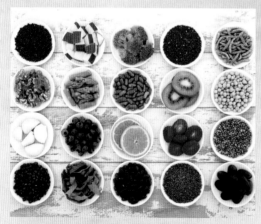

"Diet-induced weight gain" is considerd a factor in the increasing obesity epidemic.

EATING INTUITIVELY

For years I've followed my intuition to know what to eat. Over time my intuitive eating style has developed, and I am more fine-tuned to my body's own particular needs for diet and nutrition. I was delighted to find there is research to support what I've known for years about the key to eating right for you as an individual.

Research by Tracy Tylka PhD, professor of psychology at The Ohio State University, has shown that the healthiest and best way to lose weight naturally is through becoming aware of the needs of your own body and mind. This process of inner-oriented awareness is called "Intuitive Eating." According to the research, dieting interferes with your inner awareness and natural hunger signals that get switched off. By engaging in a program of Intuitive Eating, along with your appetite suppressant, you'll regain awareness and reset your inner guidance system for healthy, natural weight loss.

KEY PRINCIPLES FOR EATING INTUITIVELY

- Eat when you're hungry and whatever foods you desire.

- Eat for physical nourishment rather than emotional comfort.

- Listen to your internal hunger signals to know when and how much to eat.

HELPFUL GUIDANCE

1. The first step to healthy, natural weight loss is to be aware that you have a weight-loss issue and dieting doesn't work.

2. Make a firm commitment to healthy natural weight loss. Connect with your motivation and true desire for losing weight. Knowing the reason why you truly desire to lose weight can help you make a firm commitment to changing your belief about yourself as being overweight.

3. Understand your own overweight issue. You probably have psychological and emotional reasons for overeating that operate automatically at the subconscious level. You may believe that eating will give you comfort and help you deal with uncomfortable emotions. Eating can also be like a reward mechanism to get your emotional needs met. Becoming aware of the psychological and emotional rewards that overeating gives you can help you take your power back and disrupt the overeating "habit loop" to break an emotional eating habit.

4. Connect the dots. Becoming aware of the situations that trigger overeating helps you understand what the habit of overeating is giving you as a short-term reward. Becoming aware of the context that triggers your urge to eat helps you break the automatic emotional eating habit. When you feel the urge to eat, take a moment to think about what may have just happened to trigger the urge. Doing so will disrupt the habitual pattern of emotional eating. Write down a few notes about what you're feeling. This helps you to observe your feelings rather than repress them through emotional eating. Observing your uncomfortable feelings helps you to take your power back and to feel more in charge of your situation.

5. Develop a plan of action. Once you become aware and understand what triggers your urge to overeat, make a clear, specific plan of action for how to minimize or even eliminate your habit triggers. It could be that certain environments, people or situations trigger your urge for emotional overeating. Take stock of what supports your new natural weight loss plan and engage in those activities.

6. Be consistent and build momentum. Be the change you wish to see by visualizing yourself at the weight you desire for yourself. Research shows that more than 90 percent of your behavior and habits operate at the unconscious level; therefore, gaining the support of your subconscious mind through consistent visualization of yourself at your desired weight and seeing yourself in an environment that supports you can be very helpful.

7. Be patient and kind to yourself. Breaking an emotional eating habit can take time. Showing compassion to yourself and being your own best friend through the process has been shown to be helpful for successfully breaking any habit, including emotional eating. Becoming aware of the psychological and emotional triggers that anchor your habit of emotional eating can take time to unravel and disentangle, so be kind and patient with yourself.

Weight Loss Formula and Treatment

Over the past 20 years, obesity has reached epidemic proportions in the U.S. According to the National Center for Health Statistics, one-third of the adult population age 20 years and older—over 100 million people—are obese. Children and teenagers are also showing increased rates of obesity. According to research, obesity is now considered primarily a lifestyle issue brought on by poor choice of diet and lack of exercise. The prevalence of obesity is resulting in increased health risks and diseases among adults and children alike. The health risks include:

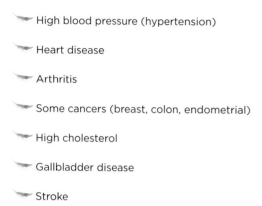

- High blood pressure (hypertension)

- Heart disease

- Arthritis

- Some cancers (breast, colon, endometrial)

- High cholesterol

- Gallbladder disease

- Stroke

I conducted a small, uncontrolled study of seven women who used a pure essential oil appetite suppressant that I formulated for them. Everyone was instructed not to diet during the use of the appetite suppressant. After 3 weeks all of the women reported weight loss with no dieting or exercise. All but one woman lost between 7–10 pounds (3–5 kg). One woman in the group lost only 1 pound (454 g). What all of the women who lost the 7–10 pounds (3–5 kg) reported was that their awareness about what they were eating significantly changed, and their desire for certain foods naturally lessened or even completely disappeared.

This is the appetite suppressant formula these women used:

To a 5-ml, colored-glass, euro-dropper bottle add:
Lemon: 35 drops
Sweet Orange: 30 drops
Grapefruit: 35 drops
Patchouli: 1 drop

Close the cap tightly and shake the bottle vigorously to thoroughly blend the essential oils. Allow to synergize for 8 or more hours before using.

Dispense 1–3 drops on a cotton ball, a smell strip or a 1-dram, colored-glass vial of Celtic salt (cap tightly and shake to disperse the oils) and inhale the aromatic vapors of your appetite suppressant blend for 10–15 seconds. You may repeat as needed. The formula is also effective diffused into the air.

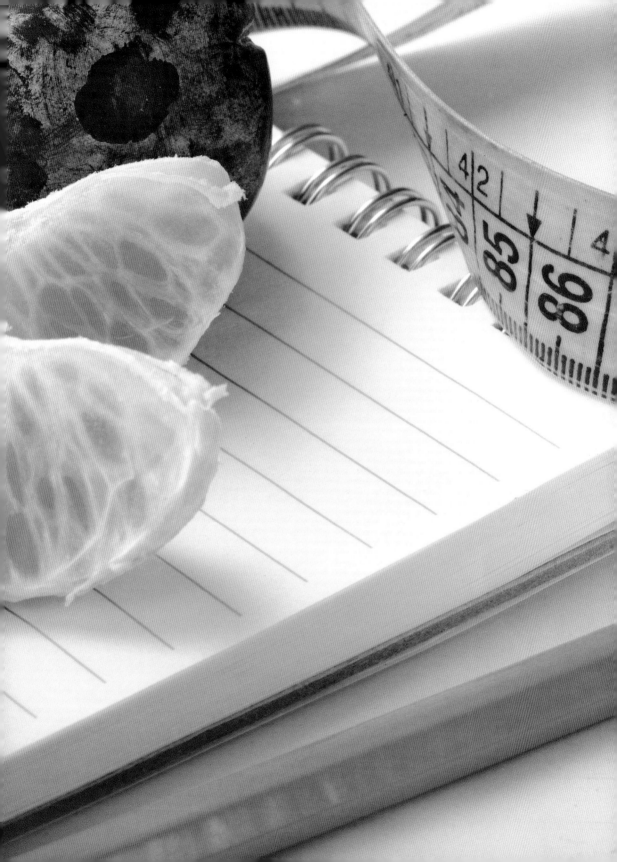

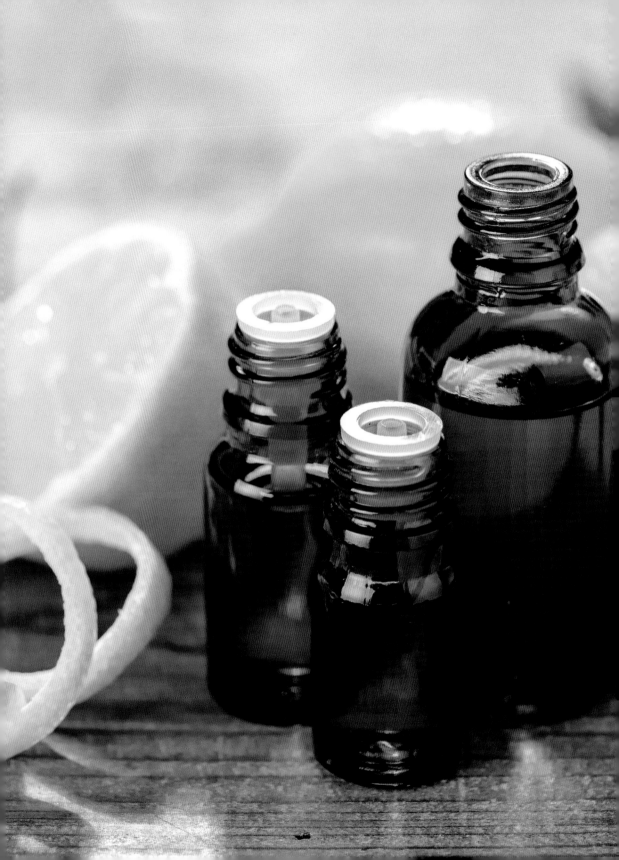

Weight Loss Formula 2

Essential oils are the pure and natural way to lose weight. You can feel great, enjoy eating the food you love and lose weight when using an appetite suppressant made with essential oils. This weight loss formula has been proven to be effective for suppressing appetite signals that may cause you to eat when you're not hungry, as well as help you control an excessive sweet tooth.

The oils in this formula are a perfect balance of aromas for curbing your appetite, as well as for increasing your fat burning and metabolism. It will help to relieve food cravings and enhance your digestion. The citrus oils are known to be natural body tonics, to have an alkalizing effect and to promote the cleansing and detoxification that are so important when losing weight. The natural detoxifying oils in this Weight Loss Formula will help free you of some of the uncomfortable side effects of losing weight like headache, fatigue and food cravings.

~~~~~~

To a 5-ml, colored-glass, euro-dropper bottle add:

Peppermint: 20 drops

Pink Grapefruit: 30 drops

Lemon: 30 drops

Sweet Orange: 20 drops

Fennel: 1–3 drops

Cap the bottle tightly and shake vigorously to blend the essential oils. Allow to synergize for 8 hours or longer before using.

Dispense 1–3 drops on a cotton ball or smell strip and inhale the aromatic vapors of your Weight Loss Formula for 10–15 seconds. You may repeat as needed. This formula is also effective when diffused into the air.

To make a ready-to-use weight loss blend, simply add 15–30 drops of your synergy blend to a 1-ounce (30-ml) bottle of your favorite carrier oil. Shake the bottle well to disperse the oils thoroughly. Apply a few drops of your ready-to-use weight loss blend to the back of your neck and upper and lower abdomen and massage in thoroughly.

Use your appetite suppressant frequently throughout the day for a minimum of 3 weeks. Inhale the scent of your appetite suppressant before you eat, go food shopping or any time you feel prone to snack or take a second helping and also when you're dining out.

Repetition (and consistency) is the key for getting results. Refer to the "Weight Loss Program" section of this book on page 220 for helpful and supportive information about how to achieve healthy and natural weight loss without dieting.

Stop Smoking Program

1. The first step to stopping smoking is to be aware that you have an addiction to smoking and that you want to stop. Some people are able to quit cold turkey, while for others it can take time and effort to break the smoking habit. Research studies show that most people may try numerous times to break the smoking habit before being successful. On a psychological and emotional level, there is an unraveling of your attachments and associations to smoking that anchor your smoking habit primarily in your subconscious mind. You believe yourself to be a smoker, and so you have a smoking habit. To break a smoking habit, you have to create a new image of yourself as a non-smoker, which can take time for some people while others can do it immediately.

2. Make a firm commitment to quit smoking. Connecting your motivation with the reason why you truly desire to quit smoking can help you make a firm decision and commit to changing your belief about yourself as being a non-smoker. Over time, with firm commitment, you build the momentum and follow-though necessary to stop smoking.

3. Understand your smoking habit. You probably have psychological and emotional anchors to your smoking habit that operate automatically. You may believe that smoking helps you relax and deal with uncomfortable emotions, problems and situations in your life. You have an association with smoking as being your friend that you look to for support and comfort when in stressful situations. Smoking can also act like a reward mechanism, and you may believe it helps you accomplish a challenging task. Becoming aware of the psychological and emotional rewards that smoking gives helps you take your power back and disrupt the smoking habit loop.

4. Connect the dots. Becoming aware of the situations that trigger smoking can help you to understand what the habit of smoking is giving you as a short-term reward. Understanding the context which triggers your urge to smoke helps you break the automatic habit. When you feel the urge to smoke, take a moment to become aware of what may have just happened to trigger it. Doing so will disrupt the habitual pattern of smoking. Write down a few notes about what you're feeling. This helps you to observe your feelings rather than repress them by habitually smoking. Observing your uncomfortable feelings helps you to take your power back and to feel more in charge of your situation.

5. Develop a plan of action. Once you become aware of and understand what triggers your urge to smoke, make a clear, specific plan of action for how to minimize or even eliminate your habit triggers. It could be certain environments, people or situations that trigger your urge to smoke. Take stock of what supports your new smoke-free habit and engage in those activities.

6. Be consistent and build momentum. Be the change you wish to see by visualizing yourself as a non-smoker. Visualizing your success has the effect of gaining the cooperation of your subconscious mind to help you to break a smoking habit. Research shows that more than 90 percent of your behavior and habits operate at the unconscious level; therefore, gaining the support of your subconscious mind through consistent visualization of yourself as a non-smoker and seeing yourself in an environment that supports being smoke-free can be very helpful.

7. Breaking a smoking habit can take time. Showing compassion for yourself and being your own best friend through the process has been shown to be helpful for successfully breaking a smoking habit. Becoming aware of the psychological and emotional triggers that anchor your smoking habit can take time to unravel and disentangle, so be kind and patient with yourself.

Research suggests that it takes a minimum of 3 weeks for your established pattern and mental image of yourself to dissolve and a new mental image as a non-smoker to be created, leading to the formation of your new habit.

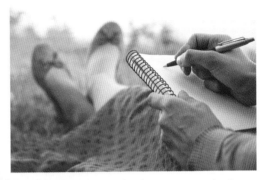

Journaling can help you develop awareness about what triggers your urge to smoke. This helps you take back your power from the addiction.

Other research suggests a minimum of 40 days, while a recent study of ninety-six people published in the *European Journal of Social Psychology* reported that it took an average of 66 days to form a new habit.

With repetition, you build momentum for your new habit to take root in your subconscious. Seeing a picture in your mind of yourself as a non-smoker feels natural and becomes automatic.

Based on this information, you want to use your Stop Smoking Formula (page 228) continuously for a minimum of 3 weeks and then as needed to maintain your new smoke-free habit.

Stop Smoking Formula and Treatment

Stopping a smoking addiction can be either cold turkey or a long-term plan that involves cutting down smoking over a period of time to eventually quit altogether. Recent psychosocial pressures and the banning of smoking in or near public facilities have resulted in a decrease in the smoking habit. Studies have shown that smoking in the U.S. has continued to decrease since 2005 and has now reached an all-time low, even though the population has increased. Worldwide statistics show that smoking is the leading cause of preventable death. The problem is that nicotine in tobacco is very addictive, and the symptoms of nicotine withdrawal when stopping smoking are very uncomfortable and include anxiety, food cravings, weight gain, agitation and depression.

Essential oils can be helpful not only in helping you to break the nicotine habit, but also in supporting the detoxification process and relieving symptoms of withdrawal.

To a 5-ml, colored-glass, euro-dropper bottle add:

Bergamot: 50 drops

Black Pepper: 40 drops

Rosemary Verbenone: 10 drops

Close the cap tightly and shake the bottle vigorously to thoroughly blend the essential oils. Allow to synergize for 8 or more hours before using.

Dispense 1–3 drops of the Stop Smoking Formula blend onto a cotton ball or smell strip and inhale the aromatic vapors for 10–15 seconds. This formula is also effective in a diffuser or as an aromatic mist. To make a ready-to-use stop smoking blend, simply add 15–30 drops of your synergy blend to a 1-ounce (30-ml) bottle of your favorite carrier oil, and shake the bottle well to disperse the oils thoroughly. Apply a few drops of your ready-to-use blend to sinus points around your nose and forehead, as well as on the back of your neck. You may repeat as needed.

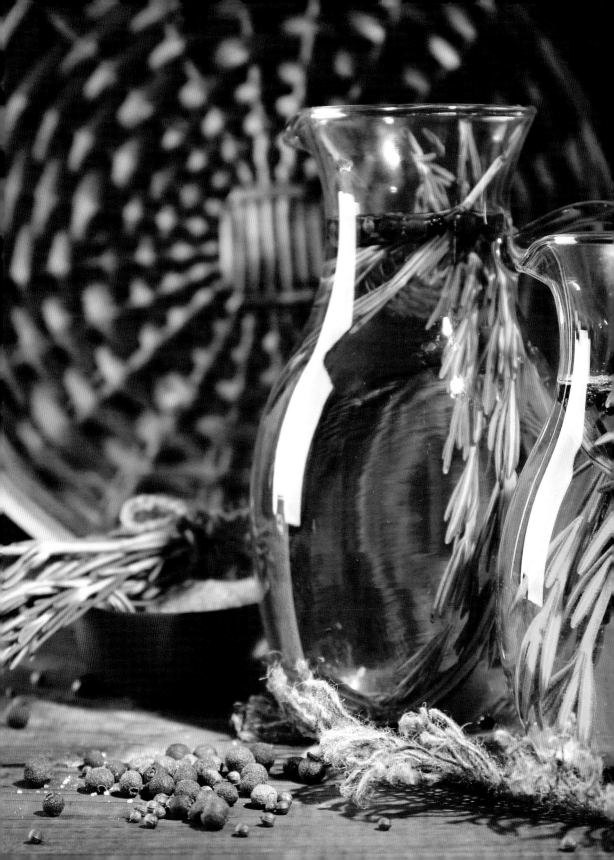

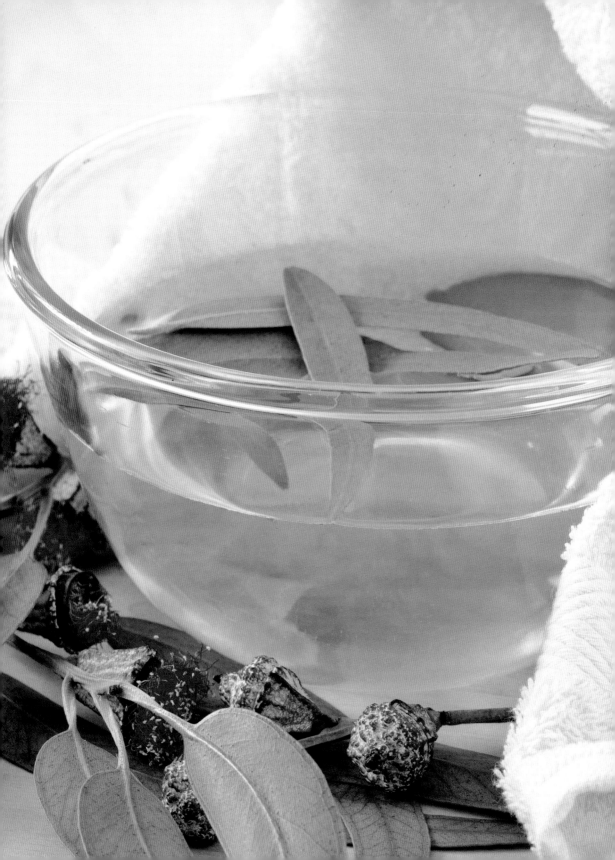

Steam Inhalation to Support Respiratory System Formula

Steam inhalation with essential oils can be most effective for supporting the respiratory system and to aid in breathing. Whether you desire relief for asthma and allergy symptoms or for treating upper or lower respiratory tract infections, steam inhalation can be a great friend in your process of healing and recovery. Upper respiratory tract infections include sinusitis, tonsillitis, laryngitis and the common cold. Research now shows that poor oral hygiene and gum disease may be a contributing factor in pneumonia.

The essential oils in the respiratory support formula contain antibacterial, antihistamine, anti-allergic, antispasmodic and bronchodilating properties that make it useful for relieving respiratory conditions and associated symptoms of swelling and itching.

~~~~~~

To a 5-ml, colored-glass, euro-dropper bottle add:
Blue Tansy: 20 drops
Hyssop: 20 drops
Frankincense: 20 drops
Lemon: 10 drops
Eucalyptus Radiata: 20 drops
Blue Yarrow: 10 drops

Close the cap tightly and shake the bottle vigorously to thoroughly blend the essential oils. Allow to synergize for 8 or more hours before using.

Use your Steam Inhalation Formula in a steam (refer to the "How to Use Essential Oils" section on page 29) or in a diffuser. Or you can dispense 1–3 drops of the respiratory blend onto a cotton ball or smell strip and inhale the aromatic vapors for 10–15 seconds. The formula is also effective as an aromatic mist. To make a ready-to-use blend, simply add 15–30 drops of your synergy blend to a 1-ounce (30-ml) bottle of your favorite carrier oil. Shake the bottle well to disperse the oils thoroughly. Apply a few drops of your ready-to-use blend to sinus points around your nose and forehead, as well as on the back of your neck. You may repeat as needed.

Oral Health Program

COMPLETE PROGRAM FOR PREVENTION AND TREATMENT OF TOOTH DECAY AND GUM DISEASE

For more than 10 years, I've practiced preventative dentistry and have used the treatments I recommend for preventing and reversing tooth decay, as well as whitening my teeth and keeping my gums healthy. Plus, I save money on dental care. When I went to my dentist for a cleaning recently, I had a full set of x-rays taken (the first I've had in 8 years). I wanted to check just in case I might have a cavity. My dentist, who supports my preventative dental care approach, gave my teeth a clean bill of health.

It is a common presumption that once you have a cavity the only way to "cure" it is to have a dentist drill out your cavity and replace it with a filling made of synthetic material. However, according to research that was published in the *British Medical Journal*, cavities and tooth decay can potentially be healed or even reversed with proper diet and nutrition.

When you remove the cause of cavities, your teeth naturally secrete new dentine to renew, repair and heal your teeth and gums. Your teeth thrive in an alkaline environment, so promoting alkalinity in your mouth through your diet and nutrition promotes the health of your teeth and gums.

I've used several different preventative dental care approaches and will share the program I've developed, which includes the use of a re-mineralizing toothpaste.

When a customer shared a type of re-mineralizing toothpaste recipe with me, I decided to give it a try myself. I adjusted the ingredients a little, so they were more to my own liking for a natural product.

After my first treatment, I noticed immediate results. I could actually feel and see a difference in the brightness of my smile and comfort level of my teeth and gums. Soon after beginning treatment, this natural re-mineralizing toothpaste had easily and effectively removed any signs of plaque buildup or stains from my teeth.

My teeth were noticeably whiter and brighter and felt stronger, healthier and happier. You know how your teeth feel after a good cleaning by the dental hygienist? That's how my teeth felt.

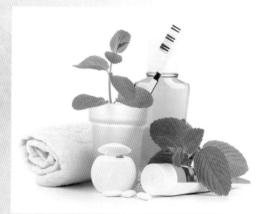

Preventative dentistry can reverse tooth decay, as well as whiten your teeth and save you time and money.

Natural Re-Mineralizing Toothpaste Formula

This natural re-mineralizing toothpaste promotes removal of plaque buildup and stains.

~~~~~~

Makes 8 ounces (237 ml):

¾ cup (175 ml) purified water, boiling

1 tbsp (15 ml) organic raw extra virgin coconut oil (kills viruses and bacteria)

¼ tsp Celtic salt (source of natural minerals)

½ tsp organic stevia leaf (green, unprocessed, dry herb and natural sweetener)

⅓ cup (75 g) bentonite green clay (draws out toxins and removes stains)

2 drops thyme oil (kills germs and bacteria, promotes healing of cavity)

2 drops oregano oil (kills germs and bacteria, promotes healing of cavity)

2 drops lemon oil (kills germs and bacteria, promotes healing of cavity)

2 drops cinnamon leaf oil (kills germs and bacteria, promotes healing of cavity)

2 drops clove bud oil (kills germs and bacteria, promotes healing of cavity)

15 drops peppermint oil (breath freshener)

In a pan, bring the water to a boil. In a ceramic bowl, add ¼ cup (60 ml) of the boiling water. Stir in the organic raw extra virgin coconut oil. Blend the Celtic salt and stevia into the liquid.

Mix the bentonite clay into the hot liquid with a stainless steel spoon. Blend the mixture together until smooth and even like a paste. Add more heated purified water if needed to make a nice smooth and consistent paste. Blend the essential oils into the paste.

Transfer the re-mineralizing toothpaste into an 8-ounce (237-ml) glass container and seal tightly with a lid. Store in a cool, dark place.

To use, wet your toothbrush and dip the bristles onto the surface of the re-mineralizing toothpaste. Apply a sufficient amount of toothpaste to brush your teeth. Be sure to thoroughly brush each tooth. I recommend that you floss before brushing. Use daily until you finish the entire 8-ounce (237-ml) jar. Continue use as needed.

CAUTION: Oregano oil is a potent, "hot" antimicrobial and should be used with extreme caution. As it is a strong irritant to the skin and mucous membranes, use a less than 1-percent dilution for safe skin application. Avoid during pregnancy and with young children and pets.

Oil Pulling

Oil pulling is a traditional folk remedy practiced in Ayurvedic medicine. Raw coconut oil contains 50 percent lauric acid, which the body converts into monolaurin, an antiviral, antibacterial and antiprotozoal agent that can destroy viruses like HIV, herpes, influenza and various other pathogens.

Oil pulling, or "oil swishing" as it is also called, is a method of swishing or holding the oil in the mouth for a period of time (20 minutes or longer). There are many claims for its improving oral and systemic health. It's thought to help various health issues like headache, migraine, asthma and acne, as well as whitening the teeth. Oil swishing of coconut oil is thought to work by "pulling out" toxins.

Oil pulling is a part of my regular dental health routine. It's a great cleanser and teeth whitener. I usually hold it in my mouth and swish it around for 30-60 minutes once a week between meals.

As part of my preventative dental program I also floss daily, brush with baking soda after meals and swish with hydrogen peroxide at least once daily. All have a therapeutically cleansing and whitening effect on the teeth and gums.

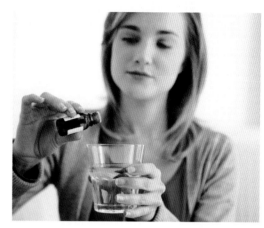

Routine oil pulling will whiten your teeth and keep your gums healthy.

Recovery After Illness Formula

A powerful tonic, astringent and immune stimulant, this Recovery After Illness Formula contains essential oils with properties known for boosting and protecting the immune system. Its action to stimulate the formation of white blood cells aids the oxygenation of tissue and the removal of toxic waste. It may be effective for restoring the immune system after prolonged illness.

To a 5-ml, colored-glass, euro-dropper bottle add:

Geranium Roseum and Graveolens: 20 drops

Myrrh: 20 drops

Frankincense: 20 drops

Lemon: 5 drops

Eucalyptus Globulus: 5 drops

Eucalyptus Radiata: 5 drops

Thyme: 5 drops

Lavender: 5 drops

Rosemary: 5 drops

Cypress: 5 drops

Ledum: 5 drops

Close the cap tightly and shake the bottle vigorously to thoroughly blend the essential oils. Allow to synergize for 8 or more hours before using.

Use in a diffuser or dispense 1–3 drops of the Recovery After Illness Formula onto a cotton ball or smell strip and inhale the aromatic vapors for 10–15 seconds. It is also effective as an aromatic mist. To make a ready-to-use Recovery After Illness blend, simply add 15–30 drops of your synergy blend to a 1-ounce (30-ml) bottle of your favorite carrier oil. Shake the bottle well to disperse the oils thoroughly. Apply a few drops of your ready-to-use blend to sinus points around your nose and forehead, as well as on the back of your neck. You may repeat as needed.

Rejuvenating and Healing Formula

A powerful, broad-spectrum tonic and immune stimulant, this Rejuvenating and Healing blend has tremendous capacity for healing. It contains nature's most potent antimicrobial oils for supporting and protecting the immune system, as well as killing viral, bacterial (especially airborne) and fungal infections.

~~~~~~

To a 5-ml, colored-glass, euro-dropper bottle add:

Clove: 10 drops

Cinnamon Leaf: 10 drops

Eucalyptus Radiata: 20 drops

Lemon: 20 drops

Thyme: 5 drops

Oregano: 10 drops

Tea Tree: 5 drops

Lavender: 5 drops

Myrrh: 10 drops

Rosemary: 5 drops

Close the cap tightly and shake the bottle vigorously to thoroughly blend the essential oils. Allow to synergize for 8 or more hours before using.

Use in a diffuser, or dispense 1–3 drops of the Rejuvenating and Healing Formula onto a cotton ball or smell strip and inhale the aromatic vapors for 10–15 seconds. This formula is also effective as an aromatic mist. To make a ready-to-use Rejuvenating and Healing blend, simply add 15–30 drops of your synergy blend to a 1-ounce (30-ml) bottle of your favorite carrier oil. Shake the bottle well to disperse the oils thoroughly. Apply a few drops of your ready-to-use blend to sinus points around your nose and forehead, as well as on the back of your neck. You may repeat as needed.

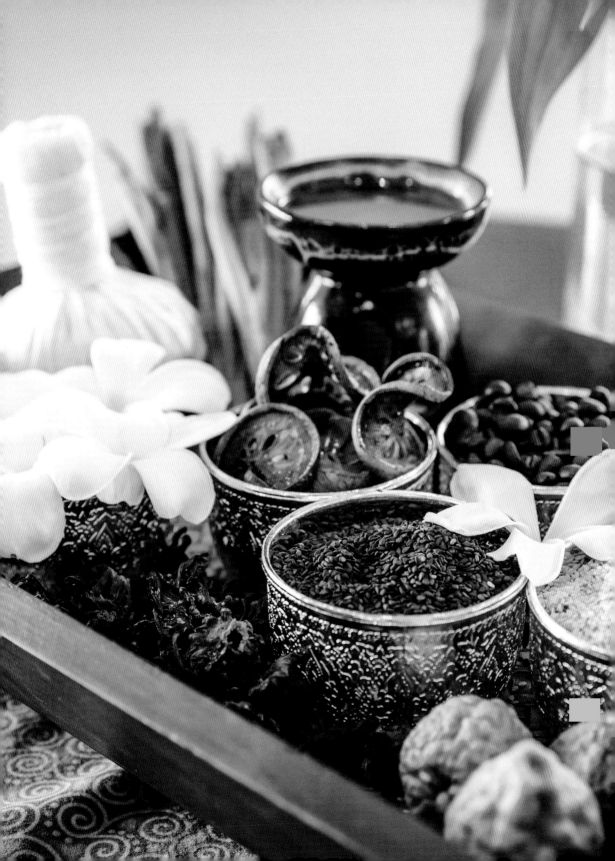

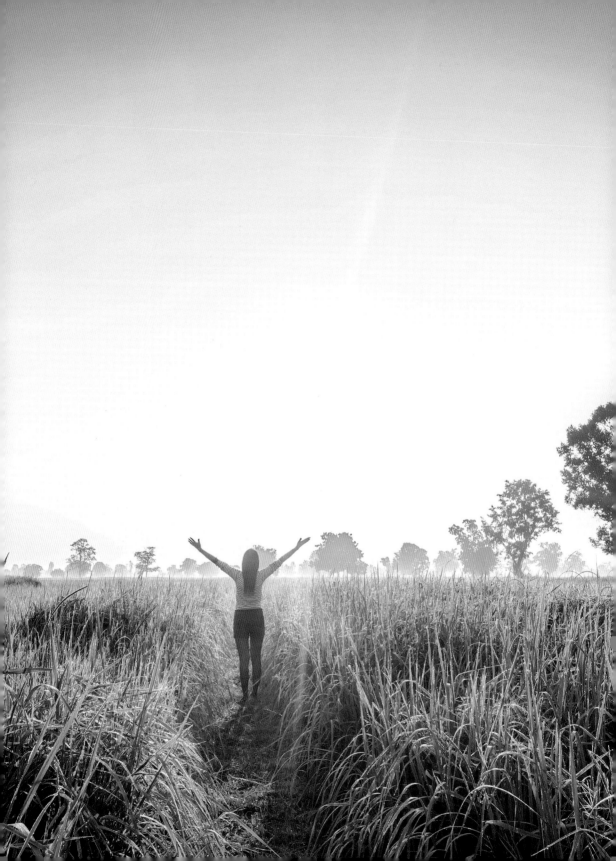

Women's Health Formulas

These women's health formulas are the result of years of experience and working with women to help them find pure and natural solutions to their health concerns.

Female Toner

The female psyche is very open and sensitive to the environment and its influences. Being in the world can deplete energy reserves that need daily replenishing with sufficient rest and recovery time. Hormonal balance plays a crucial role in a woman's sense of well-being, level of emotional comfort and security. Nourishing the hormonal system with proper nutrition, exercise and time for rest and recovery helps to keep the hormonal system naturally balanced.

The essential oils in this Female Toner formula have been shown to have a regulating and balancing effect on the hormonal system and are helpful for relieving symptoms of imbalance like menstrual tension and cramping, as well as menopausal symptoms like hot flashes, headache, sleeplessness, tearfulness, depression, irritability and mood swings.

To a 5-ml, colored-glass, euro-dropper bottle add:

Geranium (Bourbon): 20 drops

Palmarosa: 20 drops

Lavender: 20 drops

Cypress: 20 drops

Clary Sage: 10 drops

Rose: 5 drops

Frankincense: 5 drops

Close the cap tightly and shake the bottle vigorously to thoroughly blend the essential oils. Allow to synergize for 8 or more hours before using.

Dispense 1–3 drops on a cotton ball or smell strip and inhale the aromatic vapors of your Female Toner for 10–15 seconds. You may repeat as needed. Female toner may be especially effective used as a hot compress to relieve menstrual cramps.

To make a ready-to-use Female Toner blend simply add 15–30 drops of your synergy blend to a 1-ounce (30-ml) bottle of your favorite carrier oil. Shake the bottle well to disperse the oils thoroughly. Apply a few drops of your blend to sinus points around your nose and forehead, as well as on the back of your neck. Clients report that with regular use signs of hormonal imbalance diminish in severity and are less frequent or even stop completely.

Hormone Balance Formula

The endocrine glands secrete hormones (electro-chemicals) that regulate all the body's organs and systems. Some of the body functions that hormones control include digestion, metabolism, respiration, perception, sleep, excretion, lactation, stress, growth and development, movement, reproduction and mood. Nourishing the hormonal system with proper nutrition, exercise and time for rest and recovery help to keep the hormonal system naturally balanced.

The essential oils in this Hormone Balance Formula have been shown to have a regulating and balancing effect on the hormonal system and are helpful for relieving symptoms of imbalance like premenstrual tension and cramping, as well as menopausal symptoms like hot flashes, headache, sleeplessness, tearfulness, depression, irritability and mood swings.

~~~~~~

To a 5-ml, colored-glass, euro-dropper bottle add:

Geranium (Graveolens): 20 drops

Palmarosa: 20 drops

Geranium Roseum: 20 drops

Clary Sage: 20 drops

Bergamot: 20 drops

Close the cap tightly and shake the bottle vigorously to thoroughly blend the essential oils. Allow to synergize for 8 or more hours before using.

Dispense 1–3 drops on a cotton ball or smell strip and inhale the aromatic vapors of your Hormone Balance Formula for 10–15 seconds. You may repeat as needed. This is also effective when diffused into the air or used as an aromatic mist.

To make a ready-to-use Hormone Balance Formula, simply add 15–30 drops of your synergy blend to a 1-ounce (30-ml) bottle of your favorite carrier oil. Shake the bottle well to disperse the oils thoroughly. Apply a few drops of your ready-to-use blend to sinus points around your nose and forehead, as well as on the back of your neck. Clients report that with regular use signs of hormonal imbalance diminish in severity, occur less frequently or even stop completely.

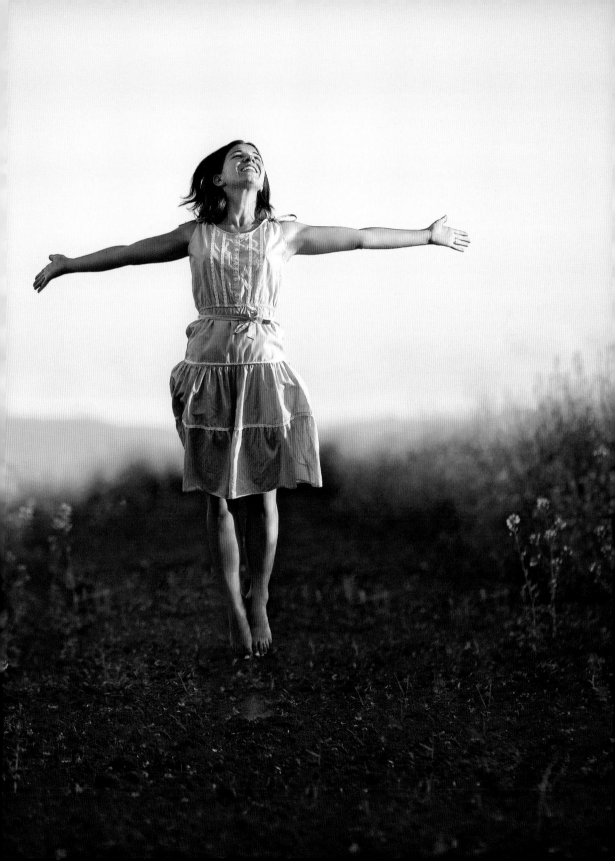

Hot Flash Relief Formula

Hot flashes are caused by fluctuations in hormones and are often associated with menopause. Symptoms include sudden intense heat, profuse sweating, visible reddening of the skin, feelings of faintness and rapid pulse. Symptoms can last for a couple of minutes or up to half an hour. Hot flashes may occur sporadically or be a common occurrence and disrupt the quality of one's life. Accompanying symptoms include night sweats (which interrupt sleep), insomnia, depression, poor mood and an inability to focus and pay attention.

The North American Menopause Society (NAMS) attributes certain foods and lifestyle habits to the aggravation of hot flashes, including hot and spicy foods, alcohol and caffeine. It's also thought that obesity issues may contribute to menopausal symptoms like hot flashes.

The essential oils in this formula have been shown to be effective as a comfort care measure to promote natural relief for symptoms of hot flashes.

To a 5-ml, colored-glass, euro-dropper bottle add:

Peppermint: 20 drops

Cypress: 20 drops

Lemon: 20 drops

Geranium Roseum and Graveolens: 5 drops each

Clary Sage: 10 drops

Palmarosa: 10 drops

Lemongrass: 10 drops

Cap the bottle tightly and shake vigorously to blend the essential oils. Allow to synergize for 8 hours or longer before using.

This formula makes a wonderfully cooling aromatic mist and is also effective diffused into the air. You may use as often as needed.

To make a ready-to-use Hot Flash Relief Formula, simply add 15–30 drops of your synergy blend to a 1-ounce (30-ml) bottle of your favorite carrier oil. Shake the bottle well to disperse the oils thoroughly. Apply a few drops of your ready-to-use blend to sinus points around your nose and forehead, as well as the back of your neck. Clients report that with regular use signs of hormonal imbalance like hot flashes diminish in severity, occur less frequently or even stop completely.

Breast Health

Breast self-awareness includes regular breast self-examination (BSE), a screening method used to detect early breast cancer. A BSE involves looking and feeling each breast for painful or swollen tissue or any distortions in tissue quality.

Though much less common, men can develop breast cancer. So breast self-awareness is not gender-specific.

A regular breast massage is a great way to develop your breast self-awareness, as well as perform your BSE.

WHY PERFORMING A REGULAR BREAST MASSAGE IS SO BENEFICIAL

- Breast massage increases your personal awareness about changes in your breasts and is considered one of the most important methods for detection of breast cancer in its early stages.

- Breast massage sends an important message of self-love and acceptance, which is fundamental to good health.

- Breast massage allows you to learn to recognize and get comfortable with normal breast changes that may include natural lumpiness of your breast tissue.

- Breast massage increases the flow of lymph drainage to remove toxins within and around the breast, encouraging the area to remain free of toxic build-up. Lymph also carries immune cells for fighting against infection and rogue tissue growth, like cancer. Unlike the circulatory system, which has the heart to pump blood, the lymph system does not have a pump to move its fluids. The continuous action of muscular contraction squeezes lymph vessels to move lymph fluid throughout the lymphatic system. If there is prolonged restriction or tightness of tissues, lymph builds up and inflammation can occur.

Much research supports the idea that when women wear bras they restrict the normal flow of lymph fluid within the breast tissue. Because the lymphatic system is responsible for the removal of toxins from your body, researchers have concluded that restricting the flow of lymph has the potential for contributing to the development of breast cancer, as well as other uncomfortable breast tissue conditions.

To ensure healthy lymph flow and drainage and to promote healthy breast tissue, regular movement, exercise and stretching are absolutely essential. It is also important to practice breast health care with a regular BSE, which can include giving yourself a regular breast massage.

BREAST MASSAGE MAY RELIEVE THESE SYMPTOMS:

- Breast tenderness

- Uneven or lumpy breast tissue

- Pre-menstrual tension and discomfort

- Swelling and pain from breast surgery

- Pectoralis muscle pain

- Mastitis

PLEASE NOTE: Your open readiness to discuss any unusual breast tissue changes you may find with your doctor is also very important.

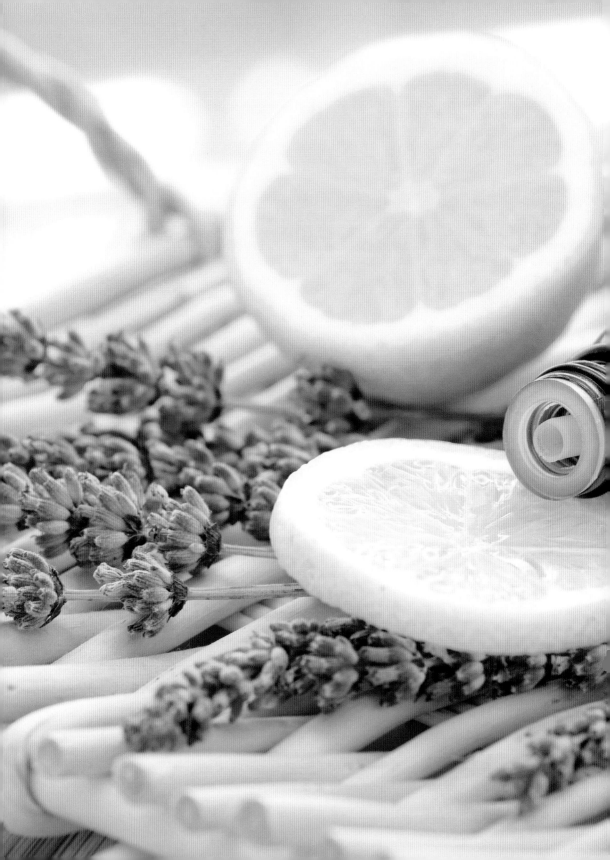

Fibroids Formula

"True health is only possible when we understand the unity of our minds, emotions, spirits and physical bodies and stop striving for perfection." —Christiane Northrup, MD

Uterine fibroids are considered benign tumors of the uterus. The medical term for a fibroid tumor is *myoma* or *fibromyoma*. Up to 80 percent of women develop fibroids by age fifty. In 2013 it was reported that 171 million women had fibroids. Fibroids are most often asymptomatic, depending upon their size and location. Symptoms may include heavy periods and frequent urination, as well as occasionally a hindrance for getting pregnant.

Though the cause of fibroids isn't clear, the tendency for getting a fibroid seems genetically linked and can run in one's family. Obesity and overeating, especially red meat, also seem to be causative factors.

Dr. Christiane Northrup, an OB/GYN physician for 25 years and the author of *Women's Bodies, Women's Wisdom*, says that many women develop uterine fibroids during the middle and later reproductive years. After menopause, fibroids usually decrease in size and even disappear. The research seems to bear this out. However, in the U.S., uterine fibroids are a common reason for surgical removal of the uterus.

The essential oils in this comfort care formula have been shown to be effective for relieving fibroid symptoms.

To a 5-ml, colored-glass, euro-dropper bottle add:

Lavender: 20 drops

Lemon: 10 drops

Juniper Berry: 10 drops

Palmarosa: 40 drops

Helichrysum: 20 drops

Cap the bottle tightly and shake vigorously to blend the essential oils. Allow to synergize for 8 hours or longer before using.

To use in a sitz bath, fill the bath with pure warm water (98°F [37°C]) and add the Fibroids Formula essential oils blend. Soak the area for 15 minutes or until the warm water cools. Repeat as needed to relieve symptoms of discomfort and to support natural healing.

You can also use a sitz bath for treatments of other ailments like Bartholin gland cysts. A sitz bath is more effective for getting results than a full bath is for cysts.

Breast Health Massage Formula

The essential oils in this Breast Health Massage Formula have been shown to be effective for relieving symptoms of nausea that may be caused by dizziness, sea sickness, motion sickness, migraine headache, stomach flu or food poisoning. The formula also offers relief from nausea resulting from side effects of many medications, including chemotherapy, as well as morning sickness in early pregnancy.

The essential oils in the Breast Health Massage Formula promote gentle penetrating action that is regenerative and healing to breast tissue.

Gently apply a small amount of the Breast Health Massage Formula onto your breast and chest areas and lightly massage in, or use in a hot compress to help relieve congestion, promote circulation and relieve acute and chronic pain.

This massage oil also makes an excellent Swedish or deep tissue massage lubricant. You may use this oil during or after subtle bodywork, such as acupuncture, Reiki or Therapeutic Touch to enhance your treatment results.

~~~~~~

To a 5-ml, colored-glass, euro-dropper bottle add:

Peppermint: 20 drops

Ginger: 20 drops

Lemon: 20 drops

Geranium Roseum: 30 drops

Clary Sage: 10 drops

Cap the bottle tightly and shake vigorously to blend the essential oils. Allow to synergize for 8 hours or longer before using.

To make a ready-to-use breast massage oil simply add 15–30 drops of your synergy blend to a 1-ounce (30-ml) bottle of your favorite carrier oil. Shake the bottle well to disperse the oils thoroughly. Dispense 1–3 drops. Inhale the scent of the oil first and then apply to the breast and massage thoroughly into the tissues.

Sitz Bath

A sitz bath will help you focus your essential oil treatment to the area of discomfort for better results.

~~~~~~

1–3 cups (500–1,500 g) Epsom or sea salts
15–18 drops Fibroids Formula (page 245)

Pour the salts into a bowl and add the essential oil. Blend together thoroughly. Cover and set aside.

Fill the sitz bath with pure warm water (98°F [37°C]), add the scented salts and blend in thoroughly. Soak in the bath for 15 minutes or until the waters cool. Repeat as needed to relieve symptoms of discomfort and to support natural healing. This formula is also effective as a warm compress over the lower belly or any area of discomfort.

You can also use a sitz bath for other treatments like for Bartholin gland cysts. A sitz bath is more effective for getting results than the full bath that we see here.

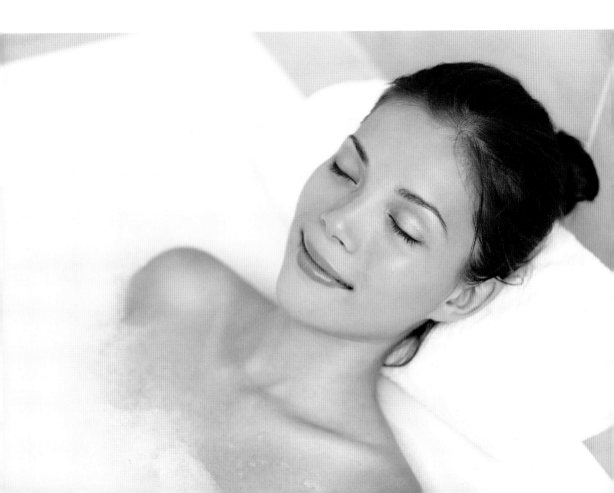

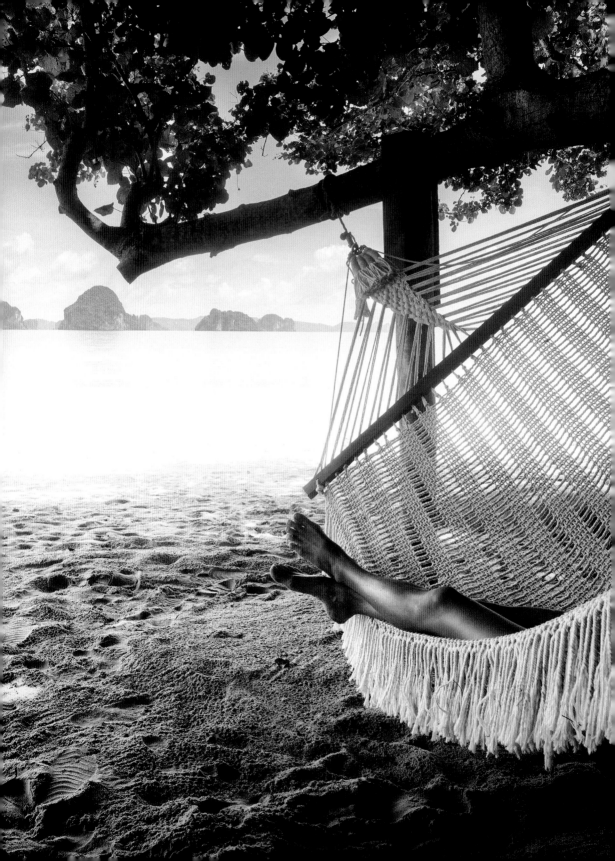

CHAPTER 13

Relaxation and Emotional Support Formulas

Enthusiasm

When one is filled with an intense enjoyment of life and the feeling of being alive, there is nothing one cannot do. You look forward to each day with renewed optimism and faith in the unseen adventures life will bring you. Many children are quite naturally filled with an enthusiastic spirit and throw themselves into every activity with wild abandon. The word "enthusiastic" was first coined by the Greeks and meant "possessed by god's essence." If you've lost your zest for life, essential oils can help renew and lift your spirits.

Lift the Spirits Formula

This Lift the Spirits Formula contains essential oils with stimulating, regulating and energizing properties that make it effective for lifting your spirits and renewing your enthusiasm for life.

To a 5-ml, colored-glass, euro-dropper bottle add:

Grapefruit: 40 drops

Peppermint: 20 drops

Lemon: 20 drops

Geranium Roseum and Graveolens: 10 drops each

Close the cap tightly and shake the bottle vigorously to thoroughly blend the essential oils. Allow to synergize for 8 or more hours before using.

Dispense 1–3 drops on a cotton ball or smell strip and inhale the aromatic vapors of your Lift the Spirits Formula for 10–15 seconds. You may repeat as needed. This formula is also effective when diffused into the air, as an aromatic mist or in the bath.

To make a ready-to-use Lift the Spirits Formula, simply add 15–30 drops of your synergy blend to a 1-ounce (30-ml) bottle of your favorite carrier oil. Shake the bottle well to disperse the oils thoroughly. Apply a few drops of your ready-to-use blend to sinus points around your nose and forehead, as well as on the back of your neck.

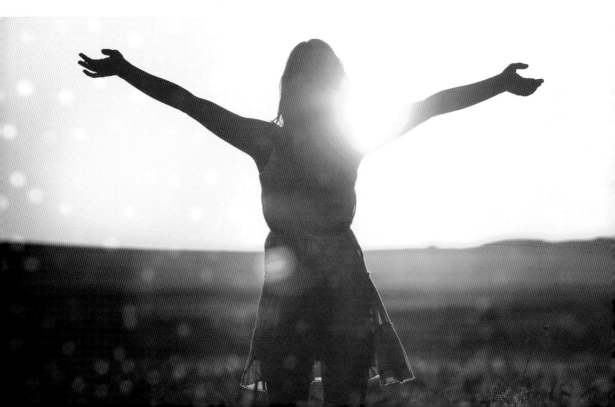

Mood

A mood is a very general emotional state that can dramatically affect how you experience life. When you're in a good mood, things seems to go your way. Whereas, when you're in a bad mood, it can feel like you have two left feet and can't seem to get in sync with your life. Sometimes you just wake up in a bad mood or something happens that triggers a bad mood. Essential oils are great for creating an ambiance that will immediately shift a bad mood—or enhance an already good one—so that you feel even better almost instantly.

Lift the Mood Formula

This Lift the Mood Formula contains essential oils with regulating properties that may be effective for shifting mental states and lifting the mood.

To a 5-ml, colored-glass, euro-dropper bottle add:

Bergamot: 40 drops

Ylang Ylang III: 20 drops

Geranium Roseum and Graveolens: 20 drops

Clary Sage: 20 drops

Close the cap tightly and shake the bottle vigorously to thoroughly blend the essential oils. Allow to synergize for 8 or more hours before using.

Dispense 1–3 drops on a cotton ball or smell strip and inhale the aromatic vapors of your Lift the Mood blend for 10–15 seconds. You may repeat as needed. This formula is also effective when diffused into the air, as an aromatic mist or in the bath.

To make a ready-to-use Lift the Mood Formula, simply add 15–30 drops of your synergy blend to a 1-ounce (30-ml) bottle of your favorite carrier oil. Shake the bottle well to disperse the oils thoroughly. Apply a few drops of your ready-to-use blend to sinus points around your nose and forehead, as well as on the back of your neck.

Meditation

Some form of meditation or mindfulness practice has been around since antiquity. Meditation may include many different practices and techniques for the purpose of calming and regulating the mind, as well as recognizing a heightened state of awareness. Becoming identified with pure consciousness while doing some form of meditation helps to free the meditator from the grip of the egoism of the mind, which is changeable and thus a source of suffering. Many health problems are now being treated with meditation, including high blood pressure, depression and anxiety. Meditation is also used to engender loving kindness and compassion for one's fellow man.

Meditation Formula

The essential oils in the Meditation Formula support meditation practice by calming and harmonizing your mind and emotions and slowing down your heart rate, breathing and cellular respiration.

To a 5-ml, colored-glass, euro-dropper bottle add:

Frankincense: 20 drops

Atlas Cedarwood: 20 drops

Myrrh: 20 drops

Spikenard: 20 drops

Ylang Ylang III: 10 drops

Bergamot: 10 drops

Close the cap tightly and shake the bottle vigorously to thoroughly blend the essential oils. Allow to synergize for 8 or more hours before using.

Dispense 1–3 drops on a cotton ball or smell strip and inhale the aromatic vapors of your Meditation blend for 10–15 seconds. You may repeat as needed. This formula is also effective when diffused into the air or as an aromatic mist.

To make a ready-to-use Meditation Formula blend, simply add 15–30 drops of your synergy blend to a 1-ounce (30-ml) bottle of your favorite carrier oil. Shake the bottle well to disperse the oils thoroughly. Apply a few drops to sinus points around your nose and forehead, as well as on the back of your neck.

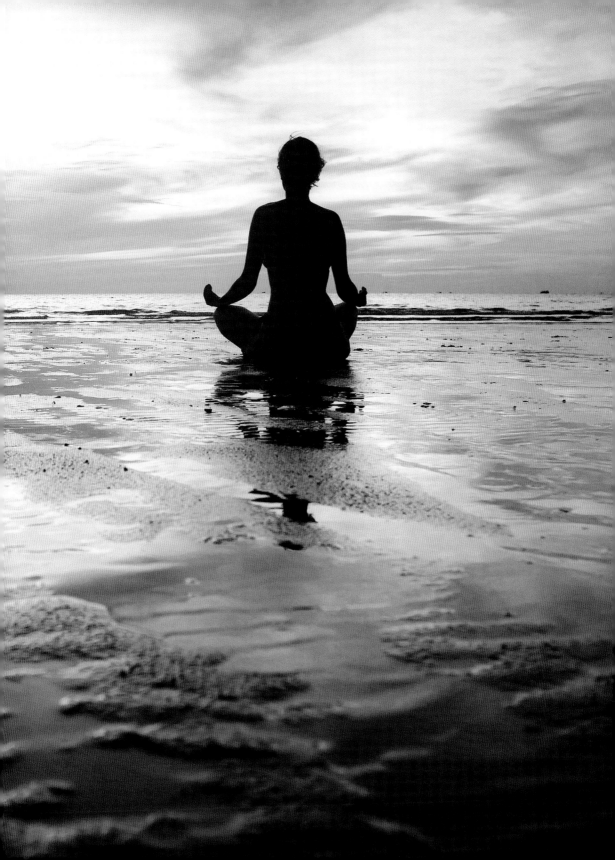

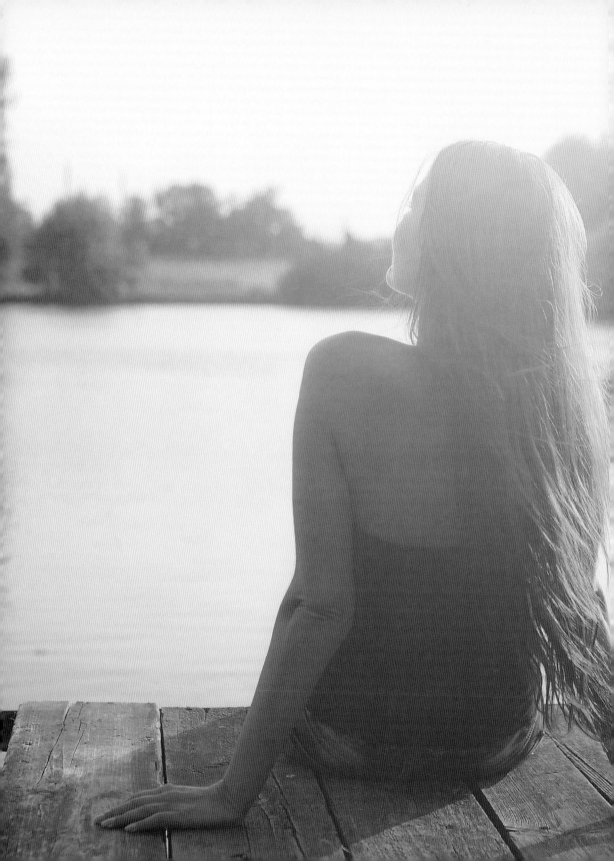

Stress Relief

The strain, effort and pressure induced by the demands of stress can be good in that stress provides an incredible stimulus to grow and reach new potentials for oneself, whether physically or psychologically. However, ongoing and long-term stress can also have a damaging effect with attributes that may be less than desirable, leading to anxiety, stroke, ulcers, heart attack, depression and nervous disorders. Essential oils can help relieve stress, as well as help you handle it better.

Stress Relief Formula

This Stress Relief Formula contains essential oils with powerful sedative action, helping to calm the emotions and an overactive and turbulent mind.

To a 5-ml, colored-glass, euro-dropper bottle add:

Vetiver: 20 drops

Spikenard: 20 drops

Chamomile: 20 drops

Geranium Roseum and Graveolens: 10 drops each

Clary Sage: 20 drops

Close the cap tightly and shake the bottle vigorously to thoroughly blend the essential oils. Allow to synergize for 8 or more hours before using.

Dispense 1–3 drops on a cotton ball or smell strip and inhale the aromatic vapors of your Stress Relief Formula for 10–15 seconds. You may repeat as needed. This formula is also effective when diffused into the air, as an aromatic mist or in the bath.

To make a ready-to-use Stress Relief Formula blend, simply add 15–30 drops of your synergy blend to a 1-ounce (30-ml) bottle of your favorite carrier oil. Shake the bottle well to disperse the oils thoroughly. Apply a few drops to sinus points around your nose and forehead, as well as on the back of your neck.

Anxiety Relief

Anxiety is a kind of fearful expectation about the future that comes from a turbulent inner mind that worries and imagines what might go wrong. It is not based on a real event that is happening but is rather the imagination running wild. It's an unpleasant state of mind that can lead to feelings of dread about what might happen in the future. Physical symptoms often accompany anxiety, such as heart palpitations, hair loss, insomnia, aches and pains, irritable bowel, OCD, loss of appetite, restlessness and an inability to focus. Everyone experiences anxiety periodically. Essential oils can help relieve simple anxiety and its related symptoms.

Anxiety Relief Formula

Helpful for letting go of stressful emotions and soothing an overactive, troubled or nervous state of mind, the essential oils in the Anxiety Relief Formula are known for their sedative action and ability to promote inner balance, peace and calm.

To a 5-ml, colored-glass, euro-dropper bottle add:

Red Mandarin: 20 drops

Bergamot: 20 drops

Ylang Ylang III: 20 drops

German Chamomile: 10 drops

Roman Chamomile: 10 drops

Spikenard: 10 drops

Vetiver: 10 drops

Close the cap tightly and shake the bottle vigorously to thoroughly blend the essential oils. Allow to synergize for 8 or more hours before using.

Dispense 1–3 drops on a cotton ball or smell strip and inhale the aromatic vapors of your Anxiety Relief Formula for 10–15 seconds. You may repeat as needed. This formula is also effective when diffused into the air or as an aromatic mist.

To make a ready-to-use Anxiety Relief Formula blend, simply add 15–30 drops of your synergy blend to a 1-ounce (30-ml) bottle of your favorite carrier oil. Shake the bottle well to disperse the oils thoroughly. Apply a few drops to sinus points around your nose and forehead, as well as on the back of your neck.

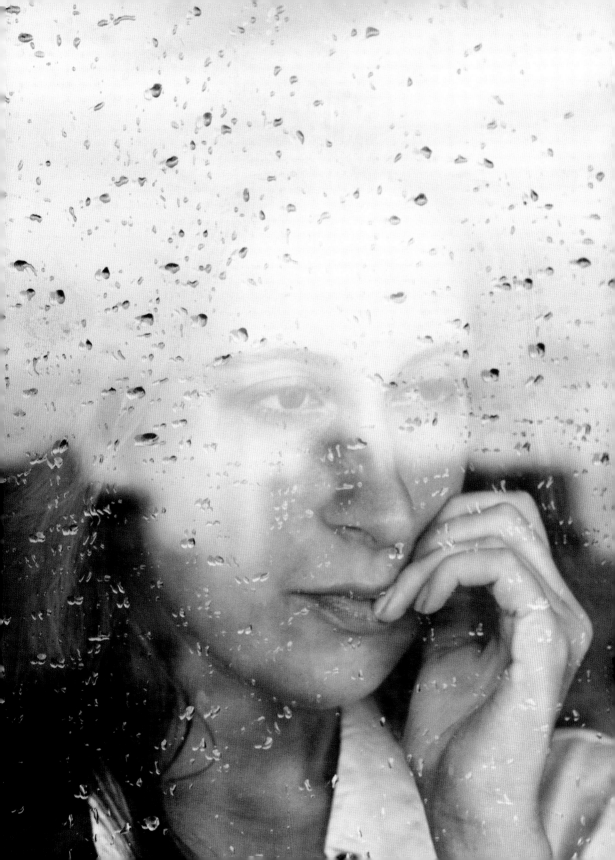

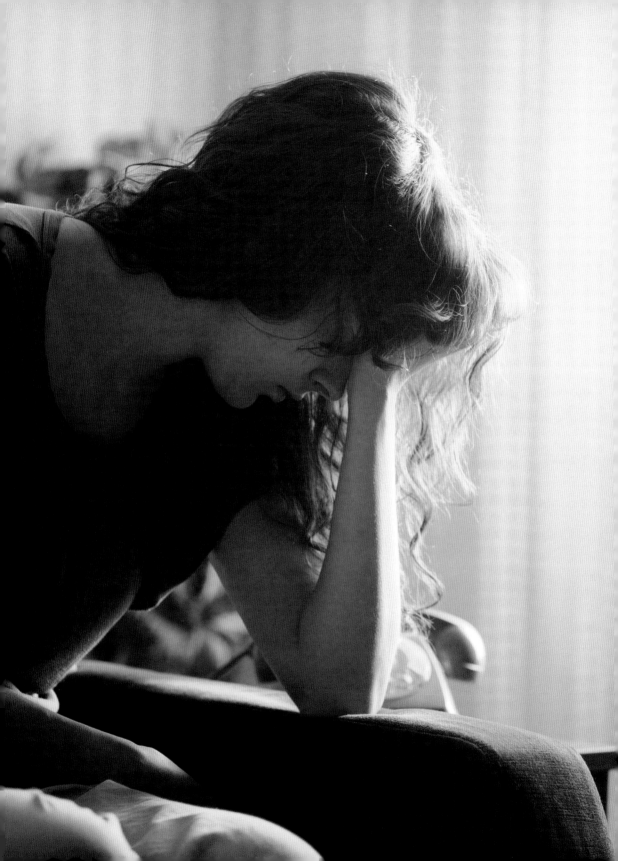

Depression Relief

When a person is depressed, they experience a lowered state of mood which affects their thoughts, feelings, behaviors and overall sense of well-being. Depression can express itself in many different ways, including feelings of sadness, anxiety, hopelessness, guilt, shame, low self-worth, loss of appetite or overeating, insomnia or sleeplessness, poor ability to focus, body aches and pain, poor digestion and low energy.

Research is showing that depression can be inherited through one's cultural conditioning and early childhood experiences. Certain medications or even foods like sugar can lead to a letdown withdrawal response that lowers the mood. Life events like the death of a loved one, the loss of a job, physical illness, a major life transition (like puberty or menopause) or feelings like anger can all contribute to depression. Depression can lead to withdrawal from daily activities and isolation from others.

Depression is most often a temporary and natural state that both men and women can experience in life at one time or another. When you accept and allow yourself to feel your feelings, you can pass on through them. Feelings are not one's identity, but rather a transitory experience everyone has. Essential oils can be used as a comfort care measure to help lift the mood and promote a happier state of mind.

Depression Relief Formula

This formula will help lift your mood and shift to a more positive mental state.

To a 5-ml, colored-glass, euro-dropper bottle add:
Lemon: 10 drops
Tangerine: 20 drops
Sweet Orange: 10 drops
Bergamot: 20 drops
Ylang Ylang: 20 drops
Geranium: 20 drops

Cap the bottle tightly and shake vigorously to blend the essential oils. Allow to synergize for 8 hours or longer before using.

Dispense 1–3 drops on a cotton ball or smell strip and inhale the aromatic vapors of your Depression Relief blend for 10–15 seconds. You may repeat as needed. This formula is also effective diffused into the air.

To make a ready-to-use Depression Relief Formula simply add 15–30 drops of your synergy blend to a 1-ounce (30-ml) bottle of your favorite carrier oil. Shake the bottle well to disperse the oils thoroughly. Dispense 1–3 drops, inhale the scent first and then apply behind both ears, as well as on the back of your neck.

Depression Relief Formula 2

A comforting and supportive tonic for your body, mind, spirit and emotions, the essential oils in the Depression Relief Formula contain properties that are known to calm the nerves, elevate the mood and relieve depressive states of mind.

~~~~~~

To a 5-ml, colored-glass, euro-dropper bottle add:

Ylang Ylang III: 40 drops

Bergamot: 40 drops

Geranium Roseum and Graveolens: 10 drops

Sweet Orange: 5 drops

Atlas Cedarwood: 5 drops

Close the cap tightly and shake the bottle vigorously to thoroughly blend the essential oils. Allow to synergize for 8 or more hours before using.

Dispense 1–3 drops on a cotton ball or smell strip and inhale the aromatic vapors of your Depression Relief Formula blend for 10–15 seconds. You may repeat as needed. This formula is also effective when diffused into the air or as an aromatic mist.

To make a ready-to-use Depression Relief Formula 2 blend, simply add 15–30 drops of your synergy blend to a 1-ounce (30-ml) bottle of your favorite carrier oil. Shake the bottle well to disperse the oils thoroughly. Apply a few drops to sinus points around your nose and forehead, as well as on the back of your neck.

Grief and Loss

Bereavement for the loss of a loved one is a very complicated process that each of us experiences in life. In a world that is continually changing, there is always some form of loss occurring in each of our lives, especially the death or loss of someone or something we have loved whole-heartedly, and it can feel extremely painful. Bonds with loved ones, formed over many years, take time to release, move on to a new phase with and this process can help out the person or thing you have had such a strong connection with. The feeling of loss can be so deep that it can be felt at all levels of our being—including our heart, mind, body and soul—in the routines of our daily life.

Grief and the loss it entails can be so pervasive that it can take time to process our loss and feel whole again. Essential oils can definitely play the role of a comforting friend. They can help with the process of grieving and letting go of a loved one and moving forward to the next stage in our life.

Grief and Loss Formula

This Grief and Loss Formula promotes the release of painful memories, regret, guilt, disappointment, anxiety, stress, emotional wounds and psychic tension. It may also be useful for overcoming addictions.

To a 5-ml, colored-glass, euro-dropper bottle add:

Red Mandarin: 20 drops

Ylang Ylang III: 20 drops

Frankincense: 20 drops

Geranium Roseum and Graveolens: 10 drops each

Bergamot: 10 drops

Helichrysum: 5 drops

Rose: 5 drops

Close the cap tightly and shake the bottle vigorously to thoroughly blend the essential oils. Allow to synergize for 8 or more hours before using.

Dispense 1–3 drops on a cotton ball or smell strip and inhale the aromatic vapors of your Grief and Loss Formula blend for 10–15 seconds. You may repeat as needed. This formula is also effective when diffused into the air, used in a bath or sprayed as an aromatic mist.

To make a ready-to-use Grief and Loss Formula 2 blend, simply add 15–30 drops of your synergy blend to a 1-ounce (30-ml) bottle of your favorite carrier oil. Shake the bottle well to disperse the oils thoroughly. Apply a few drops to sinus points around your nose and forehead, as well as on the back of your neck.

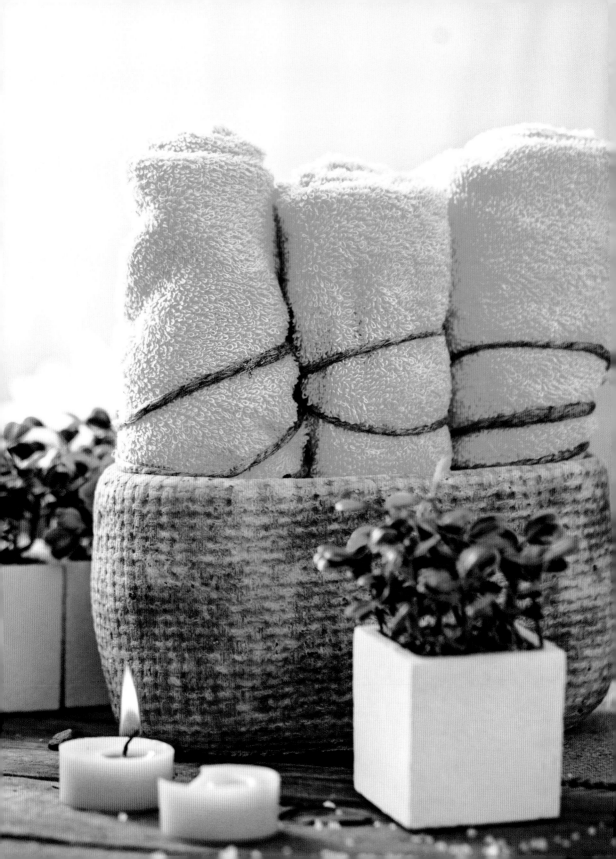

CHAPTER 14

Spa and Beauty Treatments

COMPLETE SKINCARE BEAUTY TREATMENT PROGRAM

I have to admit that I never once saw anyone in my family perform any skincare routine. Never once do I recall seeing any hygienic routines for skincare even from my mom, who was a licensed cosmetologist and really into the idea of beauty. She was always buying the latest skin lotions, creams and make-up, but cleansing did not seem to be a part of her beauty care system.

It wasn't until I reached the age of thirty that it suddenly dawned on me that a regular facial cleansing ritual might be a good idea. At this same time, I started hydrating by drinking lots of pure fresh water. This was well before the bottled drinking craze that came along several years later.

As with all of my health routines and habits, my skincare treatment program has evolved for me intuitively and naturally over time. Periodically, I'll change things up a bit, but essentially this is the complete skincare beauty treatment program that I follow. By the way, I never use any body lotions on my skin. I used to, but not anymore.

My diet has ample oils like raw extra virgin coconut and olive oils that nourish my skin from the inside so that it stays moist and supple.

For beautiful, healthy and radiant skin, try a skincare routine like this one, keeping in mind to use the skincare formulas that are right for your skin type.

- Skincare Formulas
  (once daily–page 264)

- Facial and Body Toner
  (once daily, or as needed–page 270)

- French Clay Facial Mask
  (once monthly–page 273)

- Repair Butters for Body and Face
  (as needed–page 274)

- Hair and Scalp Treatments
  (once monthly–page 279)

- Lip Balms
  (once daily or as needed–page 286)

- Salt Glow Treatments
  (once daily–page 297)

Skincare Formulas

Your skin, called the integumentary system, is your largest organ. It is made up of three layers of ectodermal tissue—ectoderm (outer layer), mesoderm (middle layer) and endoderm (deepest layer)—that protect and guard the underlying muscles, bones, ligaments and internal organs.

The skin interacts with the external environment and is your first line of defense against external conditions. For instance, the skin plays a vital role in protecting the body against foreign invaders and guards against excessive water loss. It also functions as insulation to protect against heat loss, provides ventilation to keep you cool through perspiration and gives you experiences of both pleasurable and painful sensation.

Personally, I've made all of my own skincare products for more than 20 years and have not had any skin issues since that time. I used to be troubled with regular breakouts which completely stopped after beginning to make my own skincare products. Sufficient hydration also plays a key role in healthy skin.

SKINCARE FORMULAS FOR DIFFERENT SKIN TYPES

For facial cleansing, I like to use raw, unscented, goat milk soap made fresh from the farm. If you are still washing your skin with soap made with a water base, then you're missing out on a truly great facial cleanser. It's certainly the best facial soap I've ever used to date. It is gentle, soothing and nourishing for your facial skin, and one bar lasts an incredibly long time. Raw goat's milk soap is beneficial for dry, sensitive, oily or problematic skin conditions like eczema and psoriasis or for keeping your skin healthy. I wash with either a hypoallergenic facial mitt made from flax (my preference) or a natural facial loofa to gently exfoliate my skin daily.

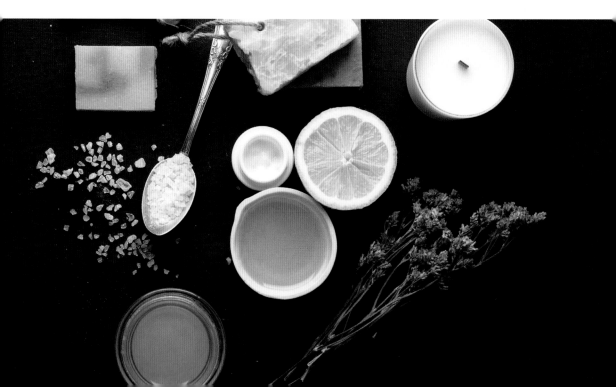

Normal to Dry Skincare Formula

Harmonizing for dry to normal skin types, the oils in this formula are known for their ability to tone, moisturize, balance and heal dry skin cells. Excellent for smoothing lines and wrinkles, use alone or add a drop to your favorite moisturizer or night cream.

To a 5-ml, colored-glass, euro-dropper bottle add:
Lavender: 10 drops
Geranium Roseum and Graveolens: 10 drops each
Palmarosa: 30 drops
Ylang Ylang: 40 drops

Close the cap tightly and shake the bottle vigorously to thoroughly blend the essential oils. Allow to synergize for 8 or more hours before using.

To make a ready-to-use Skincare Formula blend simply add 12–15 drops of your synergy blend to a 1-ounce (30-ml) bottle of your favorite carrier oil. Shake the bottle well to disperse the oils thoroughly. Apply 1–3 drops of your ready-to-use blend to your fingertips and gently apply to your face. Use upward sweeping motions to completely cover your skin. Very little is needed, and the oil should quickly absorb into your skin. If your skin feels oily or greasy after application, then you've used too much of the oil. Use once daily at the end of your regular facial cleansing routine.

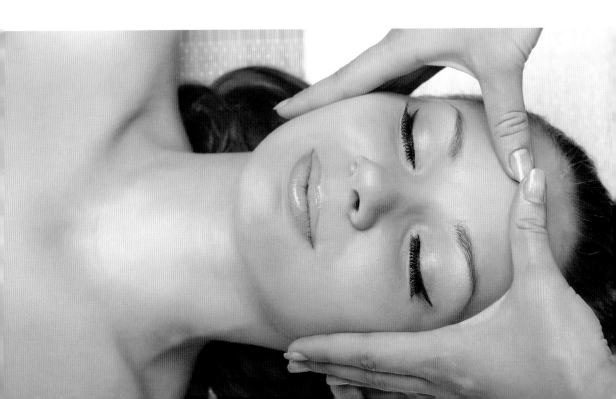

Oily Skincare Formula

This formula is harmonizing and balancing for oily skin cells. Use alone, or add a drop to your favorite skin care product.

~~~~~~

To a 5-ml, colored-glass, euro-dropper bottle add:

Cypress: 40 drops

Myrrh: 10 drops

Carrot Seed: 10 drops

Geranium: 40 drops

Rosemary Verbenone: 1–2 drops

Close the cap tightly and shake the bottle vigorously to thoroughly blend the essential oils. Allow to synergize for 8 or more hours before using.

To make a ready-to-use skincare blend, simply add 12–15 drops of your synergy blend to a 1-ounce (30-ml) bottle of your favorite carrier oil. Shake the bottle well to disperse the oils thoroughly. Apply 1–3 drops of your ready-to-use blend to your fingertips and gently apply to your face. Use upward sweeping motions to completely cover your skin. Very little is needed, and the oil should quickly absorb into your skin. If your skin feels oily or greasy after application, then you've used too much of the oil. Use once daily at the end of your regular facial cleansing routine.

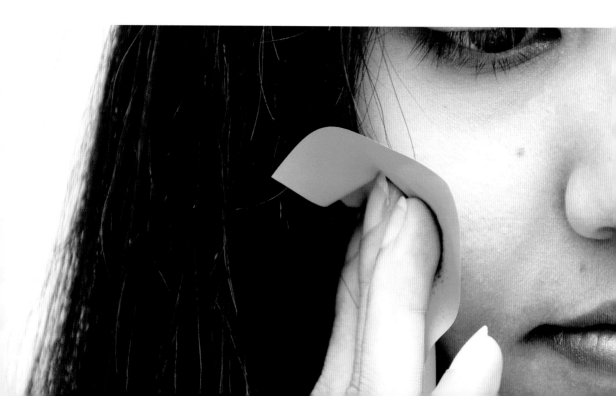

Sensitive Skincare Formula

Harmonizing for sensititive skin types, the oils in this formula are known for their ability to tone, moisturize, balance and heal sensitive skin cells. Use alone, or add a drop to your favorite moisturizer or night cream.

~~~~~~

To a 5-ml, colored-glass, euro-dropper bottle add:

German Chamomile: 40 drops

Palmarosa: 30 drops

Rose: 10 drops

Helichrysum: 10 drops

Carrot Seed: 10 drops

Galbanum: 1–2 drops

Close the cap tightly and shake the bottle vigorously to thoroughly blend the essential oils. Allow to synergize for 8 or more hours before using.

To make a ready-to-use skincare blend, simply add 12–15 drops of your synergy blend to a 1-ounce (30-ml) bottle of your favorite carrier oil. Shake the bottle well to disperse the oils thoroughly. Apply 1–3 drops of your ready-to-use blend to your fingertips and gently apply to your face. Use upward sweeping motions to completely cover your skin. Very little is needed, and the oil should quickly absorb into your skin. If your skin feels oily or greasy after application, then you've used too much of the oil. Use once daily at the end of your regular facial cleansing routine.

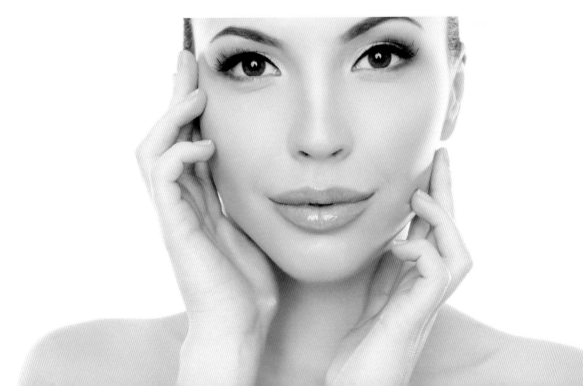

Mature Skincare Formula

This blend is harmonizing and balancing for mature skin cells and excellent for smoothing and softening facial lines and wrinkles. Use alone or add a drop to your favorite moisturizer or night cream.

To a 5-ml, colored-glass, euro-dropper bottle add:

Frankincense: 20 drops

Rose: 20 drops

Ylang Ylang: 20 drops

Geranium Roseum and Graveolens: 10 drops each

Helichrysum: 10 drops

Carrot Seed: 10 drops

Close the cap tightly and shake the bottle vigorously to thoroughly blend the essential oils. Allow to synergize for 8 or more hours before using.

To make a ready-to-use skincare blend, simply add 12–15 drops of your synergy blend to a 1-ounce (30-ml) bottle of your favorite carrier oil. Shake the bottle well to disperse the oils thoroughly. Apply 1–3 drops of your ready-to-use blend to your fingertips and gently apply to your face. Use upward sweeping motions to completely cover your skin. Very little is needed, and the oil should quickly absorb into your skin. If your skin feels oily or greasy after application, then you've used too much of the oil. Use once daily at the end of your regular facial cleansing routine.

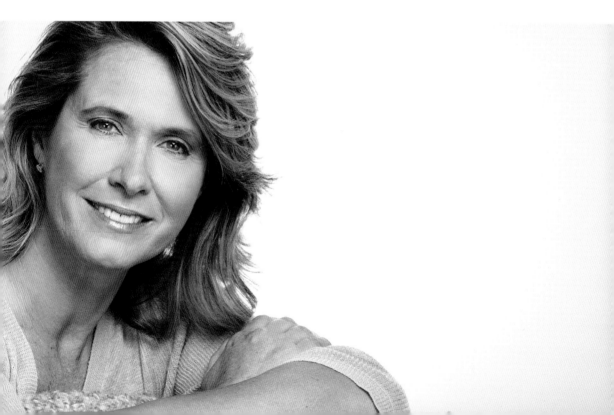

Body and Facial Skin Toners

A skin toner may be used for your body or face and is designed to cleanse and freshen your skin, as well as shrink the appearance of pores. You can use your body and facial toners by applying on cotton or to a damp woolen cloth, or you can spray directly on your face as a freshener.

Toner may be applied after your usual skin washing routine, and should be immediately followed by applying moisturizer once the toner has dried.

The mildest and most gentle form of skin toner that's suitable for all skin types, including dry and sensitive skin, uses pure fresh water and a small percentage of an astringent like alcohol or witch hazel (0–10 percent). Some kind of humectant like glycerine may also be used to hold in skin moisture, as well as to act as a preservative.

For slightly more skin-toning action that's suitable for all skin types, including oily and combination skin, use a bit more astringent (up to 20 percent) in water with a humectant, if desired.

Finally, the strongest toners are excellent for oily skin and controlling excess sebum production. These skin toners contain higher percentages of astringent (up to 60 percent) and the strongest antiseptic properties and action which helps to prevent and control acne outbreaks.

Adding an essential oil or blend to your toner—that has skin nourishing and healing properties suitable for your skin type—enhances the effectiveness of your toner. Check out the section on skincare formulas (page 264) for different skin types and for more formulas to use in your toner.

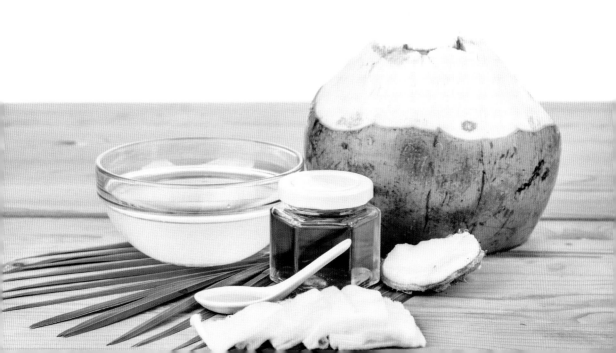

Facial and Body Toner Formula (Normal to Dry Skin)

This may be used as a facial toner or as an allover body freshener.

I recommend the following essential oils by skin type and suitability for the particular skin condition as noted:

- German chamomile (sensitive skin)
- Geranium roseum and graveolens (regulating for all skin types)
- Palmarosa (problem skin)
- Lavender (burns and sunburned skin)
- Ylang ylang (moisturizing and balancing for all skin types)
- Cypress (oily skin)
- Myrrh and patchouli (dry, cracked and chapped skin)
- Frankincense (mature skin)
- Rose (mature skin) reduces appearance of lines and wrinkles

To a 5-ml, colored-glass, euro-dropper bottle add:

Lavender: 20 drops

Ylang Ylang III: 30 drops

Geranium Roseum and Graveolens: 25 drops each

1 (2-oz [60-ml]) colored-glass misting bottle

1 tsp glycerin (optional)

Astringent (alcohol or witch hazel, 0–20 percent)

Purified or fresh spring water

8–12 drops essential oil or blend by skin type

Close the cap tightly and shake the bottle vigorously to thoroughly blend the essential oils. Allow to synergize for 8 or more hours before using.

To a 2-ounce (60-ml), colored-glass misting bottle, add your teaspoon of glycerin (if you're using it). Next, add the astringent to the bottle, cap with the atomizer top and shake the bottle vigorously to mix the glycerin and water. Add the essential oil or blend to the mixture, cap the bottle again and shake vigorously to blend the oils in the mixture. Add water to fill the bottle, making sure to leave room to insert the atomizer spray top.

As there is no true emulsifying agent in this recipe, the oils will not stay completely mixed with the glycerin, astringent and water, so you will need to shake the bottle well each time before using.

Use your facial and body toner any time. You may find it especially beneficial after your shower, bath or facial cleansing ritual. Lightly spray onto the desired skin areas to freshen, heal and tone. You may also spray toner onto a cotton or woolen pad and apply to your face and skin with gentle, upward, sweeping movements. Allow to dry thoroughly before applying a facial moisturizer or body lotion, if desired.

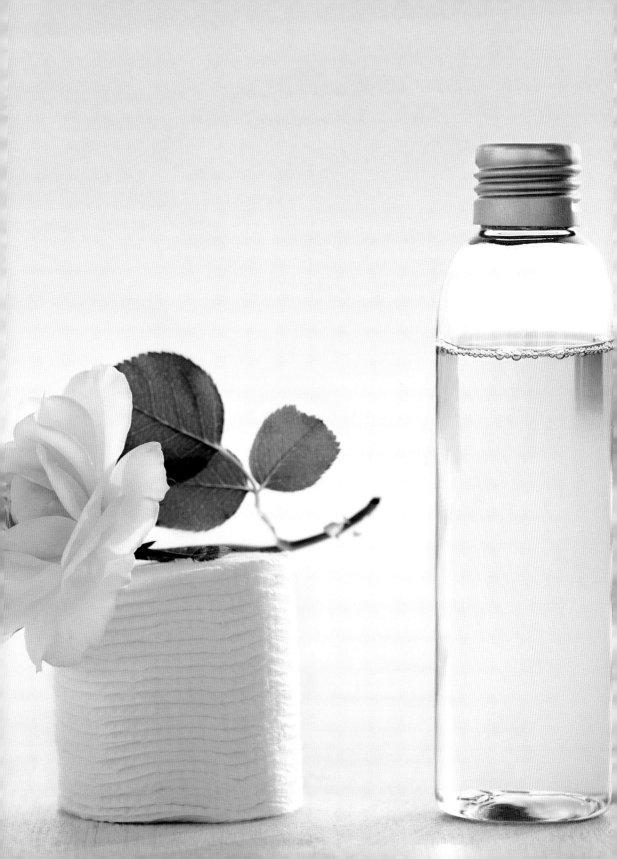

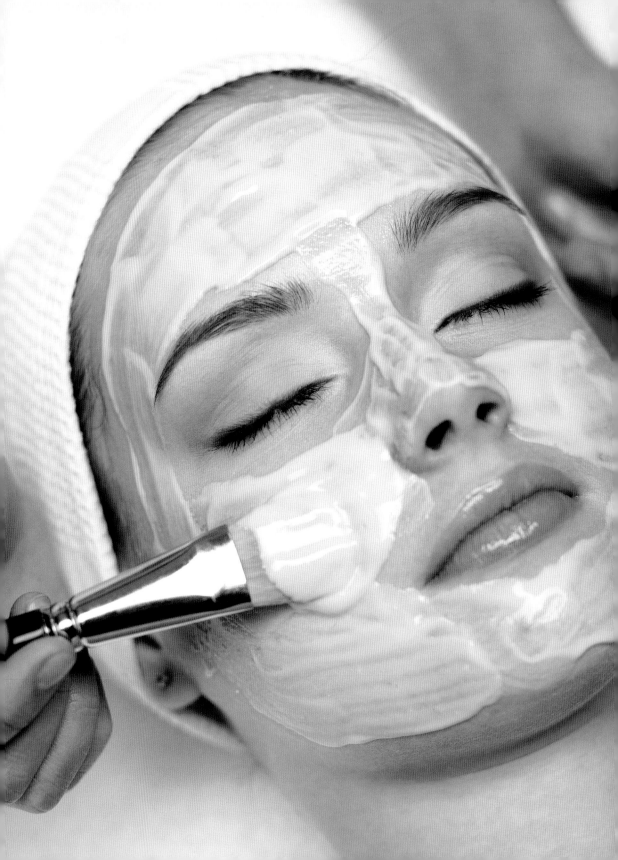

French Clay Facial Mask

Use this clay facial mask formula made with French clay and essential oils to promote cleansing and detoxification of your facial skin, as well as to improve your skin's elasticity and impart a radiant, healthy glow. Create a supportive and relaxing environment for enjoying and making the most of your time by turning off phones and electronic devices. Make the room comfortably warm for relaxing during, and for a brief time after, your facial mask. Light a candle and play gentle and soothing music in the background, or just relax and be still during and after your treatment.

~~~~~~

Rose: 30 drops (You can use a 10-percent dilution in carrier oil. If you use rose oil that has been diluted in a carrier oil, be sure to wait and add it directly to the French clay mixture, because a diluted essential oil will not synergize with other essential oils and can prevent other oils from synergizing with each other.)

Geranium Roseum and Graveolens: 20 drops each

Ylang Ylang: 20 drops

Carrot Seed: 10 drops

1 tbsp (15 g) French pink or green clay

1½–2 tbsp (7–10 ml) purified or spring water or cream

⅛ tsp light coconut oil or other suitable vegetable oil of your choice (Refer to the "Face Carrier Oils" section on page 36 for more about carrier oils)

Make a synergy blend of your essential oils in a 5-milliliter euro-dropper bottle and allow to synergize for a minimum of 24 hours. Refer to the "Aromatherapy Blending Guide" on page 157 for more about making synergy blends.

Before preparing your facial mask, wash your face with your favorite cleanser and towel dry.

In a small bowl, mix together your choice of natural French clay with the purified or spring water (or cream) and the light coconut oil to make a loose paste, but make sure it's not wet.

Add one drop of the essential oil synergy blend to the paste and blend thoroughly together.

Immediately begin applying the French Clay Facial Mask to your face using gentle upward sweeping strokes. Start with your décolletage and apply the mask evenly over your chin, both cheeks, nose and forehead. Be sure to completely cover your entire face with the mask.

After applying the mask and completely covering your face with it, take time to relax. Enjoy a refreshing glass of water with a slice of lemon as you allow the mask to dry for 10–20 minutes.

Rinse off your facial mask thoroughly with warm water, making sure the mask is completely removed. Your skin will feel soft, silky smooth, toned and refreshed. After your facial mask, you can perform your usual cleansing and moisturizing routine if you like and continue to hydrate with fresh-squeezed lemon water.

CAUTION: Clay may stain fabric, so take care.

Repair Butters for Body and Face

Repair butter is excellent for moisturizing and deep healing of skin cell tissue. Use on body parts that are weathered, dry, cracked or chapped, like the soles of feet and heels or to areas that have signs of premature aging such as face lines and wrinkles. When applied topically on skin, the waxy substance of this regenerative repair butter acts as an intensive, long-wear protective barrier to the elements. It also helps to moisturize and heal the skin.

Repair Butter Essential Oils Formula

This non-greasy and petroleum-free repair butter is formulated to moisturize and heal aging, dry or cracked skin. It's easy to make, very similar to the long-wear, intensive lip balm recipe, with the addition of shea or cocoa butter, which boosts its moisturizing capacity. It can be stored for periods of 1 year or longer when vitamin E oil is used as a natural preservative and the butter is sealed properly and stored in the refrigerator.

Makes a 1-ounce (28 g) container of repair butter:

¼ cup (60 ml) light coconut oil

1 tbsp (21 g) beeswax (Less beeswax makes your butter softer and more gives it a firmer consistency)

30–36 drops any essential oil synergy blend

1 tbsp (15 g) shea or cocoa butter

4 drops vitamin E oil

Put the beeswax into the light coconut oil and heat in a double boiler. For a homemade double boiler, use a glass measuring cup (such as Pyrex) inside a pan of water. Heat the mixture over medium-low heat until the beeswax melts.

Remove from the heat source and allow the liquid to cool slightly before adding your essential oil synergy blend. Gently blend in the oils with a sterile instrument. Immediately pour the mixture into a 1-ounce (30-ml) container and refrigerate, allowing to cool.

Apply the repair butter liberally with your fingertips to problem areas of your skin to moisturize and heal skin tissues. Use as frequently as you like; it won't build up!

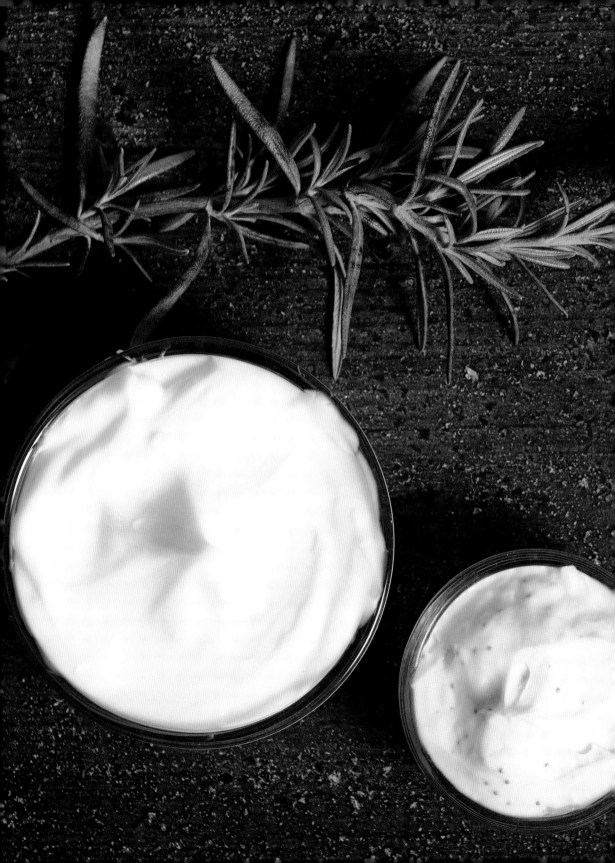

Premature Aging Skincare Formula

Regulating and harmonizing action for skin cells, this formula is known for its toning and moisturizing ability. Use alone, or add a drop to your favorite moisturizer.

To a 5-ml, colored-glass, euro-dropper bottle add:
Geranium Roseum and Graveolens: 20 drops each
Rose: 30 drops
Ylang Ylang: 30 drops

To make a ready-to-use skincare blend, simply add 12–15 drops of your synergy blend to a 1-ounce (30-ml) bottle of your favorite carrier oil. Shake the bottle well to disperse the oils thoroughly. Apply 1–3 drops of your blend to your fingertips and gently apply to your face. Use upward sweeping motions to completely cover your skin. Very little is needed, and the oil should quickly absorb into your skin. If your skin feels oily or greasy after application, then you've used too much of the oil. Use once daily at the end of your regular facial cleansing routine.

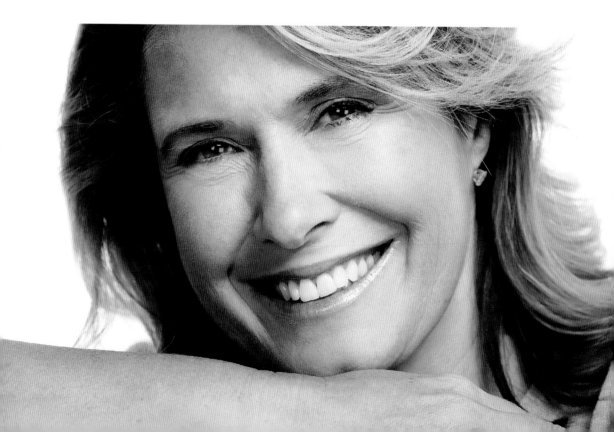

Severely Dry and Cracked Skin Formula

This blend is harmonizing and balancing for severely cracked and dry skin cell tissues. Use alone or add a drop to your favorite moisturizer or night cream.

~~~~~~

To a 5-ml, colored-glass, euro-dropper bottle add:

Myrrh: 50 drops

Spikenard: 30 drops

Helichrysum: 20 drops

Close the cap tightly and shake the bottle vigorously to thoroughly blend the essential oils. Allow to synergize for 8 or more hours before using.

To make a ready-to-use skincare blend, simply add 12–15 drops of your synergy blend to a 1-ounce (30-ml) bottle of your favorite carrier oil. Shake the bottle well to disperse the oils thoroughly. Apply 1–3 drops of your blend to your fingertips and gently apply to your face. Use upward sweeping motions to completely cover your skin. Very little is needed, and the oil should quickly absorb into your skin. If your skin feels oily or greasy after application, then you've used too much of the oil. Use once daily at the end of your regular facial cleansing routine.

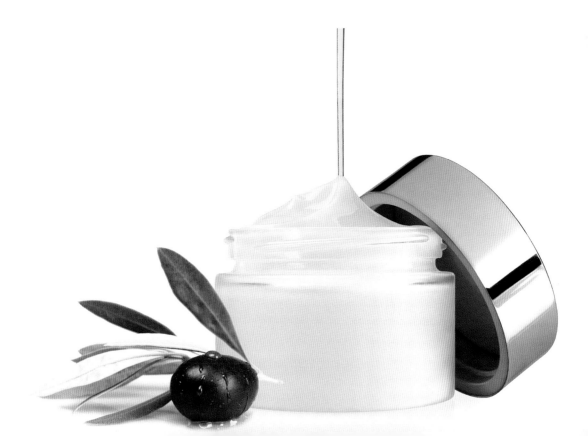

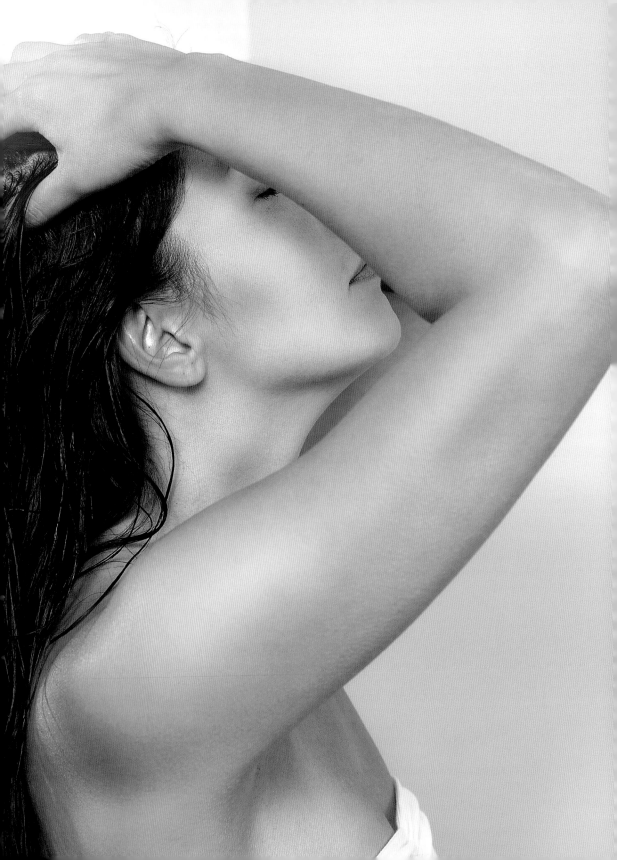

Hair and Scalp Treatments

The condition of your hair is largely dependent upon a good supply of blood carrying adequate amounts of nutrition such as amino acids, vitamins and minerals to your hair follicle. Your hair is made of keratin, a stretchable protein material manufactured by your hair follicle. Hair follicles in your scalp grow at a rate of about half an inch (1.3 cm) per month, though this rate of growth can vary.

An aromatherapy scalp massage has been shown to effectively stimulate blood flow to the scalp and the underlying hair follicles to promote healthy hair growth. It is also helpful for stopping hair loss and hair thinning, both of which are of great concern for many modern day men and women.

Research conducted in Aberdeen, Scotland by the Department of Dermatology showed successful outcomes for the use of essential oils in the treatment of alopecia. The results of the study showed aromatherapy massage to be a safe and effective treatment for alopecia areata. It also showed that treatment with essential oils was significantly more effective than treatment with a carrier oil alone.

In many ways, hair is similar to skin as it reflects your inner state of balance and health. A poor state of health can be responsible for dullness and loss of hair.

Men and women can suffer from age-related hair loss or thinning due to hormonal fluctuations during pregnancy and menopause. Research has shown that essential oils like palmarosa and geranium roseum and graveolens help to balance hormonal fluctuations that can lead to hair thinning and loss of hair.

Extreme stress can also play a significant role in hair loss for which the healing power of emotionally calming pure essential oils like clary sage, ylang ylang and German chamomile are highly recommended.

Most hair loss problems, not directly caused by imbalances of health, can usually be traced to maltreatment of the hair with excessive heat or chemical treatments like coloring and perming or washing with strong detergent-based shampoos.

These are the major causes of hair loss and can lead to dandruff and other common hair problems.

Scalp Reconditioning Formula

The Scalp Reconditioning Formula contains essential oils with stimulating, restorative and hormone-balancing properties known to be effective for stimulating new, healthy hair growth, as well as helping to stop hair loss and hair thinning.

~~~~~~

To a 5-ml, colored-glass, euro-dropper bottle add:

Vetiver: 30 drops

Ylang Ylang: 30 drops

Geranium Roseum and Graveolens: 15 drops each

Rosemary: 5 drops

Carrot Seed: 5 drops

Cap the bottle tightly and shake vigorously to blend the oils together. Allow to synergize for 24 hours or longer before using.

You can also add 1–2 drops of your Scalp Reconditioning Formula to your favorite carrier oil and use as a leave-on conditioner for up to an hour. Then shampoo your hair thoroughly afterward. Refer to the "Hair and Scalp Treatment Program" section on page 281 for more about how to use your Scalp Reconditioning Formula.

Use this formula as an invigorating Scalp Massage Oil to stop hair loss and to stimulate new hair growth. Apply daily for an invigorating scalp aromatherapy massage and leave on for about 1 hour. Shampoo thoroughly afterward.

TIP: To easily remove oil from the hair shaft, use your favorite shampoo (without the addition of water) to wash your hair. The shampoo will absorb the oil from the hair shaft. Then re-rinse the hair with warm water. Repeat if needed.

Hair and Scalp Treatment Program

Use either the "Stop Hair Loss Formula" (page 282) as a ready-to-use leave-on conditioner or the Scalp Reconditioning Formula (page 280) as an aromatherapy scalp massage daily for 10–14 days. Then, take a week break before beginning the cycle of daily application for another 10–14 days.

Follow the instructions outlined and continue your application of either formula as needed to promote restoration of your hair's natural beauty, luster and health. Experiment with both formulas to find out which formula and application works best for getting the results you desire.

Stop Hair Loss (Alopecia)

Hair loss, hair thinning or baldness are a great concern for many people. The medical term for hair loss is alopecia, and it can be either partial (*alopecia areata*) or total (*alopecia totalis*).

There is often a great deal of psychological and emotional stress caused by one's appearance by hair loss. As hair plays a large role in one's overall identity, especially for women, hair loss can be an especially sensitive issue to talk about and is often experienced as a feeling of loss of control, loss of youth and even a loss of status in the world. Hair loss can lead to feelings of low self-esteem and can result in isolation from others. For cancer patients undergoing chemotherapy treatment, hair loss has been reported to forever change one's self-image and sense of belonging in the world.

A study on male pattern baldness compared Minoxidil (an over-the-counter hair loss product) to rosemary essential oil—just one of the ingredients in the Stop Hair Loss Formula (page 282). Groups rubbed either rosemary oil or Minoxidil into the scalp daily. At six months, both groups experienced a significant increase in hair growth, with rosemary users having less itchy scalps.

Stop Hair Loss (Alopecia) Formula

To stimulate new hair growth and to prevent or stop hair loss and hair thinning use this stimulating and restorative Stop Hair Loss Formula made of pure essential oils. The essential oils in this formula are known to be helpful for relieving stress and promoting hormone balance, which studies show can be contributing factors in hair loss.

~~~~~~

To a 5-ml, colored-glass, euro-dropper bottle, add:

Blue Yarrow: 20 drops

Ylang Ylang: 20 drops

Palmarosa: 30 drops

Clary Sage: 10 drops

Cedarwood: 10 drops

Thyme: 5 drops

Rosemary Verbenone: 5 drops

Cap the bottle tightly and shake vigorously to blend the oils together. Allow to synergize for 24 hours before using.

The simplest way to use your Stop Hair Loss Formula is to add 1–2 drops of it to your favorite shampoo. Use it as your regular hair wash to stimulate new, healthy hair growth and to prevent hair loss and thinning.

To make a ready-to-use Stop Hair Loss Formula, simply add 15 drops of your synergy blend to a 1-ounce (30-ml) bottle of your favorite carrier oil. Shake the bottle well to disperse the oils thoroughly. Apply enough of your formula to cover your scalp and saturate your hair shaft. Leave on for up to an hour to allow the oils time to be completely absorbed into your scalp and hair follicles. Shampoo your hair thoroughly afterward to completely remove the oil from your hair and scalp. Refer to the "Hair and Scalp Treatment Program" sections on page 281 for more information about using essential oils to stop hair loss.

CAUTION: Please keep oils away from eyes, and do not apply oil directly on any open sores as this can cause sensitization to essential oils.

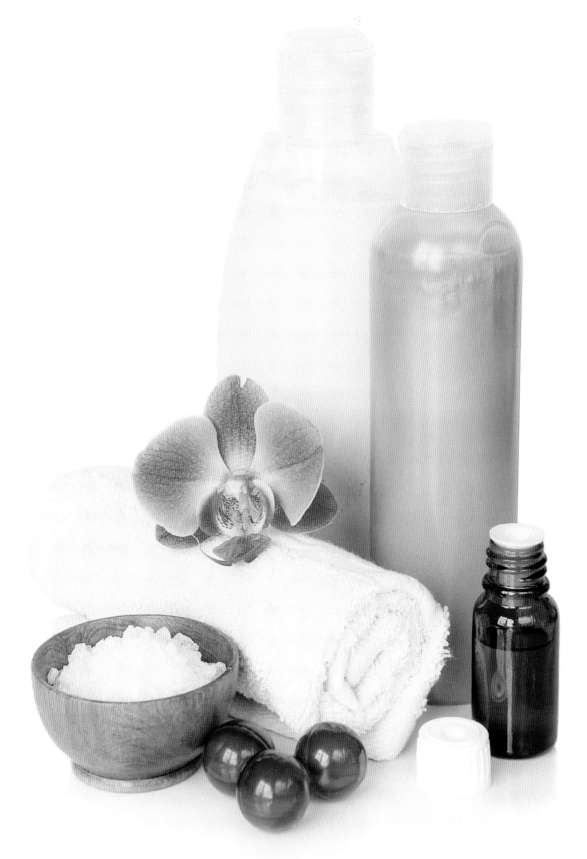

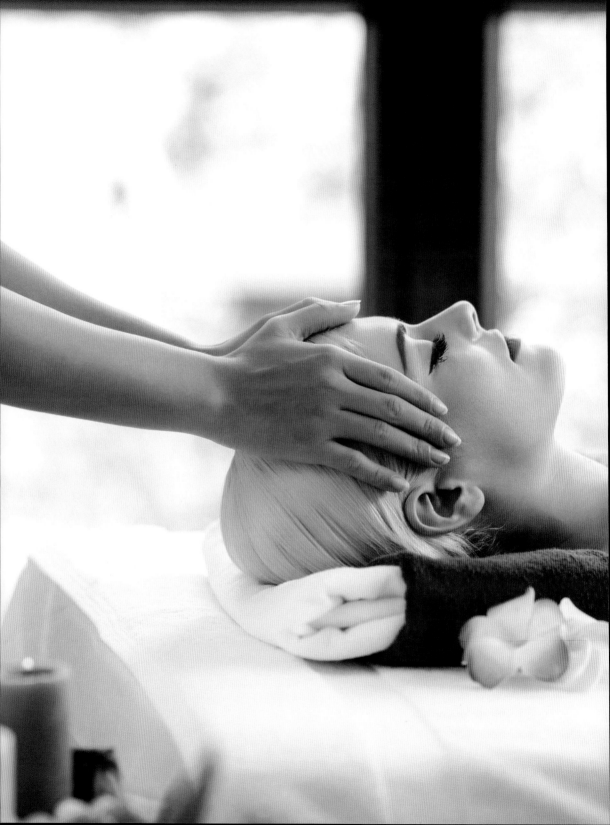

Scalp Massage Oil

Use the Scalp Reconditioning Formula as an invigorating Scalp Massage Oil to stimulate new healthy hair growth. Scalp treatments are effective for treating hair loss and hair thinning, as well as encouraging, new, healthy hair growth.

To a 5-ml, colored-glass, euro-dropper bottle add:

Cypress: 20 drops

Lemon: 20 drops

Helichrysum: 40 drops

Birch: 10 drops

Juniper Berry: 10 drops

Close the cap tightly and shake the bottle vigorously to thoroughly blend the essential oils. Allow to synergize for 8 or more hours before using.

You can add 1–2 drops of your Scalp Massage Oil to your favorite carrier oil and use as a leave-in conditioner for up to an hour. Then shampoo your hair thoroughly after.

Lip Balms

Lip balm is excellent for moisturizing and healing dry, cracked and chapped lips often caused by environmental and weather conditions or simple dehydration. The waxy substance of lip balm applied topically over your lips effectively moisturizes them, as well as sealing and protecting them from exposure to harsh environments. The first lip balm may have been inspired by Lydia Maria Child's popular book, *The American Frugal Housewife*, in which Child recommended the use of an "earwax remedy successful when others have failed."

Dry, Chapped Lips Formula

Easy to make, this lip balm can be stored for long periods of time of one year or more when using vitamin E oil as a natural preservative and when sealed properly and stored in the refrigerator. Use it it to heal dry, cracked or chapped lips and to smooth mouth wrinkles and prevent and treat cold sore outbreaks. An intensive, long-wear lip balm, this formula is non-greasy and petroleum-free. Formulated to moisturize and heal your lips, this lip balm makes a wonderful gift for friends and family members.

To a 5-ml, colored-glass, euro-dropper bottle add:

Lavender: 30 drops

Sandalwood: 50 drops

Ylang Ylang: 20 drops

Makes 8–10, ⅛-ounce (4-ml) lip balm containers:

¼ cup (60 ml) light coconut oil

1 heaping tbsp (22 g) beeswax (Less makes your lip balm softer; more beeswax makes it more firm.)

Close cap tightly and shake bottle vigorously to thoroughly blend essential oils. Allow to synergize for 8 or more hours before using.

Put the beeswax and light coconut oil into a double boiler. For a homemade double boiler, use a glass measuring cup (such as Pyrex) inside a pan of water. Heat the mixture over medium-low heat until the beeswax melts.

Remove from the heat source and allow the liquid to cool slightly before adding your essential oils. Gently blend in the essential oils with a sterile instrument. Immediately pour the mixture into your lip balm containers and refrigerate to cool.

Apply liberally to your lips with your fingertips. Use as frequently as you like.

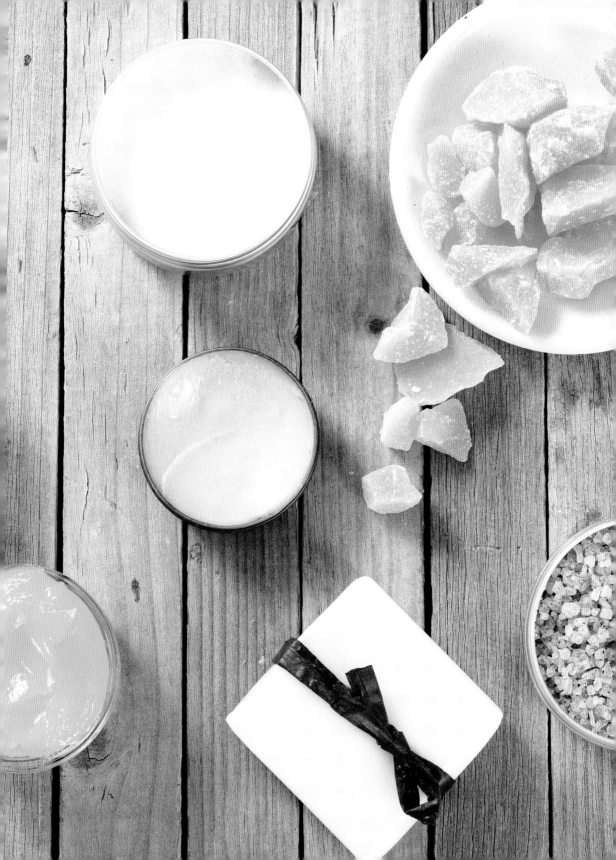

Severely Dry, Cracked, Chapped Lips

The oils in this formula are known for their ability to regulate and heal dry, cracked and chapped lips.

To a 5-ml, colored-glass, euro-dropper bottle add:

Myrrh: 50 drops

Patchouli: 30 drops

Helichrysum: 20 drops

Cap tightly and shake bottle vigorously to thoroughly blend essential oils. Allow to synergize for 8 hours or more before using.

PLEASE NOTE: This is just one of the lip balm formulas and directions for how to make lip balm are at the bottom of the the Dry, Chapped Lips Formula on page 286.

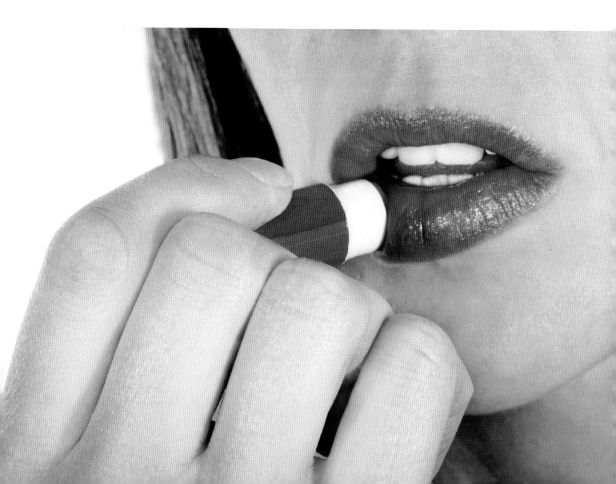

Cold Sore Formula

This Cold Sore Formula makes an intensive, long-wear lip balm, and is formulated with some of the most potent pure essential oils. These oils are beneficial for promoting fast relief and rapid healing of herpes simplex and cold sore outbreaks, and may help build your natural immunity against future outbreaks.

~~~~~~

To a 5-ml, colored-glass, euro-dropper bottle add:

Tea Tree: 20 drops

Ravensara: 30 drops

Palmarosa: 50 drops

Makes 8–10, ⅛-ounce (4-ml) lip balm containers:

¼ cup (60 ml) light coconut oil

1 heaping tbsp (22 g) beeswax (Less makes your lip balm softer; more beeswax makes it more firm.)

Close the cap tightly and shake the bottle vigorously to thoroughly blend the essential oils. Allow to synergize for 8 or more hours before using.

Put the beeswax and light coconut oil into a double boiler. For a homemade double boiler, use a glass measuring cup (such as Pyrex) inside a pan of water. Heat the mixture over medium-low heat until the beeswax melts.

Remove from the heat source and allow the liquid to cool slightly before adding your essential oils. Gently blend in the essential oils with a sterile instrument. Immediately pour the mixture into your lip balm containers and refrigerate to cool.

Apply liberally to your lips with your fingertips. Use as frequently as you like; it won't build up!

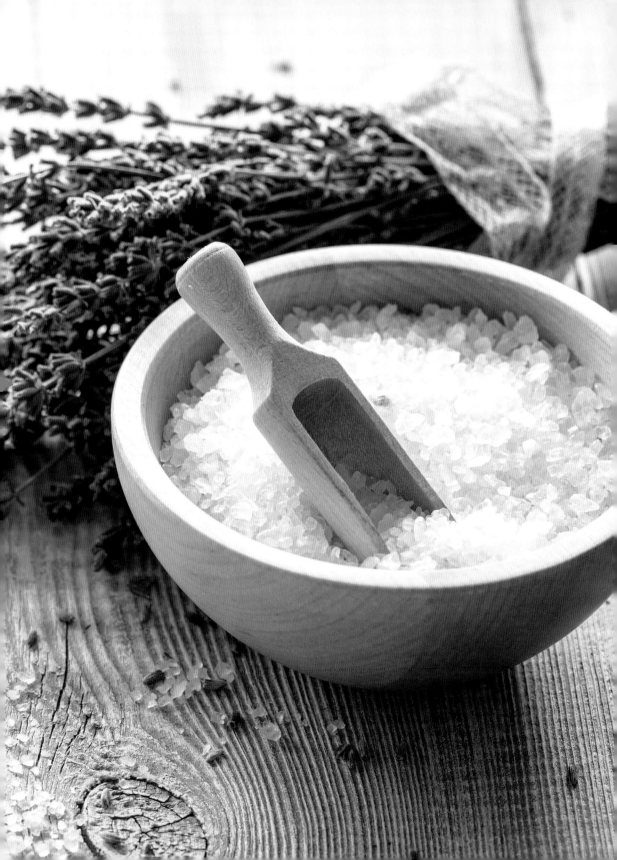

Healing Bath Salts Formula

Set the mood and ambience for a healing bath spa experience by making sure you are in a quiet space where you will not be disturbed for at least 45 minutes or longer. All phones and electronic devices should be turned off. Light a candle and play gentle and relaxing music in the background, or just relax and allow yourself to be silent.

This relaxing and rejuvenating Healing Bath Salts Formula is helpful for letting go of your cares and worries. It is soothing to an agitated state of mind. The essential oils are known for their sedative action and ability to promote inner balance, peace and calm, and are renewing to your chakra energy system.

~~~~~~

To a 5-ml, colored-glass, euro-dropper bottle add:

Red Mandarin: 40 drops

Lavender: 10 drops

Ylang Ylang III: 20 drops

Clary Sage: 10 drops

Frankincense: 20 drops

1 cup (500 g) Epsom salts (muscle relaxant, detoxifier)

1 cup (275 g) Celtic (grey) salts (rich in minerals)

1 cup (520 g) baking soda (skin softener)

Optional ingredient: ½ cup (115 g) green or pink clay

5–12 drops Healing Bath Salts Formula

Close the cap tightly and shake the bottle vigorously to thoroughly blend the essential oils. Allow to synergize for 8 or more hours before using.

Blend together your Epsom and Celtic sea salts, baking soda and choice of clay, if desired, in a small ceramic bowl.

Add 5–12 drops of the Healing Bath Salts Formula to the salts and thoroughly blend the ingredients together.

Add 1–3 cups (500–1500 g) of the scented bath salts mixture to your bathtub filled with warm water (preferably under 101°F [38°C]).

Soak for 20–30 minutes for a healing and rejuvenating bath spa experience.

After the soak, rinse off in a warm shower and towel dry. Then wrap yourself in a warm, snuggly robe and rest for 10–15 minutes in a comfortable lounging chair, or lie down for a nap in your bed.

(continued)

Healing Bath Salts Formula (Continued)

Be sure to hydrate well during and after the bath. Water with fresh squeezed lemon or lime is perfect for revitalizing your adrenals and other organs.

Natural sea salts are rich in minerals and charged with electrical and healing properties that you can especially benefit from in a warm bath. A sea salt bath with pure essential oils is an effective way to cleanse and restore your chakras and auric energy field. You can purchase natural sea salt in your local health-food store in the spice section. For even more about baths, check out the "How to Use Essential Oils" section (page 29).

PLEASE NOTE: Essential oils are not water-soluble. You must use a dispersant when adding them to a bath. Water may cause the oils to penetrate your system more quickly or cause irritation to sensitive or damaged skin (such as blemishes, sores or rash).

Exfoliating Sugar Scrubs

This natural exfoliating treatment is quick and easy to make. You can use a single essential oil in your sugar scrub, which is recommended if you have sensitive or problem skin. You can also use a blend of oils when you desire to achieve a broader spectrum of application and benefits. Use your sugar scrub before your bath or shower.

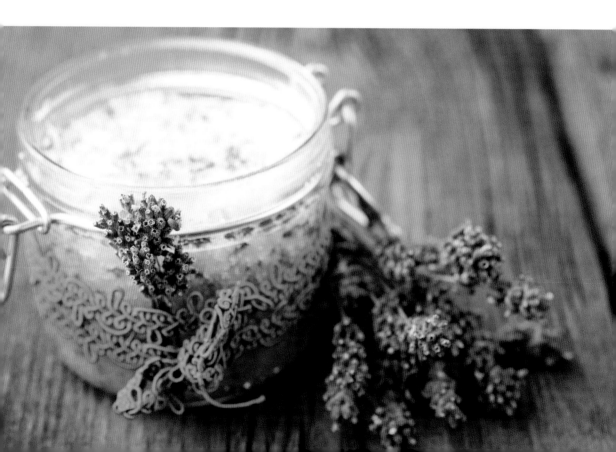

Exfoliating Sugar Scrub Oil Formula

An invigorating experience that will renew body, mind and soul.

~~~~~~

1 cup (200 g) cane sugar, fine grain (exfoliating pore polish)

Substitute: 1 cup (200 g) raw brown sugar (aggressive exfoliation)

1–4 tsp (5–20 ml) favorite carrier oil (rose hip, light coconut or jojoba recommended)

1 drop pure essential oil

In a small ceramic bowl, mix together the sugar and your chosen carrier oil until thoroughly blended. Add one drop of pure essential oil or blend to the mixture and blend thoroughly. Add more carrier oil as desired if you prefer a loose, wet action for your sugar scrub.

Stand over a large bath towel or on a non-slip bath mat inside your tub. You can also lie on a plastic spa sheet as you begin to apply the sugar scrub. Rub the skin gently, using upward sweeping strokes, starting at the toes and working upward to the abdomen. Then begin to stroke upward from the fingertips to the shoulders.

After finishing your extremities, begin rubbing the sugar scrub onto the front side of your torso and then the backside.

You can rinse off the sugar scrub in a warm and soothing shower or take a steaming hot bath afterward.

After the sugar scrub, your skin will feel silky smooth and will have the appearance of being lustrous and more youthful!

pH Balancing Honey Lemon Sugar Facial Scrub Formula

One's pH balance is the key to having great skin. The letters pH stand for "potential hydrogen" and refer to the ratio of acid to alkaline balance of your body and skin. This ranges from 1 (most acidic) to 14 (most alkaline). A pH imbalance is the cause for almost every skin problem or issue, from acne to premature aging and wrinkling. There is a simple and easy fix for balancing your skin's pH, and it's the Honey Lemon Sugar Facial Scrub. According to dermatologist Patricia Wexler MD, "The skin's barrier, which is known as the acid mantle, is responsible for keeping in lipids and moisture while blocking germs, pollution, toxins and bacteria. To work its best, the acid mantle should be slightly acidic, at a 5.5 pH balance. When it's too alkaline, skin becomes dry and sensitive; you may even get eczema. You may also experience inflammation, which inhibits the skin's ability to ward off matrix metalloproteinases [MMPs], the enzymes that destroy collagen and cause wrinkles and sagging."

This lovely mixture of honey, sugar, coconut oil and lemon pure essential oil will gently exfoliate your skin while balancing your skin's pH, leaving it feeling soft and silky smooth. It will also restore its natural luster and shine. Lemon pure essential oil boosts the cleansing and skin tonic effects of this facial scrub. It's also a delightfully aromatic spa treatment for the brain as it relieves confusion and brings clarity, as well as calms anxiety and stress.

½ cup (100 g) sugar (raw brown or white)

½ cup (108 g) light coconut oil (or favorite carrier oil)

4 tbsp (60 ml) raw honey

4 tsp (20 ml) lemon juice (fresh squeezed)

1 drop lemon pure essential oil

In a small ceramic bowl, blend the sugar and coconut oil (or other carrier oil). Then add honey, blending the mixture thoroughly together. Finally, add the fresh-squeezed lemon juice and lemon essential oil to the mixture and blend thoroughly.

With your fingertips, slowly and gently begin to apply the honey and lemon exfoliating scrub to your facial skin and polish the skin with it, making small, gentle circular movements. Begin at your décolletage and move upward, being sure to exfoliate your entire face, from the chin, over both cheeks and to the nose and forehead.

Be sure to use light, even pressure (10–60 seconds in each area) in small circular movements (clockwise and counter-clockwise) to remove old skin cells and cellular debris.

Rinse your face thoroughly with lukewarm water after you're done. Facial skin will feel invigorated and renewed and have a more youthful and radiant glow.

After your pH Balancing Honey Lemon Sugar Facial Scrub, drink plenty of pure, fresh water. You may wish to infuse your water with lemon pure essential oil diluted in a natural sweetener like stevia, honey or maple syrup. Drinking this throughout the day after your sugar scrub will help to keep your skin hydrated, your energy and stamina humming and your intellect switched on.

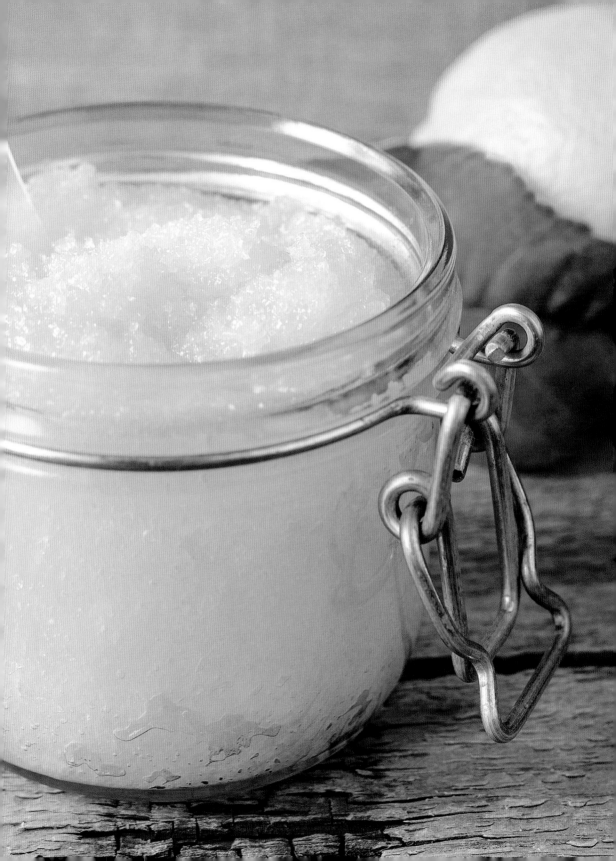

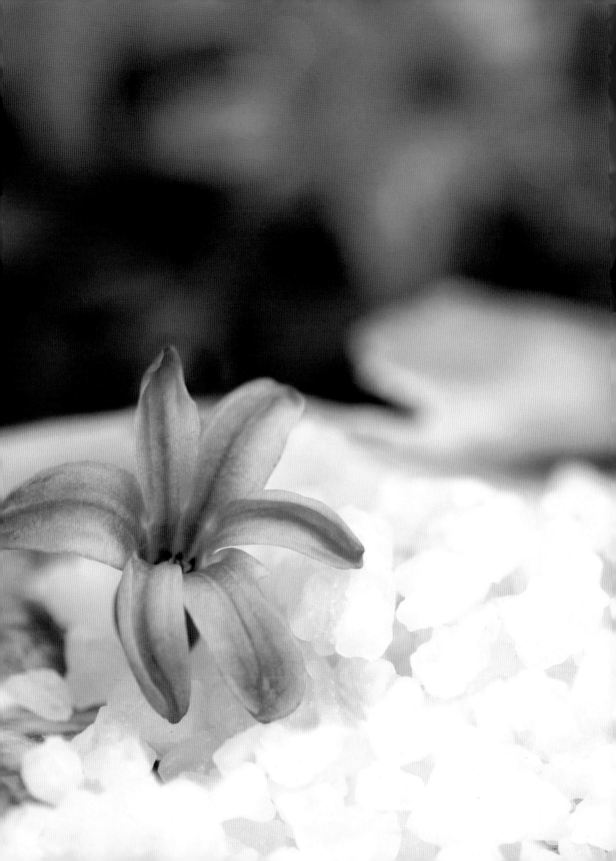

Salt Glow Treatments

A Salt Glow Treatment is an invigorating massage experience and is made with either sea salts or Epsom salts. This is one of the most inexpensive spa treatments you can use for deep exfoliation. Salt Glow Treatments renew and freshen your skin cell tissue and take only minutes to do, making them very easy to integrate into a busy and hectic lifestyle. Exfoliation is known to enhance circulation, as well as promote detoxification.

Each nourishing treatment is made with the pure essential oils known for balancing a particular skin type or condition, and all have the ability to freshen, tone and renew skin cell tissue. Use the following essential oil formulas by skin type or for balancing and healing a particular skin condition as noted.

Skin Healing and Regeneration Formula

If you tend to get blemishes frequently or have an uneven complexion, this is the formula for you.

To a 5-ml, colored-glass, euro-dropper bottle add:

Carrot Seed: 40 drops

Geranium Roseum and Graveolens: 40 drops

Helichrysum: 20 drops

1 cup (500 g) Celtic (fine grind) or regular sea salt (detoxifier)

1–4 tsp (5–20 ml) favorite carrier oil (light coconut oil, jojoba or rose hip recommended)

Close the cap tightly and shake the bottle vigorously to thoroughly blend the essential oils. Allow to synergize for 8 or more hours before using.

Add the salt and carrier oil to a bowl, and then blend together until thoroughly mixed. Add 1–3 drops of the oil blend to the mixture and blend thoroughly. Add more carrier oil if you prefer a looser, more wet action for your salt glow.

Stand over a large bath towel or on a non-slip bath mat. Begin to apply your salt glow. Rub your skin gently using upward sweeping strokes. Start at your toes and work upward to your abdomen. Then begin to stroke upward from your fingertips to your shoulders.

After finishing your extremities, begin rubbing your salt glow onto the front side of your torso and then your backside. Use gentle circular movements on your upper torso, including your abdomen, chest, buttocks, backside and upper thighs.

After gently massaging your entire upper torso with the salt glow, you can rinse off in a warm and soothing shower. You can also relax in a steaming hot bath, steam room or sauna afterward. The salt glow will leave your skin feeling soft, supple and silky smooth, with a youthful appearance.

PLEASE NOTE: Essential oils are not water-soluble, and you must use a dispersant when adding them to a bath. The water may cause the oils to penetrate your system more quickly or cause irritation to sensitive or damaged skin (such as open wounds, blemishes, sores or rashes).

Regulating All Skin Types Formula

This is the best all-around salt glow formula to use for any skin type. It's a great place to start if you've never experienced a salt glow.

~~~~~~

To a 5-ml, colored-glass, euro-dropper bottle add:

Geranium Bourbon: 40 drops

Carrot Seed: 20 drops

Ylang Ylang: 20 drops

Lavender: 20 drops

1 cup (500 g) Celtic (fine grind) or regular sea salt (detoxifier)

1–4 tsp (5–20 ml) favorite carrier oil (light coconut oil, jojoba or rose hip recommended)

Close the cap tightly and shake the bottle vigorously to thoroughly blend the essential oils. Allow to synergize for 8 or more hours before using.

Add the salt and carrier oil to a bowl, and then blend together until thoroughly mixed. Add 1–3 drops of the oil blend to the mixture and blend thoroughly. Add more carrier oil if you prefer a looser, more wet action for your salt glow.

Stand over a large bath towel or on a non-slip bath mat. Begin to apply your salt glow. Rub your skin gently using upward sweeping strokes. Start at your toes and work upward to your abdomen.

Then begin to stroke upward from your fingertips to your shoulders.

After finishing your extremities, begin rubbing your salt glow onto the front side of your torso and then your backside. Use gentle circular movements on your upper torso, including your abdomen, chest, buttocks, backside and upper thighs.

After gently massaging your entire upper torso with the salt glow, you can rinse off in a warm and soothing shower. You can also relax in a steaming hot bath, steam room or sauna afterward.

The salt glow will leave your skin feeling soft, supple and silky smooth, with a youthful appearance.

PLEASE NOTE: Essential oils are not water-soluble, and you must use a dispersant when adding them to a bath. The water may cause the oils to penetrate your system more quickly or cause irritation to sensitive or damaged skin (such as open wounds, blemishes, sores or rashes).

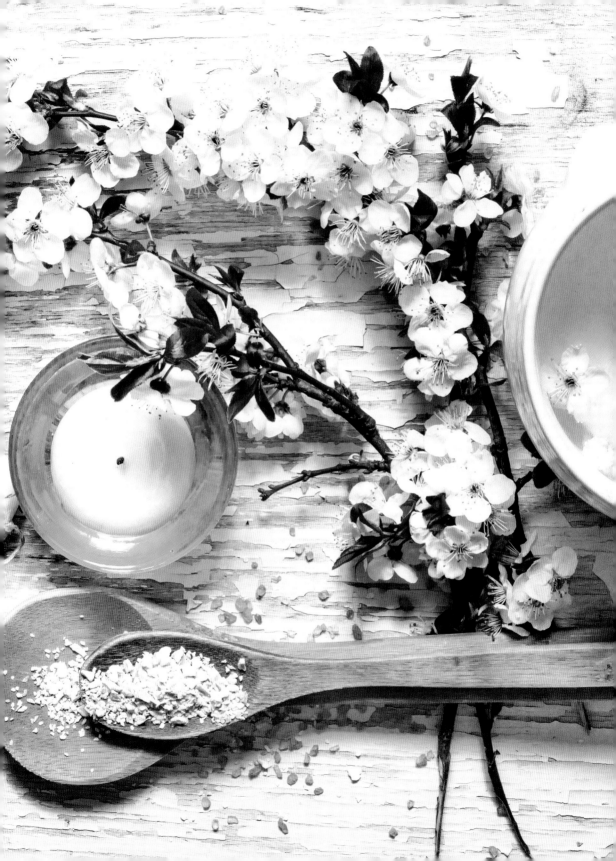

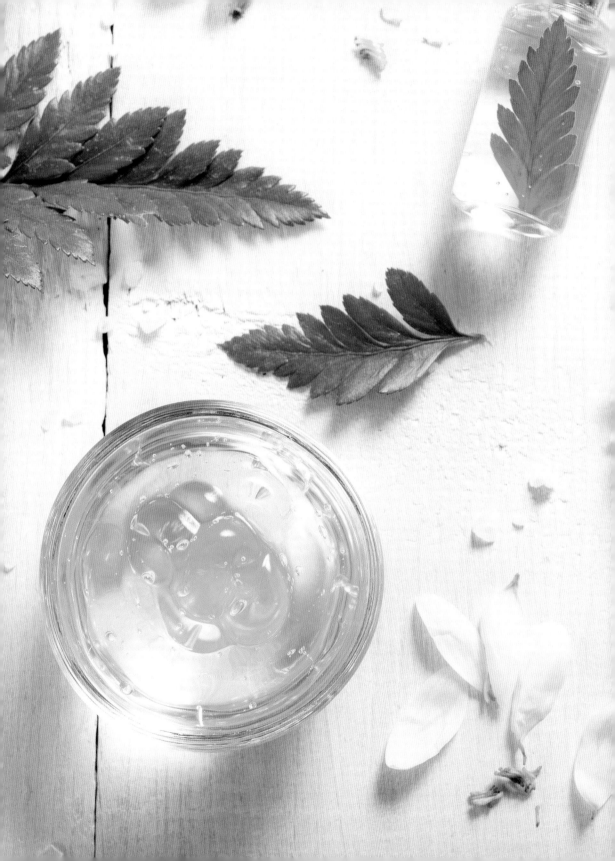

Chronic Skin Conditions Formula

If you have a chronic skin condition (such as eczema, rosacea, rash, dermatitis or psoriasis), this is the best skin formula to use to bring balance and harmony to skin cell tissue.

~~~~~~

To a 5-ml, colored-glass, euro-dropper bottle add:

Palma Rosa: 40 drops

German Chamomile: 20 drops

Helichrysum: 20 drops

Spikenard: 20 drops

1 cup (500 g) Celtic (fine grind) or regular sea salt (detoxifier)

1–4 tsp (5–20 ml) favorite carrier oil (light coconut oil, jojoba or rose hip recommended)

Close the cap tightly and shake the bottle vigorously to thoroughly blend the essential oils. Allow to synergize for 8 or more hours before using.

Add salt and carrier oil to a bowl, and then blend together until thoroughly mixed. Add 1–3 drops of the oil blend to the mixture and blend thoroughly. Add more carrier oil if you prefer a looser, more wet action for your salt glow.

Stand over a large bath towel or on a non-slip bath mat. Begin to apply your salt glow. Rub your skin gently using upward sweeping strokes. Start at your toes and work upward to your abdomen.

Then begin to stroke upward from your fingertips to your shoulders.

After finishing your extremities, begin rubbing your salt glow onto the front side of your torso and then your backside. Use gentle circular movements on your upper torso, including your abdomen, chest, buttocks, backside and upper thighs.

After gently massaging your entire upper torso with the salt glow, you can rinse off in a warm and soothing shower. You can also relax in a steaming hot bath, steam room or sauna afterwards.

The salt glow will leave your skin feeling soft, supple and silky smooth, with a youthful appearance.

PLEASE NOTE: Essential oils are not water-soluble, and you must use a dispersant when adding them to a bath. The water may cause the oils to penetrate your system more quickly or cause irritation to sensitive or damaged skin (such as open wounds, blemishes, sores or rashes).

Regulating and Balancing, Wound Healing, Problem Skin Formula

If you have acne outbreaks, combination skin, problem skin or sensitive skin, this is the salt glow formula for you to use.

~~~~~~

To a 5-ml, colored-glass, euro-dropper bottle add:

Blue Yarrow: 40 drops

Palmarosa: 40 drops

Helichrysum: 10 drops

Geranium Roseum and Graveolens: 5 drops each

1 cup (500 g) Celtic (fine grind) or regular sea salt (detoxifier)

1–4 tsp (5–20 ml) favorite carrier oil (light coconut oil, jojoba or rose hip recommended)

Close the cap tightly and shake the bottle vigorously to thoroughly blend the essential oils. Allow to synergize for 8 or more hours before using.

Add the salt and carrier oil to a bowl, and then blend together until thoroughly mixed. Add 1–3 drops of the oil blend to the mixture and blend thoroughly. Add more carrier oil if you prefer a looser, more wet action for your salt glow.

Stand over a large bath towel or on a non-slip bath mat. Begin to apply your salt glow. Rub your skin gently using upward sweeping strokes. Start at your toes and work upwards to your abdomen.

Then begin to stroke upward from your fingertips to your shoulders.

After finishing your extremities, begin rubbing your salt glow onto the front side of your torso and then your backside. Use gentle circular movements on your upper torso, including your abdomen, chest, buttocks, backside and upper thighs.

After gently massaging your entire upper torso with the salt glow, you can rinse off in a warm and soothing shower. You can also relax in a steaming hot bath, steam room or sauna afterward.

The salt glow will leave your skin feeling soft, supple and silky smooth, with a youthful appearance.

PLEASE NOTE: Essential oils are not water-soluble, and you must use a dispersant when adding them to a bath. The water may cause the oils to penetrate your system more quickly or cause irritation to sensitive or damaged skin (such as open wounds, blemishes, sores or rashes).

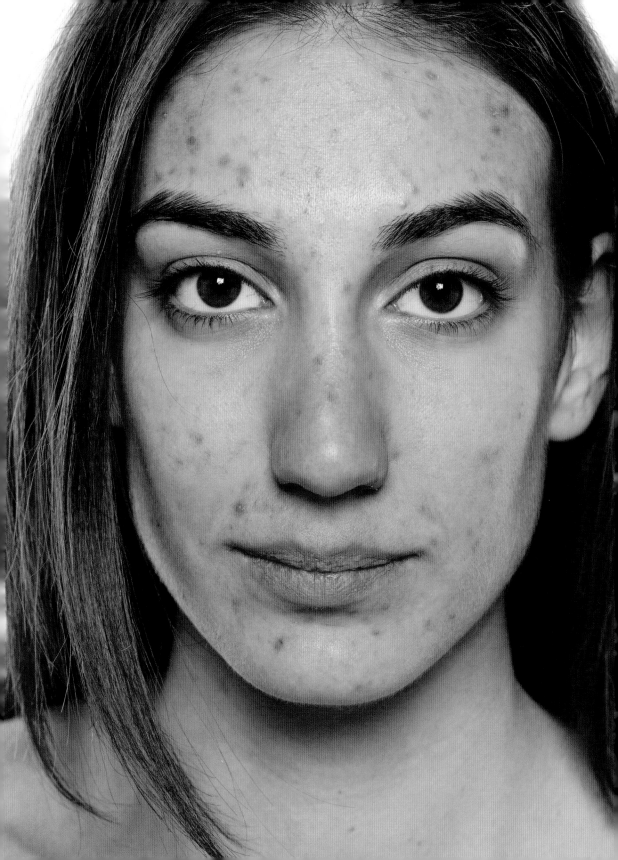

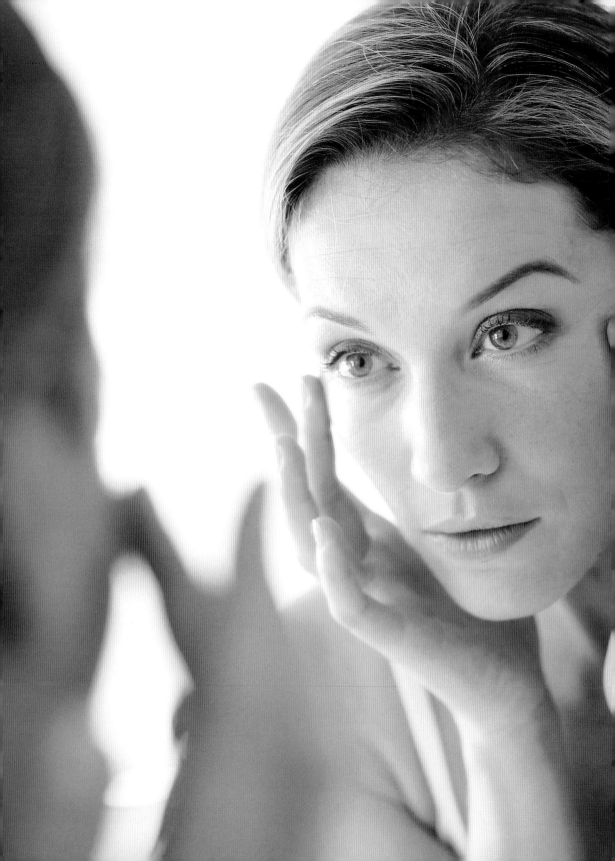

Moisture Balancing and Healing for All Skin Types Formula

An ideal beauty formula for all skin types.

~~~~~~

To a 5-ml, colored-glass, euro-dropper bottle add:

Spikenard: 40 drops

Lavender: 20 drops

Ylang Ylang III: 20 drops

Carrot Seed: 20 drops

1 cup (500 g) Celtic (fine grind) or regular sea salt (detoxifier)

1–4 tsp (5–20 ml) favorite carrier oil (light coconut oil, jojoba or rose hip recommended)

Close the cap tightly and shake the bottle vigorously to thoroughly blend the essential oils. Allow to synergize for 8 or more hours before using.

Add the salt and carrier oil to a bowl, and then blend together until thoroughly mixed. Add 1–3 drops of the oil blend to the mixture and blend thoroughly. Add more carrier oil if you prefer a looser, more wet action for your salt glow.

Stand over a large bath towel or on a non-slip bath mat. Begin to apply your salt glow. Rub your skin gently using upward sweeping strokes. Start at your toes and work upward to your abdomen.

Then begin to stroke upward from your fingertips to your shoulders.

After finishing your extremities, begin rubbing your salt glow onto the front side of your torso and then your backside. Use gentle circular movements on your upper torso, including your abdomen, chest, buttocks, backside and upper thighs.

After gently massaging your entire upper torso with the salt glow, you can rinse off in a warm and soothing shower. You can also relax in a steaming hot bath, steam room or sauna afterward.

The salt glow will leave your skin feeling soft, supple and silky smooth, with a youthful appearance.

PLEASE NOTE: Essential oils are not water-soluble, and you must use a dispersant when adding them to a bath. The water may cause the oils to penetrate your system more quickly or cause irritation to sensitive or damaged skin (such as open wounds, blemishes, sores or rashes).

Oily Skin Formula

The essential oils in this formula are ideal for regulating and balancing oily skin types.

~~~~~~

To a 5-ml, colored-glass, euro-dropper bottle add:

Cypress: 40 drops

Lemon: 20 drops

Palmarosa: 20 drops

Helichrysum: 10 drops

Geranium Roseum and Graveolens: 5 drops each

1 cup (500 g) Celtic (fine grind) or regular sea salt (detoxifier)

1–4 tsp (5–20 ml) favorite carrier oil (light coconut oil, jojoba or rose hip recommended)

Close the cap tightly and shake the bottle vigorously to thoroughly blend the essential oils. Allow to synergize for 8 or more hours before using.

Add the salt and carrier oil to a bowl, and then blend together until thoroughly mixed. Add 1–3 drops of the oil blend to the mixture and blend thoroughly. Add more carrier oil if you prefer a looser, more wet action for your salt glow.

Stand over a large bath towel or on a non-slip bath mat. Begin to apply your salt glow. Rub your skin gently using upward sweeping strokes. Start at your toes and work upward to your abdomen.

Then begin to stroke upward from your fingertips to your shoulders.

After finishing your extremities, begin rubbing your salt glow onto the front side of your torso and then your backside. Use gentle circular movements on your upper torso, including your abdomen, chest, buttocks, backside and upper thighs.

After gently massaging your entire upper torso with the salt glow, you can rinse off in a warm and soothing shower. You can also relax in a steaming hot bath, steam room or sauna afterward.

The salt glow will leave your skin feeling soft, supple and silky smooth, with a youthful appearance.

PLEASE NOTE: Essential oils are not water-soluble, and you must use a dispersant when adding them to a bath. The water may cause the oils to penetrate your system more quickly or cause irritation to sensitive or damaged skin (such as open wounds, blemishes, sores or rashes).

Dry and Mature Skin Formula

The oils in this formula help regulate and moisturize dry and mature skin cells.

~~~~~~

To a 5-ml, colored-glass, euro-dropper bottle add:

Palmarosa: 60 drops

Helichrysum: 20 drops

Geranium Roseum and Graveolens: 5 drops each

Rosemary Verbenone: 10 drops

1 cup (500 g) Celtic (fine grind) or regular sea salt (detoxifier)

1–4 tsp (5–20 ml) favorite carrier oil (light coconut oil, jojoba or rose hip recommended)

Close the cap tightly and shake the bottle vigorously to thoroughly blend the essential oils. Allow to synergize for 8 or more hours before using.

Add the salt and carrier oil to a bowl, and then blend together until thoroughly mixed. Add 1–3 drops of the oil blend to the mixture and blend thoroughly. Add more carrier oil if you prefer a looser, more wet action for your salt glow.

Stand over a large bath towel or on a non-slip bath mat. Begin to apply your salt glow. Rub your skin gently using upward sweeping strokes. Start at your toes and work upward to your abdomen.

Then begin to stroke upward from your fingertips to your shoulders.

After finishing your extremities, begin rubbing your salt glow onto the front side of your torso and then your backside. Use gentle circular movements on your upper torso, including your abdomen, chest, buttocks, backside and upper thighs.

After gently massaging your entire upper torso with the salt glow, you can rinse off in a warm and soothing shower. You can also relax in a steaming hot bath, steam room or sauna afterward.

The salt glow will leave your skin feeling soft, supple and silky smooth, with a youthful appearance.

PLEASE NOTE: Essential oils are not water-soluble, and you must use a dispersant when adding them to a bath. The water may cause the oils to penetrate your system more quickly or cause irritation to sensitive or damaged skin (such as open wounds, blemishes, sores or rashes).

Additional Body Treatments

Complete your spa treatments with a French Clay Body Mask and some Healing and Regenerative Body Butter (page 311) for the ultimate spa experience.

French Clay Body Mask Formula

This clay body mask made with French clay and pure essential oils will cleanse, detoxify and improve your skin elasticity. Create a nice ambience for your French Clay Body Mask experience by turning off all phones and electronic devices. Make sure the room is comfortably warm, but not hot. Light a candle and play gentle and relaxing music in the background, or just relax and allow yourself to be silent during your treatment.

To a 5-ml, colored-glass, euro-dropper bottle add:

Lavender: 40 drops

Ylang Ylang III: 40 drops

Carrot Seed: 15 drops

Rosemary Verbenone: 5 drops

½–1½ cups (120–363 g) French pink or green clay* (partial or full body mask)

½–1½ cups (118–355 ml) purified water or cream (partial or full body mask)

1–4 drops French Clay Body Mask Formula

For a partial body mask: Add 1 drop of the essential oil blend to the clay

For a full body mask: Add 3–4 drops of the essential oil blend to the clay

*Clay can stain fabric so take care to use a plastic covering to prevent staining.

Close the cap tightly and shake the bottle vigorously to thoroughly blend the essential oils. Allow to synergize for 8 or more hours before using.

Add your choice of natural French clay to a bowl. Then begin to blend in purified water or cream to make a loose paste, but make sure it's not totally wet. When the clay paste is the desired wetness, add your essential oil blend and mix in thoroughly.

Stand over a large bath towel or on a slip-proof bath mat and immediately begin applying the French clay mixture to a body part or to the entire body using gentle, upward sweeping strokes.

(continued)

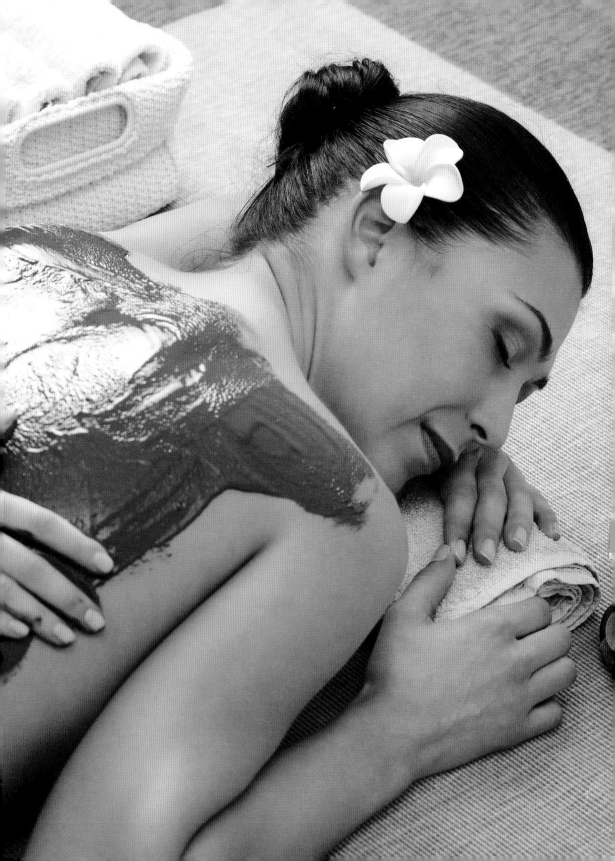

French Clay Body Mask Formula (Continued)

After you've finished applying the clay mask, it's time to relax and allow the mask to dry. You can lie down in a dry tub and drape the large bath towel lightly over you if needed, so you don't get chilled. Or you can lie down on a large bath towel or plastic spa sheet and cover yourself lightly with another large bath towel. You want air to circulate around your skin, so the clay will dry and produce the drawing effect on your skin tissues to pull out toxins and exfoliate, but you don't want to get chilled either. The best way to do this is by making sure the room is comfortably warm before starting your treatment.

Allow the mask to dry for 10–20 minutes, and then rinse off in a warm shower. Towel dry with a soft towel. Wrap yourself in a snuggly robe and relax for 10–15 minutes afterward in a lounging chair, or lie down in your bed. Be sure to hydrate during and after your treatment by drinking pure, fresh water with a slice of lemon or lime.

Your skin will feel soft, refreshed and toned after the mask.

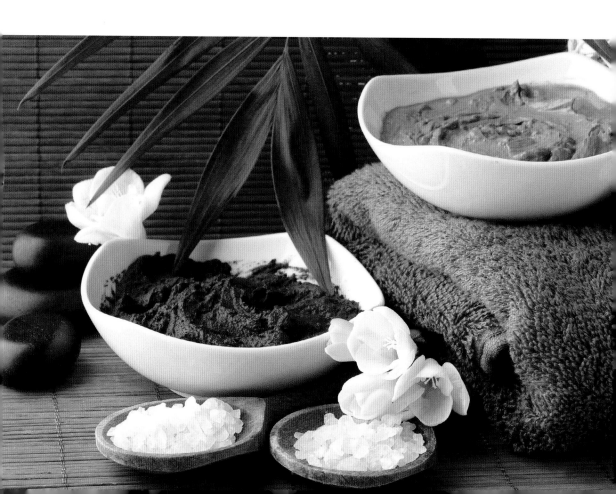

Healing and Regenerative Body Butter Formula

This healing and regenerative body butter made with pure essential oil is absolutely exquisite for balancing and nourishing your skin cell tissues. Use this youth-enhancing, healing and regenerative body butter as an anti-aging preventative treatment, as well as to smooth the appearance of deep lines and wrinkles.

Each of the recommended pure essential oils has a long history of use for skincare. Effective for renewing mature, aged or weathered skin and fading age spots, its notable balancing, moisturizing, rejuvenating and anti-inflammatory properties make it excellent for treating an assortment of skin issues.

Try the Healing and Regenerative Body Butter Formula for relieving these skin conditions:

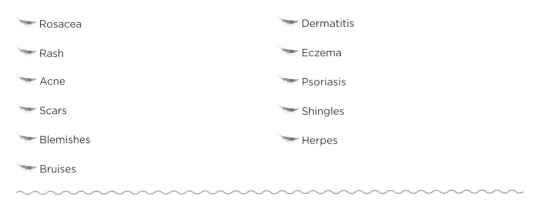

- Rosacea
- Rash
- Acne
- Scars
- Blemishes
- Bruises

- Dermatitis
- Eczema
- Psoriasis
- Shingles
- Herpes

Recipe makes approximately 4 ounces (120 ml)
Use organic ingredients if available.

2 tbsp (27 g) pure shea and/or cocoa butter (moisturizer)
1 tbsp (14 g) beeswax
4 tbsp (54 g) light fractionated coconut oil
1 tbsp (19 g) vegetable glycerin (improves smoothness and lubrication)
60 drops sandalwood essential oil
60 drops helichrysum essential oil
60–90 drops one or more pure essential oils of your choice (lavender, ylang ylang, rose or geranium)
4-oz (120-ml), colored-glass jar with tight-fitting lid
Optional: 4–6 drops vitamin E oil (natural preservative)

(continued)

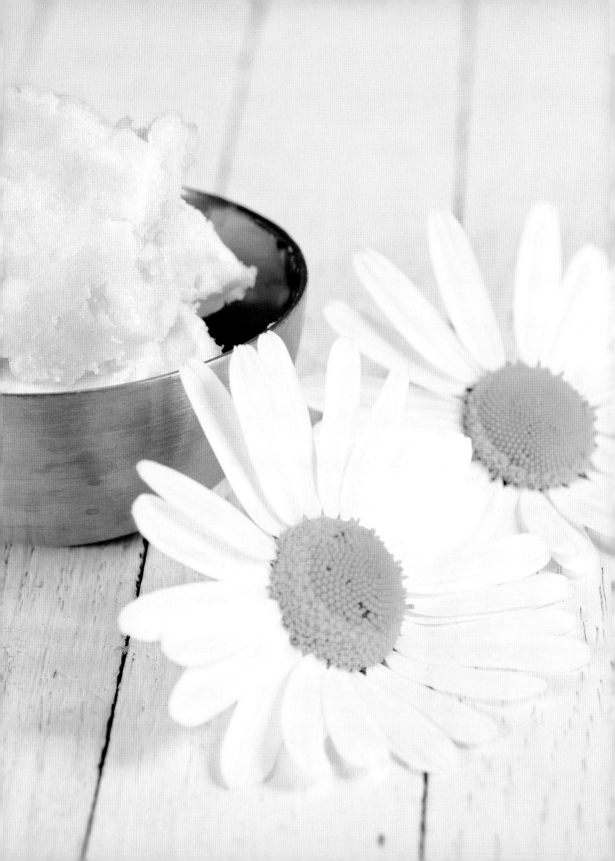

Healing and Regenerative Body Butter Formula (Continued)

Put shea or cocoa butter, or a combination of both, along with the beeswax, into the light fractionated coconut oil. Heat in a double boiler or in your homemade double boiler. (A glass measuring cup inside a pan of water, over medium-low heat.)

Heat this mixture until the shea and/or cocoa butter and beeswax are melted thoroughly together.

Remove the melted ingredients from the double boiler or take the glass measuring cup from the pan. Add vegetable glycerin and blend the mixture together with a sterile instrument.

After cooling the butter mixture slightly, add in your essential oil blend gently with a sterile instrument.

Pour the butter into your colored-glass jar and allow to set completely before using. Seal tightly with a lid and store in a cool, dry place.

Body butter will keep for 6 months or longer if properly sealed and stored.

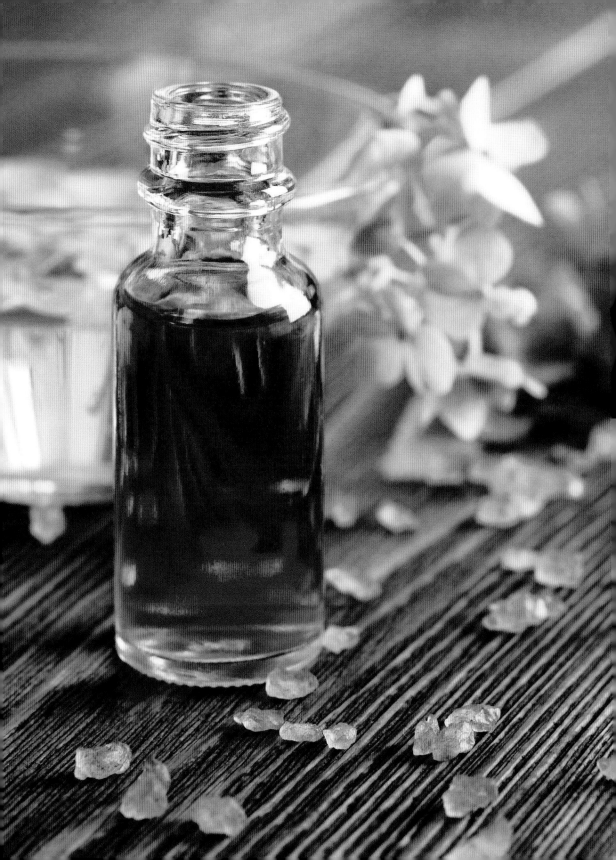

CHAPTER 15

Love and Romance Blends

Aphrodite Perfume Oil Formula

The Aphrodite Perfume Oil Formula stimulates your inner Aphrodite, the Greek goddess of love and beauty. This perfume is a celebration of passion, pleasure and procreation. In the Roman pantheon of gods and goddesses, she is the goddess Venus and is also associated with the planet of the same name.

~~~~~~

To a 5-ml, colored-glass, euro-dropper bottle add:

Ylang Ylang III: 20 drops

Rose: 20 drops

Bergamot: 10 drops

Sweet Orange: 10 drops

Sandalwood: 10 drops

Frankincense: 5 drops

Myrrh: 5 drops

Patchouli: 5 drops

Ginger: 5 drops

Cinnamon: 5 drops

Black Spruce: 1–2 drops

Dispense 1–3 drops on a cotton ball or smell strip and inhale the aromatic vapors of your Aphrodite Perfume Oil Formula for 10-15 seconds. You may repeat as needed. This formula is also effective when diffused into the air or used as an aromatic mist.

To make a ready-to-use Aphrodite Perfume Oil Formula blend, simply add 15–30 drops or more of your synergy blend to a 1-ounce (30-ml) bottle of your favorite carrier oil. Shake the bottle well to disperse the oils thoroughly. Apply a few drops of your ready-to-use blend behind both ears, as well as on the back of your neck.

Eros Aphrodisiac Formula

The Eros Aphrodisiac Formula is a celebration of intimate and romantic love. Use it to stimulate your powers of desire and attraction, as well as to enhance your creative life force energy and experience of universal love.

~~~~~~

To a 5-ml, colored-glass, euro-dropper bottle add:

Sandalwood: 40 drops

Neroli: 40 drops

Rose: 10 drops

Ylang Ylang III: 10 drops

Dispense 1–3 drops on a cotton ball or smell strip and inhale the aromatic vapors of your Eros Aphrodisiac Formula blend for 10–15 seconds. You may repeat as needed. This formula is also effective when diffused into the air or used as an aromatic mist.

To make a ready-to-use Eros Aphrodisiac Formula blend, simply add 15–30 drops or more of your synergy blend to a 1-ounce (30-ml) bottle of your favorite carrier oil. Shake the bottle well to disperse the oils thoroughly. Apply a few drops of your ready-to-use blend to your heart area, as well as on the back of your neck and behind both ears.

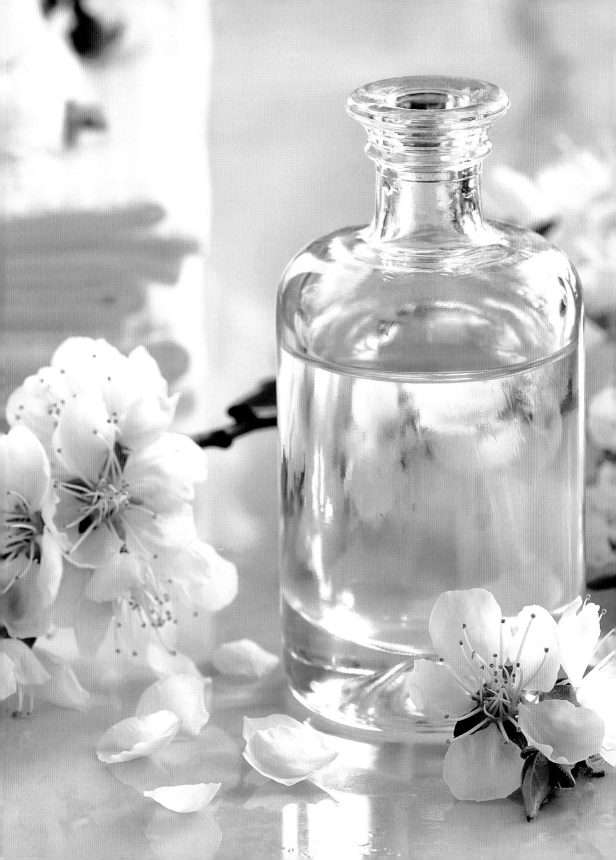

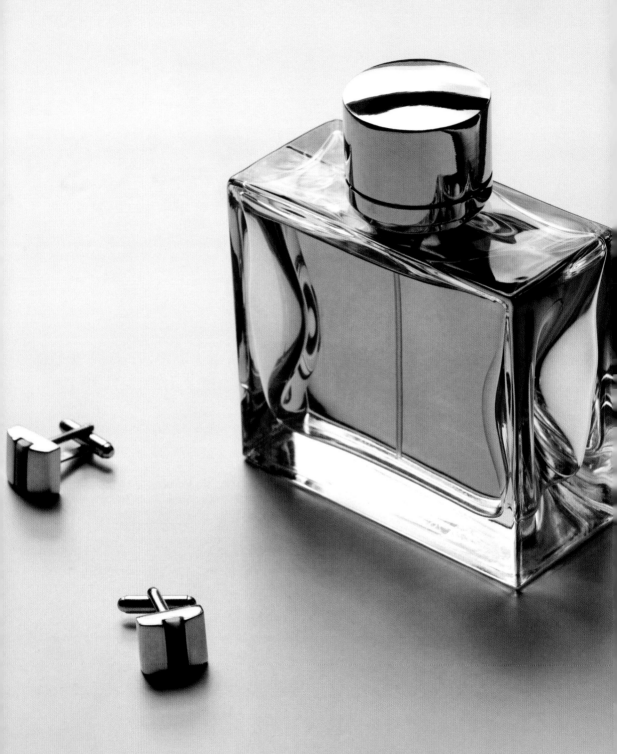

Audacity Men's Cologne Formula

The essential oils in the Audacity Men's Cologne Formula will help you find the pluck and courage you need to do what you fear to do and face any ordeal that requires strength of character.

To a 5-ml, colored-glass, euro-dropper bottle add:

Sandalwood: 30–34 drops

Atlas Cedarwood: 20 drops

Patchouli: 20 drops

Ylang Ylang III: 10 drops

Black Spruce: 1–2 drops

Ginger: 10 drops

Black Pepper: 5 drops

To promote your ability to do something that frightens you and the strength to face any pain, sorrow or grief, dispense 1–3 drops of your Audacity Blend on a cotton ball or smell strip and inhale the aromatic vapors for 10–15 seconds. You may repeat as needed. This formula is also effective when diffused into the air or used as an aromatic mist.

To make a ready-to-use Audacity Blend, simply add 15–30 drops or more of your synergy blend to a 1-ounce (30-ml) bottle of your favorite carrier oil. Shake the bottle well to disperse the oils thoroughly. Apply a few drops of your ready-to-use blend at your heart area, as well as behind both ears and on the back of your neck.

Although adding your audacity blend to alcohol or spirits will alter its chemical structure, you may wish to use your blend as a cologne.

To make a men's cologne with essentials oils use the following dilution amount:

Half fill a 5-milliliter, euro-dropper bottle with 100 percent vodka or spirits (70–80 drops). Then add 10–20 drops of your Audacity Men's Cologne Formula.

Shake the ingredients vigorously to make sure the essential oil formula is thoroughly blended with the vodka or spirits. Allow to synergize for a minimum of 24–48 hours. Then, top off the bottle with vodka or spirits and purified or spring water (10 drops). Shake vigorously to thoroughly blend the ingredients together. Allow to rest for up to 48 hours before using.

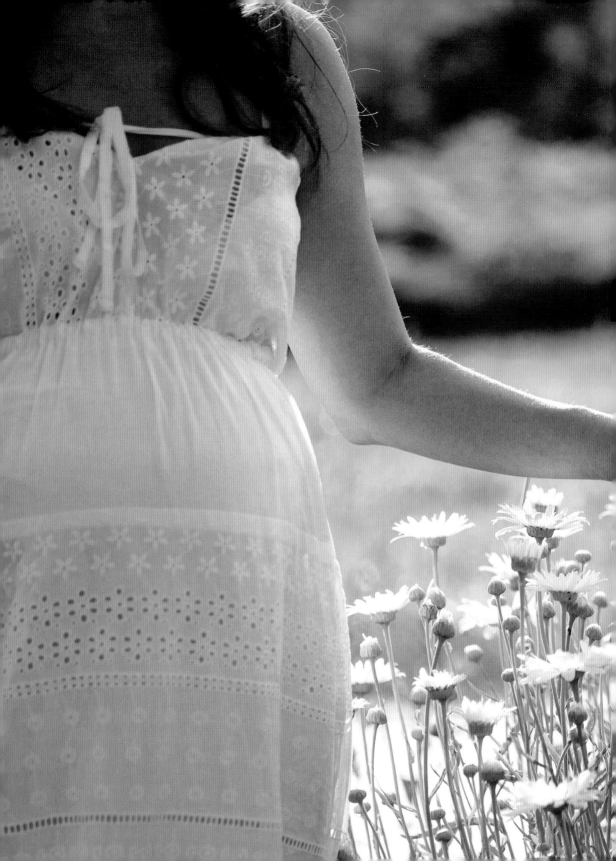

CHAPTER 16

Babies and New Mommies

Pregnancy

Essential oils can be especially useful during pregnancy and may be helpful for promoting rest and relaxation, as well relieving symptoms associated with pregnancy such as increased sensitivity, nervousness, sleep loss, lowered energy levels, nausea and frequent urination.

The two essential oils I recommend most often during pregnancy, with good results, are red mandarin and German chamomile. Both have a very gentle action and can be used safely to relieve many of the discomforts associated with pregnancy.

Childbirth, Labor and Delivery

Childbirth is experienced by many women as an intense event when powerful and sometimes overwhelming emotions can surface. Just prior to birth, in the later stages of gestation, there is an increase in the bonding hormone oxytocin. Oxytocin helps reduce feelings of anxiety and stimulates feelings of contentment and well-being.

Another common experience among new mothers is the "baby blues." Reports indicate that nearly 80 percent of women experience some feeling of sadness after giving birth. Essential oils have been used successfully by midwives and nurses in birthing centers and hospital labor rooms to help soothe the intense, and sometimes confusing, emotions that the birthing mother may experience during and after labor. Essential oils are also helpful for relieving symptoms associated with postpartum depression.

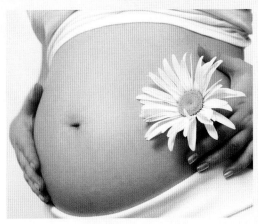

Both German chamomile and red mandarin essential oils have a long history of safe use and are reported to be highly effective.

ESSENTIAL OILS THAT HAVE BEEN USED TO ASSIST WITH LABOR PAINS, THROUGH TRANSITION AND TO THE DELIVERY OF THE BABY INCLUDE:

- Clary sage: may help soothe worry, restlessness, tension and stress
- Frankincense: assists with breathing during the labor and delivery
- Neroli: helps mothers to be calm, centered and peaceful
- Geranium roseum and graveolens: may reduce cramps
- Bergamot: soothes tension and anxiety, combats fatigue and is encouraging and balancing to the spirit
- Roman chamomile: promotes calm, soothes and relaxes tension
- German chamomile: calms nervous tension and quiets fears
- Red mandarin: relaxing, calming and regulating
- Vetiver: mild sedative action and may be useful for relieving stress
- Lavender: good for tension, restlessness, anxiety, worry and stress
- Sandalwood: relaxes stress and soothes tension
- Spikenard: contributes to inner balance and promotes peace and calm

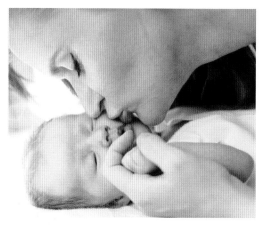

Sleep deprivation is a common issue after childbirth. German chamomile is helpful for fussy babies, so the whole family can get a good night's sleep.

Sleep Remedies and Formulas

Statistics have shown that a new baby results in an average of 400–750 hours of lost sleep for parents in the first year. As serious accidents are often associated with sleep deprivation, getting a good night's sleep is an absolute top priority for you and your entire family.

SLEEP REMEDIES

German chamomile is a traditional aromatherapy remedy for fussy newborns and babies. It has been shown to be helpful for:

- Colic
- Intestinal cramps
- Gas
- Diaper rash
- Restful sleep
- Teething pain

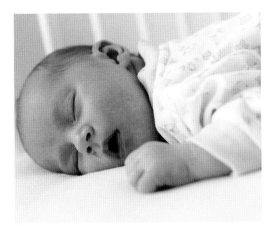

Diaper rash needn't be a concern—simply use German chamomile safely diluted in your favorite carrier oil as a massage oil.

SLEEP FORMULA

Use German chamomile diluted in a suitable vegetable carrier oil of 1 percent or less. I recommend pure light coconut oil or jojoba oil.

The ratio of pure essential oil to carrier oil should be less than 1 percent; that's about one to two drops of pure essential oil per 1 ounce (30 ml) of carrier oil.

Add your pure essential oil of German chamomile to a 1-ounce (30-ml) dispensing bottle filled halfway with your carrier oil. After adding your pure essential oil, top the bottle off with carrier oil. Then shake the bottle to thoroughly blend the pure essential oil into the carrier oil.

Use your baby massage oil topically as needed to promote deep and restful sleep. It may also be used to soothe and comfort your baby when showing any signs of distress such as colic, intestinal cramps, gas, teething pain and diaper rash. Use sparingly as a tiny amount is all that's needed for results.

Baby Massage

Easily one of the most powerful hands-on healing massage techniques I've ever used in my more than 30 years of practice as a practitioner, this kind of baby massage is very simple to do and easy to learn. I've used it to soothe newborn babies, and I've also taught it to new parents to perform with their babies with remarkable results reported.

HELPFUL FOR:

- Colic
- Intestinal cramps
- Gas
- Teething pain
- Deep and restful sleep
- Healthy functioning of organs and systems
- Promotes bonding between parents or caregivers and the baby

Parents enjoy feeling empowered by alleviating signs of their baby's discomfort, as well as helping the baby sleep through the night.

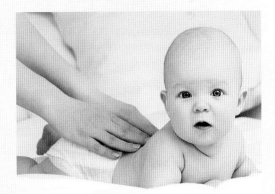

Alleviate many symptoms of your baby's discomfort with this simple, yet highly effective baby massage technique.

RESEARCH

The baby massage you're about to learn was developed by the late Tom Bowen of Perth, Australia. It has been used by thousands of moms, dads, nurses, nannies and caregivers around the world to quickly and safely relieve symptoms of discomfort common to newborn babies.

Border College of Natural Therapies in Australia conducted a research study of the effects of Bowen therapy using Medical Thermal Imaging.

Thermography uses infrared thermal imaging to see and measure thermal energy emitted from an object. The higher the object's temperature, the greater the infrared radiation emitted. Infrared measurements allow us to see what our eyes cannot.

Subjects screened before and after receiving Bowen therapy showed conclusively that Bowen therapy had an immediate, dramatic and sustained effect on lowering infrared radiation from the test subjects.

Through applying a few gentle, yet powerful, movements that take only seconds to perform, you'll be able to relieve the symptoms of discomfort your baby may experience as a newborn.

Baby Massage Technique

The baby massage technique consists of seven gentle, light-touch moves for stimulating balance in your baby's autonomic nervous system (ANS). The ANS is the control system that regulates the body's functions like heart and respiratory rate, digestion, pupillary response, urination and sexual arousal and acts primarily at the unconscious level. The ANS is also the primary control center of the fight-or-flight stress response mechanism.

Along with the Sleep Formula essential oil blend on page 232, gentle stimulation of the ANS with the baby massage technique has been shown to relieve a baby's symptoms of colic, intestinal cramps, gas and teething pain and to enhance their overall health and well-being. Parents have reported their babies being in the 75th–95th percentile for their age group when tested.

HOW OFTEN

For the first 6 weeks after birth, you may perform the baby massage as often as needed at the first sign of a baby's discomfort or weekly for general baby care.

The first four baby massage moves are made on your baby's back, between their shoulder blades.

Lay your baby down on his or her stomach with the face turned to one side. If there are two people providing the massage, one may hold the baby with the baby's chest facing you, while the other caregiver performs the first two baby massage moves. Do the best you can to gently perform the natural baby massage, and you will achieve good results.

BABY MASSAGE MOVE ONE: Always begin by doing your first baby massage move on the left side.

Place the pad of your right thumb flat on top of the muscles lying along the left side of your baby's spine. Your right thumb is just above the bottom angle of your baby's left shoulder blade, thumb tip facing down toward the outside of your baby's body.

Gently pull the flat pad of your right thumb toward the outside, moving the skin away from your baby's spine as far as it will go, like drawing the string of a bow. Gently press down and in, holding this position for 3 seconds.

Then pull your right thumb toward your baby's spine, move slowly with even, gentle pressure across the muscles. The pad of your right thumb flattens as you perform the baby massage move.

BABY MASSAGE MOVE TWO: Then, immediately perform the next baby massage move on the right side of your baby's spinal column, just above the bottom angle of your baby's left shoulder blade by placing the pad of your left thumb atop the muscles alongside the right side of your baby's spine. The thumb tip is facing the outside of your baby's body.

Gently push outside with the pad of your left thumb away from your baby's spine as far as it will go.

Gently press down and in, holding this position for 3 seconds. Then, with the pad of your left thumb, pull your thumb toward your baby's spine, moving slowly with even, gentle pressure across the muscles. The pad of your left thumb will flatten as you perform the move.

BABY MASSAGE MOVE THREE: You will immediately follow these first two moves with two more in the same exact sequence and locations except in the opposite direction, toward your baby's spine.

Place the pad of your left thumb flat on top of the muscles along the left side of your baby's spine. The thumb tip should be facing baby's spine. Push the skin and muscle beneath it towards your baby's spine, as far as it will go.

Gently press down and in, holding this position for 3 seconds. Then, with the pad of your left thumb, pull away from your baby's spine, moving slowly with even, gentle pressure across the muscles as far as you can go. Your left thumb will flatten as you perform the move.

BABY MASSAGE MOVE FOUR: Then, immediately perform the next baby massage move by placing the pad of your right thumb atop the muscles along the right side of your baby's spine.

Gently pulling with the pad of your right thumb with your thumb tip facing baby's spine, move the skin and muscle beneath it toward your baby's spine as far as it will go.

Gently press down and in, holding this position for 3 seconds. Then, with the pad of your right thumb, pull away from your baby's spine, moving slowly with even, gentle pressure across the muscles as far as you can go. Your right thumb will flatten as you perform the move.

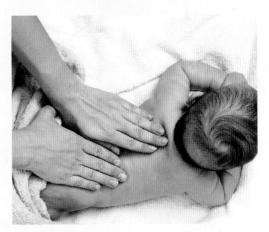

Use baby massage to relieve colic, teething pain and gas, as well as promote deep and restful sleep and increase bonding between baby and parents.

BABY MASSAGE MOVES, PART II

Your last three Baby Massage Moves are made with your baby lying flat on their back. If there are two of you, one can hold the baby facing outward as the other performs the moves.

HOLDING POINT

With the middle finger of your left hand, apply gentle pressure just below the tip of cartilage at the end of your baby's breastbone. This is called the xiphoid process.

Maintain this holding point with gentle pressure while performing the following two baby massage moves.

BABY MASSAGE MOVE FIVE: Place the pad of your right thumb mid-way along the border of your baby's left rib cage, thumb tip facing upward toward the xiphoid process. Slowly move the skin with your right thumb upward, along the border edge of your baby's rib cage as far as the skin can go.

Then slip the edge of your right thumb pad slightly under the angle of your baby's rib, and with a very gentle, light touch and pressure, move your right thumb downward in one long smooth movement following along the angle of your baby's rib as far as you can. Flatten your thumb.

BABY MASSAGE MOVE SIX: Repeat this move on the right side of your baby's rib cage, this time using the pad of your right thumb, with your fingertip facing the xiphoid process. Position your right thumb mid-way along the border of your baby's rib cage, move the skin and tissue beneath upward along the border of the right side of your baby's rib cage as far as it will go.

Then slip the edge of your right thumb slightly under the angle of your baby's rib and with a gentle, light touch and pressure move the skin and tissue beneath it with your right thumb moving downward in one long smooth movement, following along the angle of your baby's right lower rib as far as it will go. Flatten your thumb.

BABY MASSAGE MOVE SEVEN: Take your left middle finger off the Holding Point. Place the pad of your right middle finger about 1 inch (2.5 cm) below your baby's xiphoid process.

With the right pad of your middle finger, gently draw your baby's skin up toward the tip of their xiphoid process. Then, press gently down and in. Pull downward with a gentle, light touch and even pressure as far as you can. Then flatten your finger.

That's it! Allow the baby massage moves time to work. Sometimes the results are almost immediate. Allow at least 15 minutes before repeating the baby massage moves.

Teething Solutions

German chamomile oil in a dilution of carrier oil of less than 1 percent (about one to two drops per ounce of carrier oil) can be used as a massage oil to relieve teething pain.

TEETHING SOLUTIONS FORMULA

Add one to two drops of German chamomile oil to a 1-ounce (30-ml) dispensing bottle filled halfway with your carrier oil. After adding your essential oil, top the bottle off with carrier oil and then shake the bottle to thoroughly blend the pure essential oil into the carrier oil.

BABY MASSAGE TO RELIEVE TEETHING PAIN

To soothe teething pain, dispense a drop of your diluted German chamomile baby massage oil onto your fingertip, applying more diluted German chamomile oil as needed to your fingertip throughout the massage. You'll massage the area of greatest teething pain last.

The following is a protocol of massage to use for teething pain. You can follow as a guide, always being sure to leave the areas of greatest teething pain or discomfort until last. Begin at the bottom jaw line away from your baby's most tender side of teething pain or area of discomfort.

Gently make contact with the skin as you begin making small circular movements towards the midline of your baby's mouth. Work your way from the outer bottom jaw to the front of the mouth.

Now work the outer, lower jaw of the other side of the mouth. Using gentle circular movements, move toward the front of the mouth. Next, begin massaging the upper part of the mouth starting from the outer side of the jaw to the front of the mouth.

Finally, gently massage the area of the mouth of greatest teething pain or discomfort.

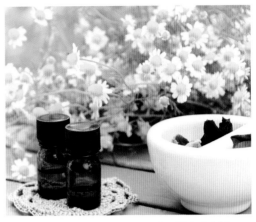

A massage with German chamomile oil is helpful for relieving baby's teething pain.

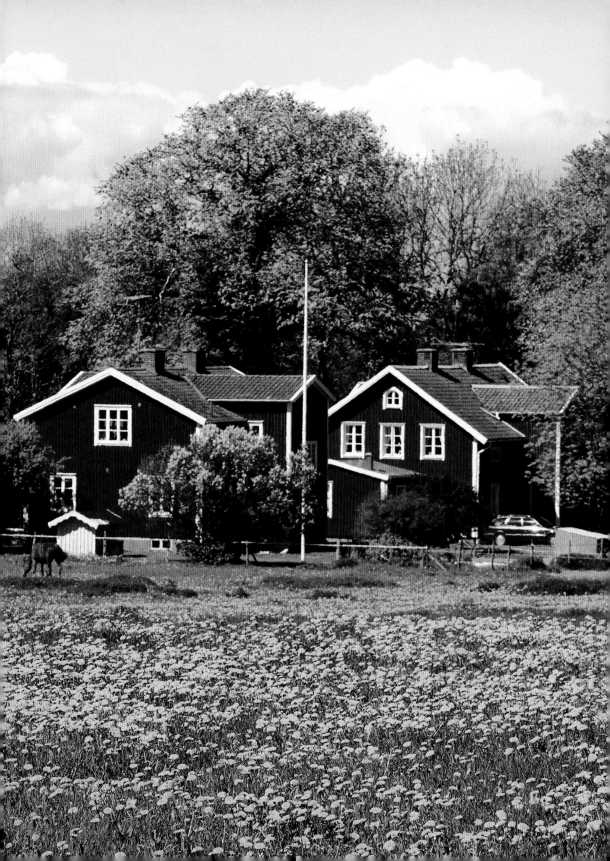

Around the House

Clear Stagnant Energy

We've all been in environments and around certain people or situations that afterward we can't seem to shake off their influence. It's like we've picked up "bad vibes," and they've stuck to us.

Quantum mechanics has now shown that negativity or bad vibes is a measure of quantum entanglement, which can easily be computed.

Since ancient times, energy medicine practitioners, natural healers and shamans from around the world have been practicing energy

clearing techniques. Plant aromatics have a long history of use for this purpose. The scent of plant aromatics has been used effectively to clear negative and stagnant energy from a house or room, as well from the auric field of a person.

The essential oils traditionally used and recommended for clearing negative energy all have highly astringent properties, which when used on surface objects are known to breakdown sticky substances like gum, built up dirt and stubborn grime. The oils recommended for energy clearing also have a powerfully refreshing and restorative effect on the mind and emotions, as well as strong antimicrobial action.

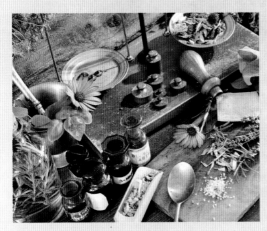

Research has shown that "bad vibes" exist. Negative energy can be easily measured and spread via quantum entanglement.

Energy Clearing Formula

Use to clean floors, walls and all surfaces and countertops, as well as to clear and freshen the atmosphere of a room. You can also use the energy clearing formula to clear the aura or energy field of a person.

~~~~~~

To a 5-ml, colored-glass, euro-dropper bottle add:

Lemon: 20 drops

Peppermint: 20 drops

Cypress: 20 drops

Cinnamon Leaf: 20 drops

Frankincense: 5 drops

Myrrh: 5 drops

Black Pepper: 5 drops

Juniper Berry: 5 drops

Close the cap tightly and shake the bottle vigorously to thoroughly blend the essential oils. Allow to synergize for 8 or more hours before using.

This formula is effective when diffused into the air or used as an aromatic room mist. For general, all-purpose cleaning, dilute the Energy Clearing Formula blend in warm soapy water to clean floors and walls, shampoo rugs and clean surfaces and countertops. This formula will also clear and freshen the atmosphere of a room. Be especially mindful to clean any darkened corners and thresholds. Dispose of dirty cleaning waters down a toilet.

To make a ready-to-use blend that you can wear as a perfume oil blend, simply add 15–30 drops of your synergy blend to a 1-ounce (30-ml) bottle of your favorite carrier oil. Shake the bottle well to disperse the oils thoroughly. Apply a few drops of your ready-to-use blend to your heart area, sinus points around your nose and forehead, as well as on the back of your neck and behind both ears.

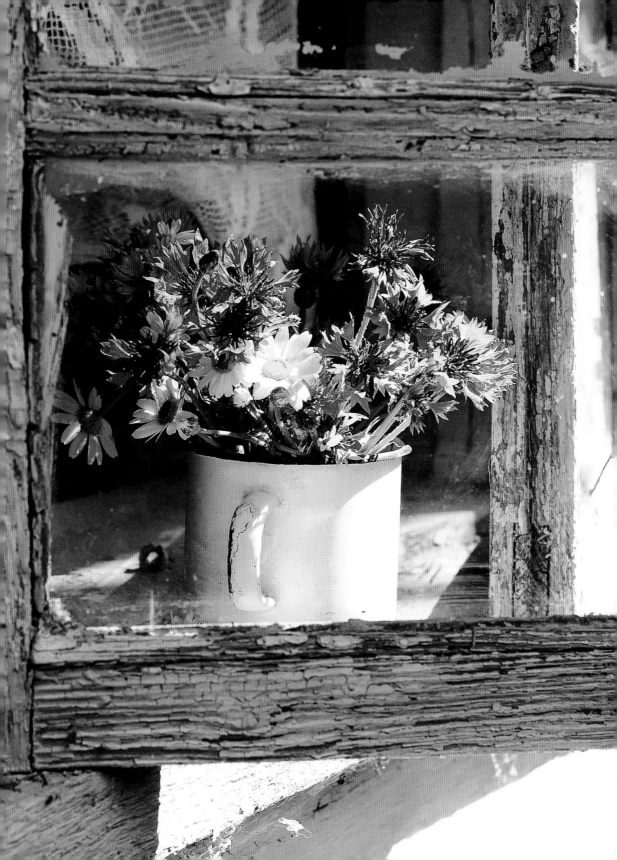

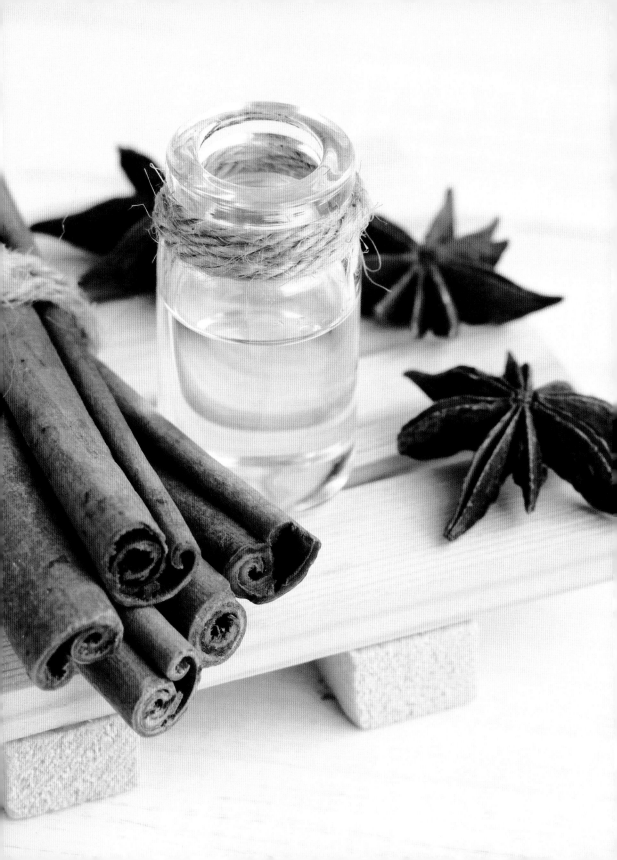

Eliminate Odors

The synthetic fragrance industry is a booming business. Most of the fragrances available on the world market simply mask odors, but do not actually eliminate them. Additionally, petroleum-based fragrances can cause reactions and are thought to result in the development of allergies.

However, essential oils, unlike synthetic fragrances, are not only natural substances, but they seldom cause reactions or sensitization when used properly.

Essential oils are chemical chelators. They make chemicals nontoxic by fracturing their molecular structure. European scientists have found that essential oils work as natural chelators, bonding to metals and chemicals and ferrying them out of the body. In this same way they act to break down and eliminate odors.

This same ability to fracture molecular structure gives essential oils the ability to break down odor molecules and eliminate odors completely.

Deodorizer Formula

For odor-free air that is also pollution-free and safe to breathe, use the Deodorizer Formula. Essential oils can deodorize stale and bad odors caused by mold and mildew, smoke, skunk, rotten eggs, food, the garbage can, compost and foot and body odor, just to name a few.

To a 5-ml, colored-glass, euro-dropper bottle add:

Black Spruce: 30 drops

Lemon: 20 drops

Cinnamon Leaf: 20 drops

Peppermint: 20 drops

Cypress: 10 drops

Close the cap tightly and shake the bottle vigorously to thoroughly blend the essential oils. Allow to synergize for 8 or more hours before using.

This formula is effective when diffused into the air or used as an aromatic room mist. For general, all-purpose deodorizing, add the deodorizer blend to warm soapy water and use to clean floors and walls, shampoo rugs and clean surfaces and countertops. This formula will also deodorize, clear and freshen the atmosphere of a room. Be especially mindful to clean any darkened corners and thresholds. Dispose of dirty cleaning waters down a toilet.

To make a simple cleaner, add the deodorizer blend to either white vinegar or baking soda and use as an air freshener in your refrigerator and underneath sinks to effectively remove odors.

Air Freshener

Because of their ability to fracture the molecular structure of chemicals, essential oils are highly prized in the air freshener industry. Removing the source or cause of an offensive aroma is, of course, preferable to masking it from human perception for brief periods of time.

Like a breath of fresh air, essential oils will help you maintain the indoor air quality of your home and quickly eliminate unpleasant and unwanted odors.

Air Freshener Formula

Use to freshen a stale room, eliminate odors in areas with poor ventilation and enhance the ambience of any room with odor-free air that is also pollution-free and safe to breathe.

~~~~~~

To a 5-ml, colored-glass, euro-dropper bottle add:

Lemongrass: 40 drops

Lemon: 20 drops

Peppermint: 20 drops

Cypress: 10 drops

Cinnamon Leaf: 10 drops

Black Spruce: 1–5 drops

Close the cap tightly and shake the bottle vigorously to thoroughly blend the essential oils. Allow to synergize for 8 or more hours before using.

This formula is effective when diffused into the air or used as an aromatic room mist. To make a simple cleaner, add the Air Freshener Formula to either white vinegar or baking soda and use as an air freshener in your refrigerator and underneath sinks to effectively remove odors.

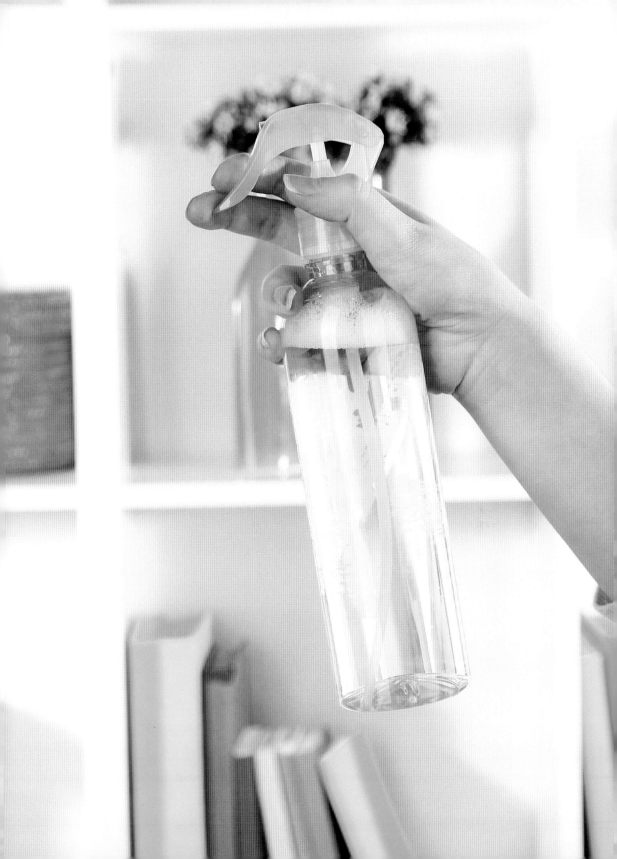

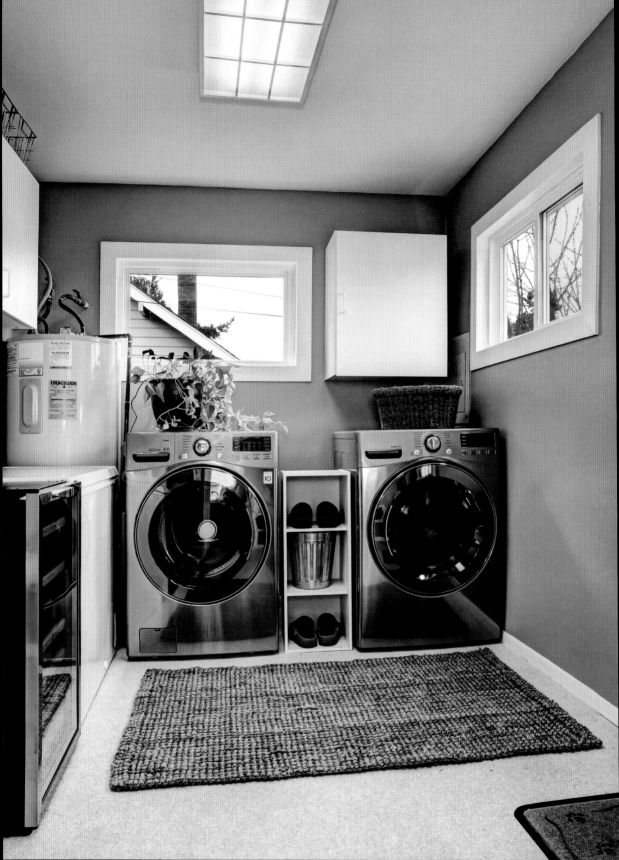

Laundry Care

Personal hygiene is the foundation of your health, which is easily your most valuable asset. A high standard of cleaning and laundry care for all of your clothing and linens gives you the added protection and support needed in today's toxic world that is filled with harsh chemicals and pollutants. Use essential oils in your laundry to keep your health robust and to stay well and happy year-round.

Washer Formula

This formula is suitable for all your washing needs to freshen and sanitize.

To a 5-ml, colored-glass, euro-dropper bottle add:

Lemon: 50 drops

Peppermint: 20 drops

Eucalyptus: 20 drops

Oregano: 10 drops

Close the cap tightly and shake the bottle vigorously to thoroughly blend the essential oils. Allow to synergize for 8 or more hours before using.

Add 3–4 drops of the Washer Formula blend to your laundry detergent at the start of your washing cycle. For those who are allergic to dust mites, eucalyptus globulus may kill dust mites in bedding.

PLEASE NOTE: Excessive use of essential oils in your washer may damage plastic or hard rubber parts.

Dryer Formula

Leaves your clothes and linens smelling fresh and like new.

Lavender: 50 drops

Lemon: 30 drops

Peppermint: 20 drops

Close the cap tightly and shake the bottle vigorously to thoroughly blend the essential oils. Allow to synergize for 8 or more hours before using.

Add 3–4 drops of the dryer blend to a cotton cloth or pad and place in your dryer during the cool down, air fluff or wrinkle release cycle. Lavender oil will give your bedding and towels a clean, fresh scent and promote relaxation and calm, while lemon and peppermint remove greasy and oily smells and grime from your laundry.

Eco-Friendly Cleaning Supplies

Adding essential oils known for their antibacterial and antiviral powers to your dishpan or scrub bucket will kill germs and leave your home and living environments smelling clean and fresh. Eco-friendly cleaning supplies made with pure essential oils also have the added benefit of eliminating odors for pollution-free air that is safer to breathe.

All-Purpose Household Surface Cleaner Formula

Use to clean all surfaces and countertops of grease and grime and to remove oily stains, sticky substances, grime and dirty residue.

To a 5-ml, colored-glass, euro-dropper bottle add:

Lemon: 40 drops

Peppermint: 20 drops

Cypress: 20 drops

Black Pepper: 10 drops

Juniper Berry: 10 drops

Close the cap tightly and shake the bottle vigorously to thoroughly blend the essential oils. Allow to synergize for 8 or more hours before using.

For use as a powerful, general, all-purpose household cleaner, dilute 4–8 drops of the surface cleaner blend in a dish pan or sink filled with warm soapy water and use to clean all surfaces. Wipe down kitchen counters and bathroom surfaces with these cleansing, germicidal oils.

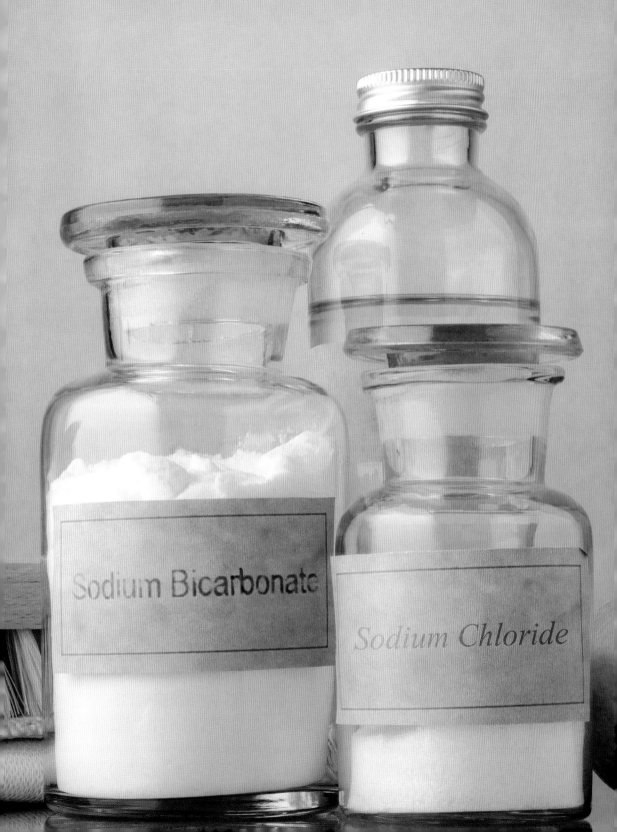

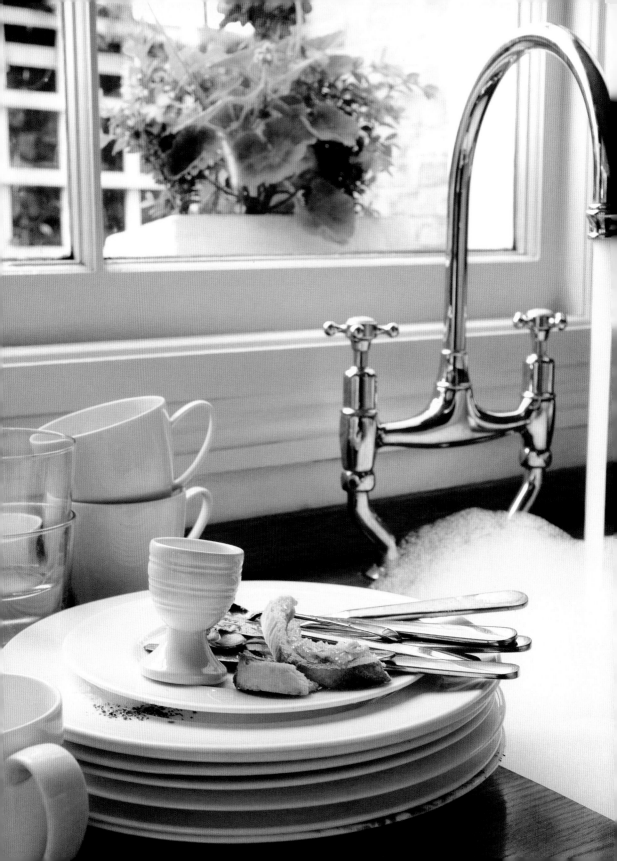

Dish Wash Formula

Use to wash your dishes, to cut grease and remove built-up grime, oily stains, sticky substances and dirty residue.

~~~~~~

To a 5-ml, colored-glass, euro-dropper bottle add:

Lemon: 40 drops

Lavender: 20 drops

Cypress: 20 drops

Tea Tree: 20 drops

Close the cap tightly and shake the bottle vigorously to thoroughly blend the essential oils. Allow to synergize for 8 or more hours before using.

For use as a powerful dish-washing and all-purpose cleansing and germicidal agent, dilute 4–8 drops of the dish wash blend in a dish pan or sink filled with warm soapy water. Use to wash dishes and as a general, all-purpose cleanser. This formula is also great for cleaning stubborn and burnt food particles from pots and pans.

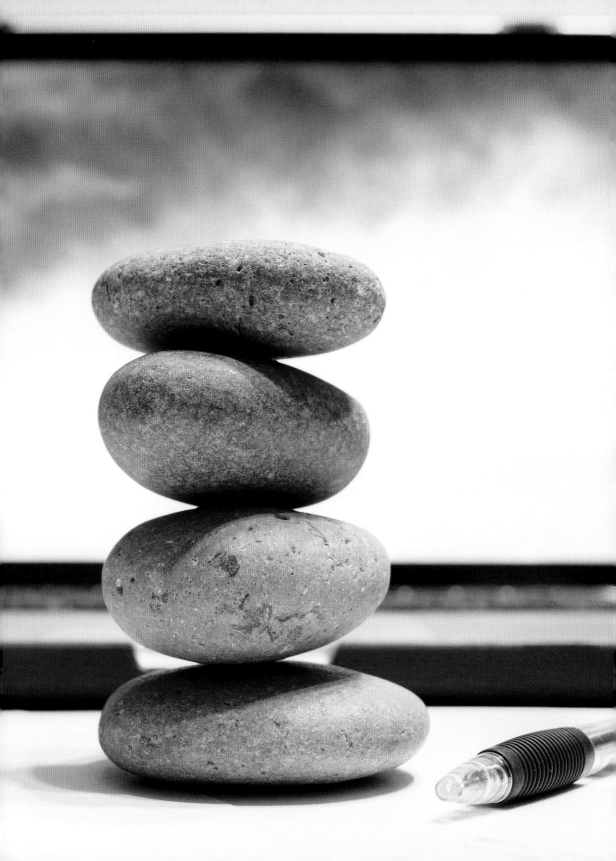

CHAPTER 18

Essential Oils in the Workplace and Daily Life

Introducing Essential Oils into Your Professional Practice, Home or Workplace

When introducing pure essential oils and aromatherapy into your daily life—whether at home, in your professional practice or in your workplace—always remember that less is more. Pure essential oils are extremely concentrated; one drop of pure essential oil is generally equal to 3-4 cups (700-945 ml) of plant matter. Even a drop or two can produce significant and immediate results upon inhalation or application.

Slowly introduce your oils, whether using them for yourself or with others, and observe the response to a single essential oil first before introducing more complex aromatherapy blends.

Listen to and watch for signs of sensitivity or displeasure for a particular scent. An essential oil may have the chemical constituents to produce the desired results, but its aroma may not be well tolerated. Remember the greatest benefits of aromatherapy can be enjoyed simply through inhaling their aroma, so it's essential to choose oils that are enjoyed for their aromatic scent, as well as the benefits of their chemical properties.

As the nose becomes accustomed to a wide spectrum of aromas for enjoyment, the response to different essential oils will change over time. When you are first learning, it's advisable to keep notes in your aromatherapy journal about how you, or someone you are administering essential oils to, is responding and being affected. This will help to expand your knowledge about aromatherapy and discover the best methods of application for obtaining consistently good results in practice. Through keeping an aromatherapy journal you will also develop your intuition for which aromas or blends to use when treating a wide variety of conditions.

Improve Productivity

Productivity, whether at home or work, is a major concern for most of us. We want to make the best and most efficient use of our time to achieve the things we value most and are our top priorities in life. Whether you're a student completing a homework assignment or project, a busy mom caring for your home and family or an executive managing hundreds of employees, the need to be productive is of great importance to you. Productivity is always connected with achieving your bottom line, whatever that might be for you.

Research has shown essential oils help to increase productivity by as much as 54 percent when diffused into the workroom. There are many courses available, and corporations spend thousands of dollars to learn how to become more productive. Essential oils can help you become more productive just by inhaling their scent for a nominal cost.

Improve Productivity Formula

This may be the perfect solution when you need help focusing for prolonged periods on work projects, homework, arts and crafts and various daily routines. Use this blend of stimulating essential oils when you need to focus on a task with your complete attention, as well as to aid memory retention. This formula may also be helpful for children diagnosed with ADD.

To a 5-ml, colored-glass, euro-dropper bottle add:

Peppermint: 50 drops

Lemon: 20 drops

Cinnamon Leaf: 20 drops

Basil: 1–3 drops

Rosemary Verbenone: 1–3 drops

Black Spruce: 1–3 drops

Atlas Cedarwood: 10 drops

Close the cap tightly and shake the bottle vigorously to thoroughly blend the essential oils. Allow to synergize for 8 or more hours before using.

Dispense 1–3 drops on a cotton ball or smell strip and inhale the aromatic vapors of your Improve Productivity Formula blend for 10–15 seconds. You may repeat as needed. This blend may also be effective as an aromatic mist.

To make a ready-to-use Improve Productivity Formula blend that you can wear like a perfume oil, simply add 15–30 drops of your synergy blend to a 1-ounce (30-ml) bottle of your favorite carrier oil. Shake the bottle well to disperse the oils thoroughly. Apply a few drops of your ready-to-use blend to sinus points around your nose and forehead, as well as on the back of your neck.

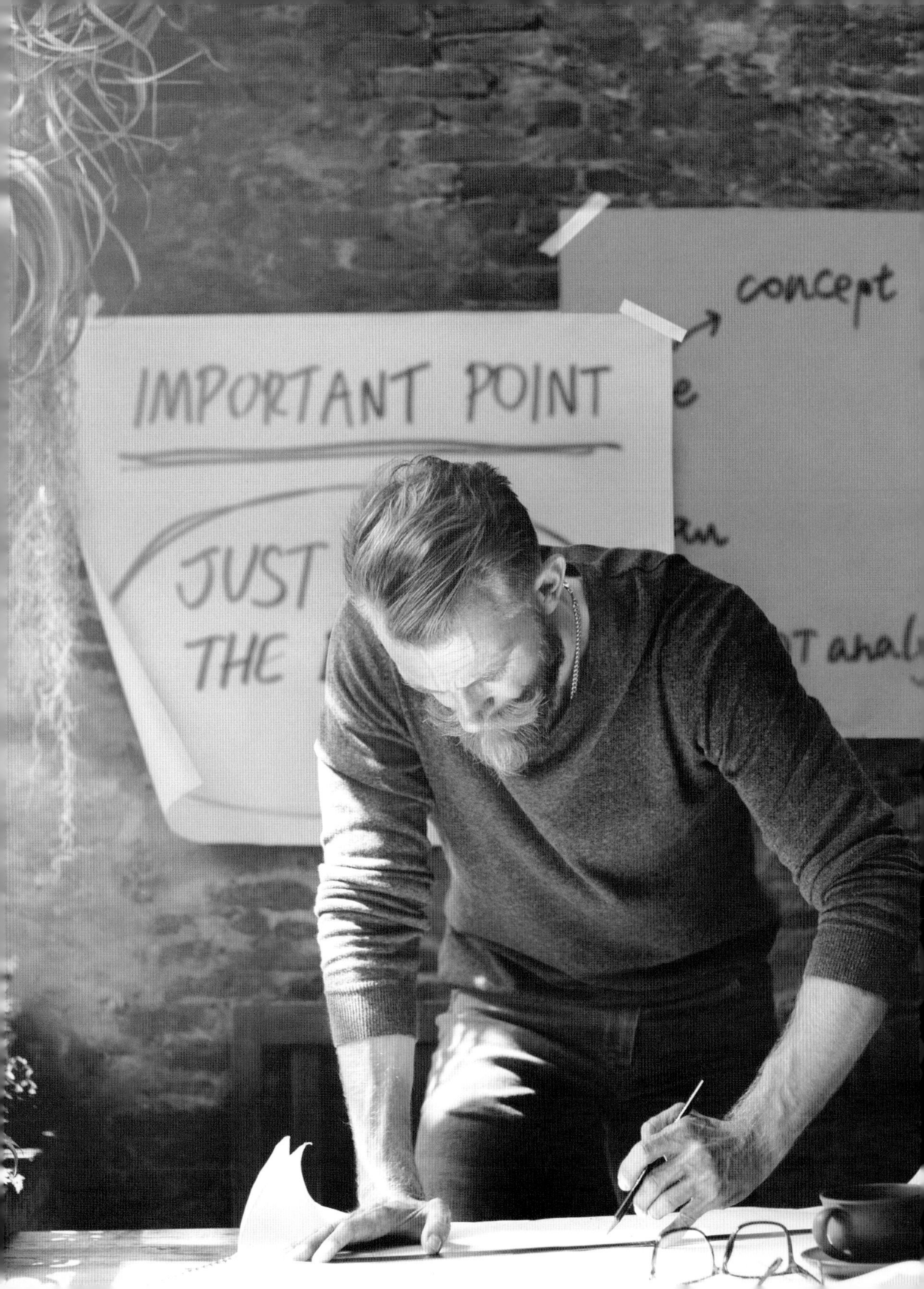
IMPORTANT POINT
JUST
THE
concept

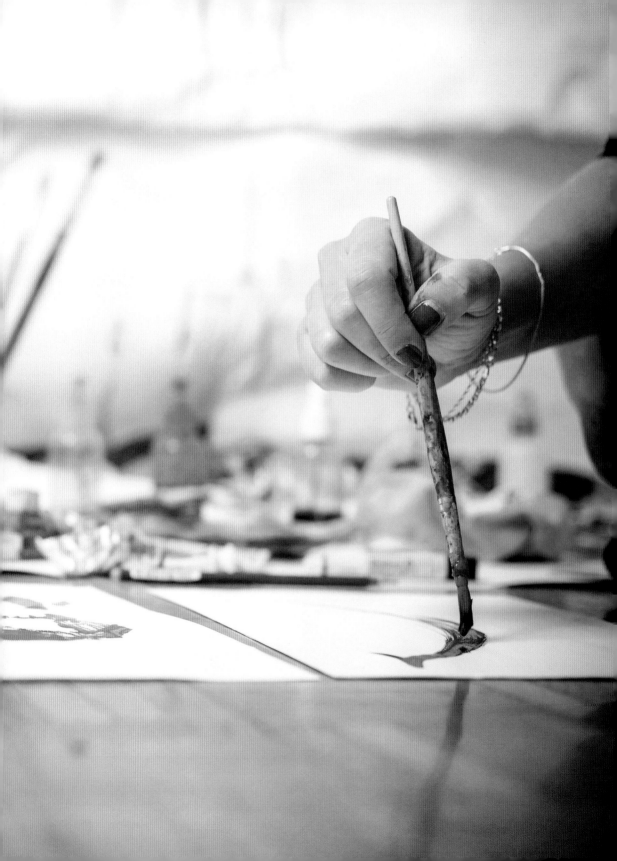

Stimulate Curiosity and Creativity

As children, we seem to have an infinite capacity for being creative and curious about everything. Your favorite word as a child may have been "why." Your "why" is at the heart of taking action to do anything. "Why" is the motivating factor that connects you with the enthusiasm needed for doing anything in life. Find a big enough "why" and you will persevere to overcome any obstacle on the way to accomplishing your goal. If you want to create change in your life circumstances, it is very important that you ask new questions to get different results. In other words, you must be curious about what's not working in your life to begin to see patterns at work that you need to change to get different results. If you keep doing what you've been doing, you'll keep getting the same results. That's great if you are 100 percent happy with your results in life; however, most of us are not.

Another key question to ask when increasing your capacity for creativity and curiosity is the question, "What else could this mean?" Motivation expert Tony Robbins, a master of creating transformation and change, reminds us to ask the question, "What else could this mean?" continually. Research has now shown that we don't see the world as it is, but as we are. We filter out anything that is happening that does not fit into our belief system. So, there you have two of the most important questions to begin asking when working to increase your capacity for curiosity and creativity and to make changes for the better in your life.

Stimulate Curiosity and Creativity Formula

This formula helps to renew your creative drive.

To a 5-ml, colored-glass, euro-dropper bottle add:

Grapefruit: 20 drops

Lemongrass: 40 drops

Palmarosa: 10 drops

Cinnamon Leaf: 10 drops

Spikenard: 10 drops

Frankincense: 10 drops

Black Pepper: 1–3 drops

Close the cap tightly and shake the bottle vigorously to thoroughly blend the essential oils. Allow to synergize for 8 or more hours before using.

Dispense 1–3 drops on a cotton ball or smell strip and inhale the aromatic vapors of your Stimulate Curiosity and Creativity Formula blend for 10–15 seconds. You may repeat as needed. This blend may also be effective as an aromatic mist.

To make a ready-to-use blend you can wear like a perfume oil, simply add 15–30 drops of your synergy blend to a 1-ounce (30-ml) bottle of your favorite carrier oil. Shake the bottle well to disperse the oils thoroughly. Apply a few drops of your ready-to-use blend to sinus points around your nose and forehead, as well as on the back of your neck.

Focus Support and Pay Attention Formula

Essential oils can help you to develop your ability to control the focus of your attention and shift into a positive emotional state at will.

Most educators and psychologists agree that your ability to focus on a task without distraction and pay attention is absolutely essential for achieving your goals.

A study conducted on 232 pairs of twins showed there was a direct correlation between temperament (frequency and intensity of temper tantrums, crying, moodiness and demanding attention) and attention span. The study showed that the twin with the most ability for absorption of an activity was much less temperamental.

Another study of 2,600 children also showed that "early exposure to television (around age two) was associated with later attention issues such as impulsiveness, disorganization and distractibility at age seven."

To a 5-ml, colored-glass, euro-dropper bottle add:

Peppermint: 40 drops

Rosemary: 1–2 drops

Lemon: 40 drops (or 80 drops if you don't want to use peppermint in your recipe)

Basil: 1–2 drops

Cedarwood: 20 drops

Close the cap tightly and shake the bottle vigorously to thoroughly blend the essential oils. Allow to synergize for 8 or more hours before using.

ADULT DIRECTIONS

Dispense 1–3 drops on a smell strip, cotton ball or tissue and inhale.

This blend may also be used in a diffuser and diffused into a room.

Use your Focus Support and Pay Attention Formula as needed for focus support, to pay attention and to stay alert naturally.

CHILDREN DIRECTIONS

Allow children to self-select the oils to use alone or in a synergy blend. Pure essential oils may be too strong for their sensitive nervous systems, and you may wish to dilute the oils to 1–10 percent in a vegetable carrier oil like pure fractionated coconut oil.

CAUTION: Research indicates that peppermint oil may aggravate GERD (gastro esophageal reflux disease), a type of heartburn. Due to its strong cooling action, peppermint should not be used by children under two and a half years of age.

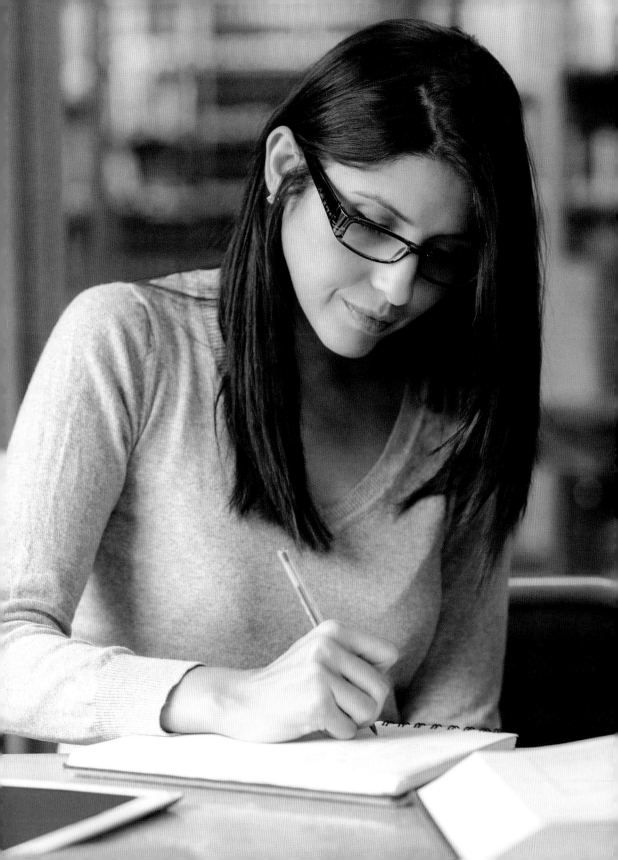

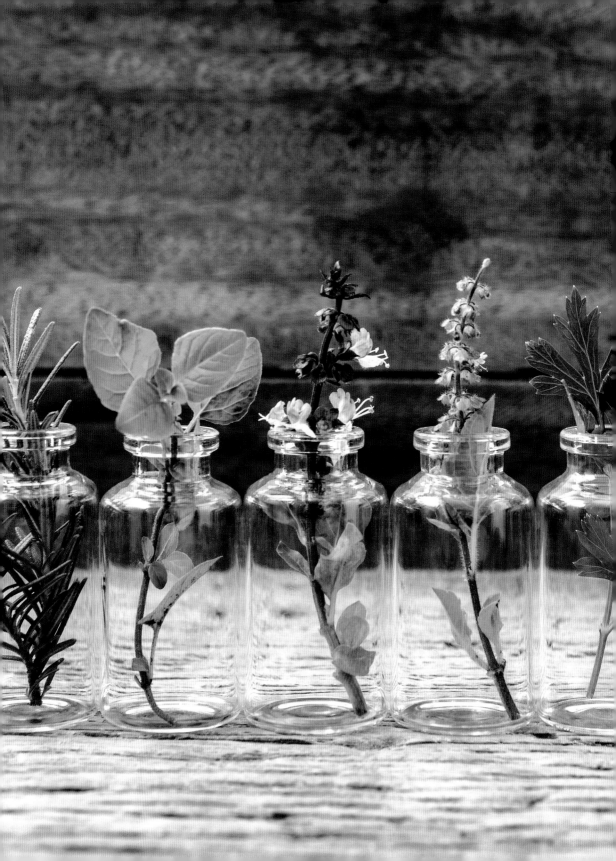

CHAPTER 19

Cooking with Essential Oils

Culinary Wellness Oils and Blends

COOKING WITH ESSENTIAL OILS FOR HEALTH AND WELL-BEING

Pure essential oils have a wide range of therapeutic uses and benefits. With a little practice, you'll be able to incorporate essential oils into every aspect of your everyday healthy lifestyle, including all of your cooking and baking needs. By doing so, you'll not only benefit from the healing properties of the oils to support your health and well-being, but also enjoy the flavorful difference cooking with essential oils can impart to all of your cuisine.

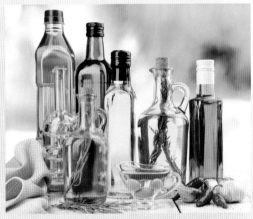

Essential oils can be an integral and flavorful component of your healthy lifestyle.

Essential Oils for Your Culinary Cabinet

- Peppermint
- Lemon
- Cinnamon
- Clove
- Ginger
- Nutmeg
- Sweet orange
- Lime
- Lemongrass
- Lavender
- Black pepper
- Sweet basil

- Sweet marjoram
- Rosemary verbenone
- Oregano
- Cardamom
- Coriander
- Cumin
- Cassia
- Holy basil
- Turmeric
- Sage
- Thyme

As essential oils are very concentrated, it's useful to make particular blends to impart the flavor you want for a dish, rather than individual single oils.

Here are a few culinary blends to get you started.

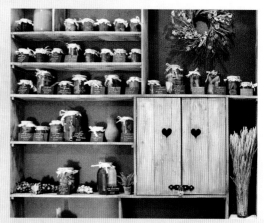

Culinary blends are a safe, easy and effective way to use your essential oils for all of your cooking and baking needs.

Italian Blend

Experience a memorable renaissance of sweet, spicy, full-bodied and intense flavor and aroma with this blend of oils. Plus, enjoy all the health benefits of powerful antimicrobial action these oils impart.

Makes 100 individual servings

To a 5-ml, colored-glass, euro-dropper bottle add:

Sweet Basil: 20 drops

Sweet Marjoram: 10 drops

Oregano: 30 drops

Rosemary: 20 drops

Thyme: 20 drops

Close the cap tightly and shake the bottle vigorously to thoroughly blend the essential oils. Allow to synergize for 8 or more hours before using. Add 1–3 drops at the end of the cooking process (if possible). This may replace all or a portion of the herbs and spices you usually use in your dish.

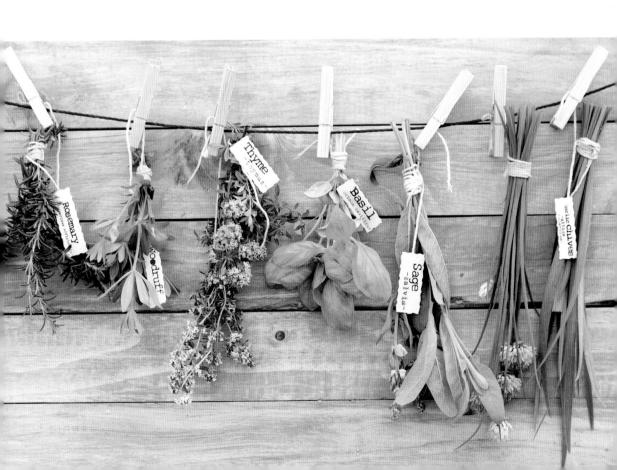

Thai Pepper Lemongrass Blend

For those who love flavorful Thai-style cooking with its spicy heat and lemongrass appeal, this intensely flavorful blend is sure to please. These oils will refresh and stimulate and leave you feeling satisfied.

Makes 100 individual servings

~~~~~~

To a 5-ml, colored-glass, euro-dropper bottle add:

Holy Basil: 15 drops

Lemongrass: 15 drops

Lime: 15 drops

Ginger: 15 drops

Peppermint: 15 drops

Black Pepper: 15 drops, or more (more makes the blend spicier)

Cumin: 5 drops

Close the cap tightly and shake the bottle vigorously to thoroughly blend the essential oils. Allow to synergize for 8 or more hours before using. Add 1–3 drops, to taste, at the end of the cooking process (if possible). This may replace all or a portion of the herbs and spices you usually use in your dish.

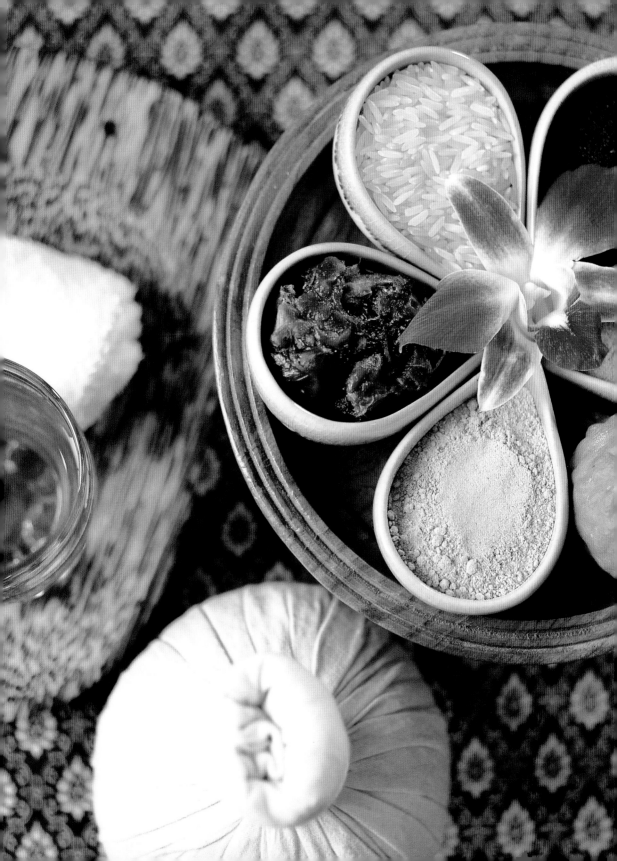

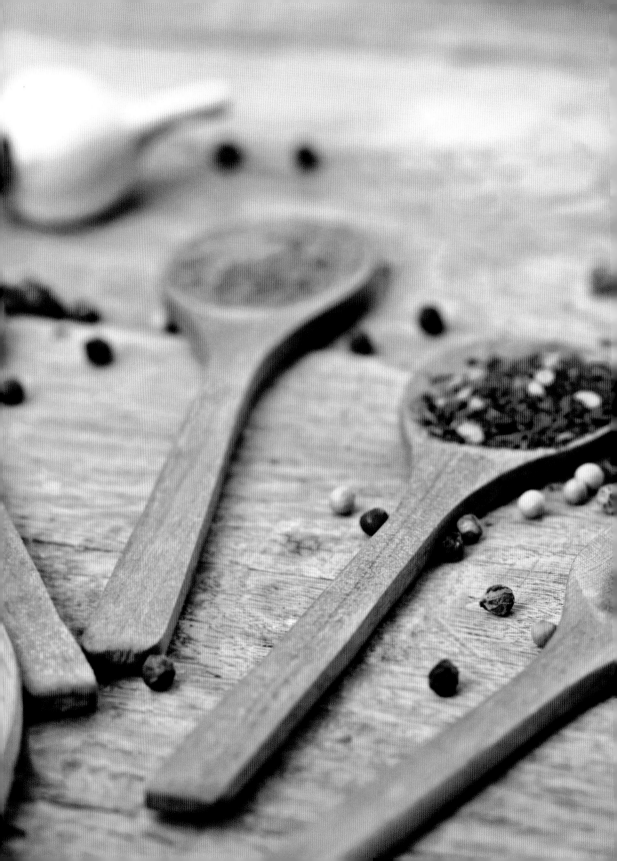

Indian Spice Blend

A vibrant, inspired blend infused with a mix of sweet and fragrant spice oils that will make your Indian dishes famous among your friends. This blend contains powerful germ-killing essential oils.

Makes 100 individual servings

~~~~~~

To a 5-ml, colored-glass, euro-dropper bottle add:

Holy Basil: **20 drops**

Coriander: **10 drops**

Cumin: **5 drops**

Cardamon: **10 drops**

Clove: **5 drops**

Cinnamon: **10 drops**

Black Pepper: **20 drops**

Turmeric: **10 drops**

Ginger: **10 drops**

Close the cap tightly and shake the bottle vigorously to thoroughly blend the essential oils. Allow to synergize for 8 or more hours before using. Add 1–3 drops, to taste, at the end of the cooking process (if possible). This may replace all or a portion of the herbs and spices you usually use in your dish.

Mexican Spice Blend

A satisfying blend of herbal and spice oils with a hint of lime that gives this blend authentic homemade Mexican flavor and aroma. A refreshing blend with all the health of these oils, including powerful antiseptic action.

Makes 100 individual servings

To a 5-ml, colored-glass, euro-dropper bottle add:

Lime: **25 drops**

Cumin: **25 drops**

Black Pepper: **40 drops**

Turmeric: **5 drops**

Thyme: **5 drops**

Close the cap tightly and shake the bottle vigorously to thoroughly blend the essential oils. Allow to synergize for 8 or more hours before using. Add 1–3 drops, to taste, at the end of the cooking process (if possible). This may replace all or a portion of the herbs and spices you usually use in your dish.

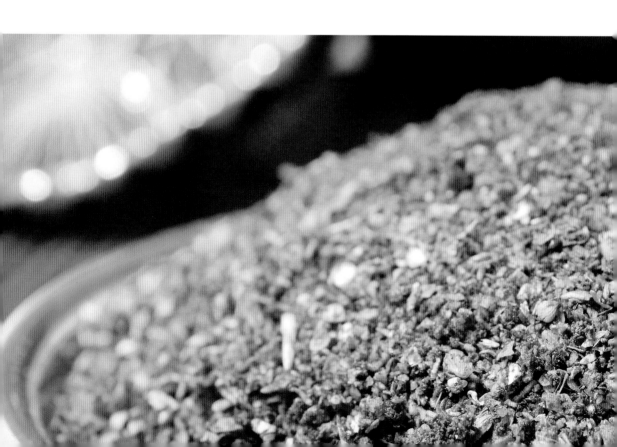

Greek Spice Blend

This aromatic blend of flavors will make your Mediterranean dishes sing with all the romance and exciting flavors of a Grecian island. Plus, enjoy the multitude of health benefits of these oils, including powerful antibacterial action.

Makes 100 individual servings

To a 5-ml, colored-glass, euro-dropper bottle add:

Sweet Basil: 20 drops

Oregano: 20 drops

Cinnamon: 10 drops

Black Pepper: 10 drops

Rosemary: 10 drops

Sweet Marjoram: 15 drops

Thyme: 10 drops

Nutmeg: 5 drops

Close the cap tightly and shake the bottle vigorously to thoroughly blend the essential oils. Allow to synergize for 8 or more hours before using. Add 1–3 drops, to taste, at the end of the cooking process (if possible). This may replace all or a portion of the herbs and spices you usually use in your dish.

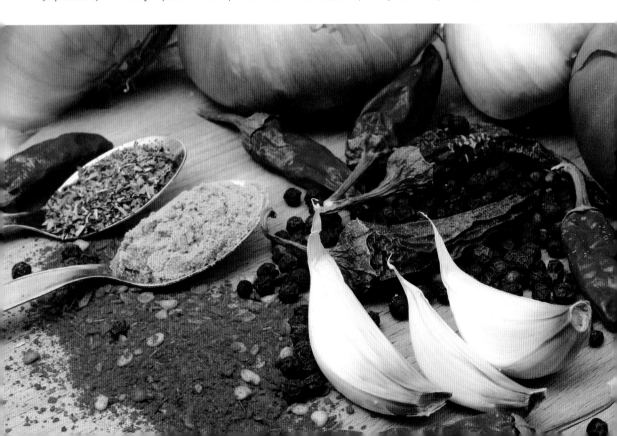

Citrus and Spice Blend

A medley of bold, exotic flavors adds a sweet and savory balance that will brighten and refresh any palate. This is probably the most potent of all the culinary blends with both citrus and spice that taste delicious.

Makes 100 individual servings

To a 5-ml, colored-glass, euro-dropper bottle add:

Sweet Orange: 20 drops

Lime: 10 drops

Lemon: 15 drops

Cinnamon Leaf: 20 drops

Clove: 10 drops

Cassia: 10 drops

Ginger: 10 drops

Nutmeg: 5 drops

Close the cap tightly and shake the bottle vigorously to thoroughly blend the essential oils. Allow to synergize for 8 or more hours before using. Add 1–3 drops, to taste, at the end of the cooking process (if possible). This may replace all or a portion of the herbs and spices you usually use in your dish.

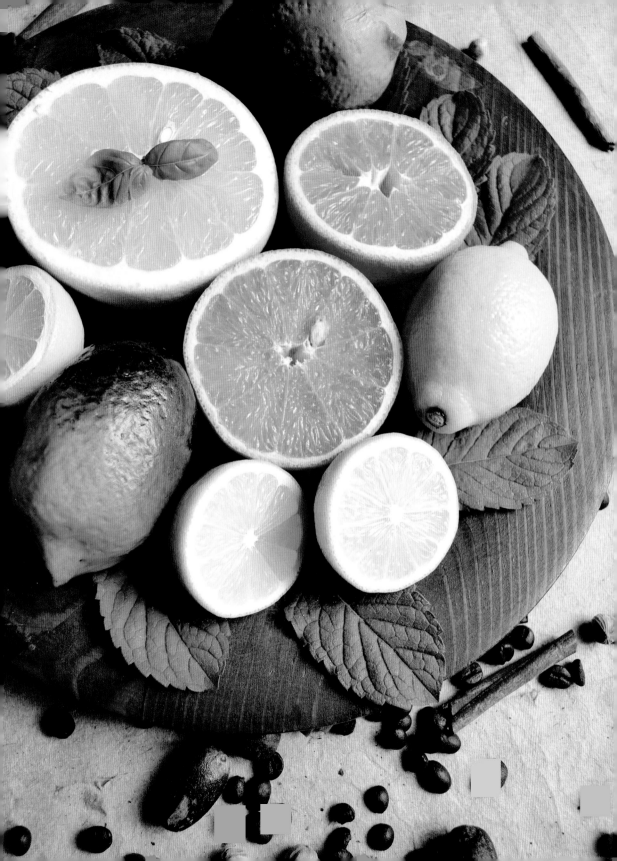

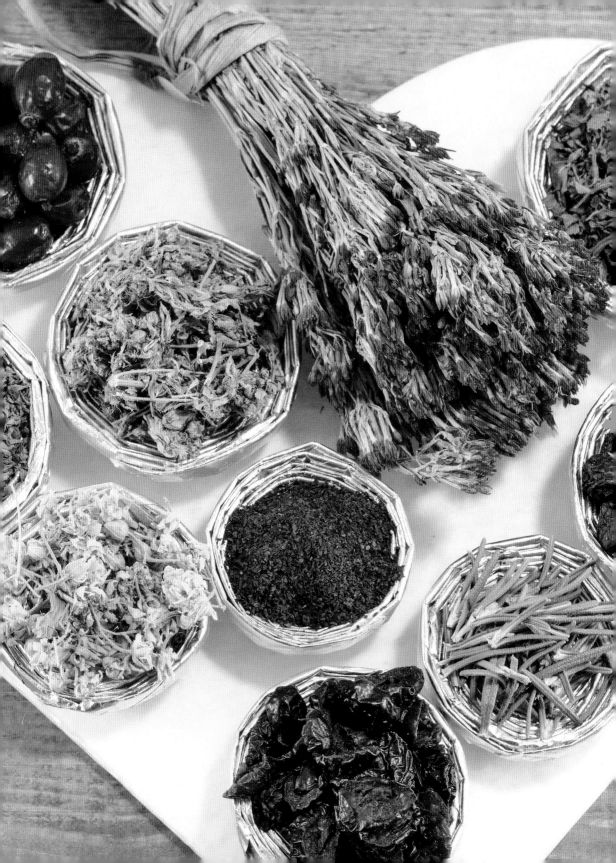

All-Purpose Herbal Blend

Enjoy the freshness of this classic herbal blend that's filled with the warm and inviting goodness of spice and umami, reminiscent of fresh picked herbs from your summer garden. This blend carries all-purpose antimicrobial action for your health.

Makes 100 individual servings

~~~~~~

To a 5-ml, colored-glass, euro-dropper bottle add:

Sweet Basil: 20 drops

Black Pepper: 20 drops

Rosemary: 5 drops

Sweet Marjoram: 10 drops

Coriander: 20 drops

Cumin: 5 drops

Thyme: 5 drops

Turmeric: 10 drops

Sage: 5 drops

Close the cap tightly and shake the bottle vigorously to thoroughly blend the essential oils. Allow to synergize for 8 or more hours before using. Add 1–3 drops, to taste, at the end of the cooking process. This may replace all or a portion of the herbs you usually use in your dish.

Breakfast and Brunch Recipes

These breakfast and brunch recipes are easy, delicious and nutritious.

Zucchini Citrus and Spice Muffins

This moist, sweet and tangy creation is packed with vegetable goodness. It is wonderful alone to brighten your morning or as a late night snack. The Citrus and Spice Blend contains excellent digestive aids and the citrus oils lend additional tart appeal for a truly delightful culinary experience.

Makes 6 large muffins

½ tsp light coconut oil

2 medium zucchinis, grated

⅓ cup (80 ml) raw honey

⅔ cup (160 ml) pure maple syrup

⅔ cup (160 ml) coconut oil

2–4 drops Citrus and Spice Blend (page 360)

2 tsp (10 ml) pure vanilla extract

2 large eggs, beaten

1½ cups (180 g) whole-wheat flour

1½ cups (190 g) all-purpose flour, sifted

1 tsp baking powder

1 tsp baking soda

½ tsp salt

Preheat the oven to 350°F (177°C). Lightly grease a six-muffin tin with light coconut oil and set aside. Grate the zucchinis with the side of your grater that has the largest holes; set aside.

In a large bowl, blend together the honey, maple syrup and coconut oil with the essential oil blend, vanilla and eggs. In a small bowl, blend together the flours, baking powder, baking soda and salt. Add the flour mixture to the egg mixture, and stir to combine. Stir in the grated zucchini. To keep the muffins moist, do not over mix.

Pour the batter into the oiled muffin tin, and spread the batter evenly. Bake 20–25 minutes, until the muffin tops are golden brown, springy to the touch and a toothpick inserted in the center comes out clean. Cool the muffins in the pan before removing. They are moist and flavorful eaten alone or can be enjoyed spread with butter and your favorite jam.

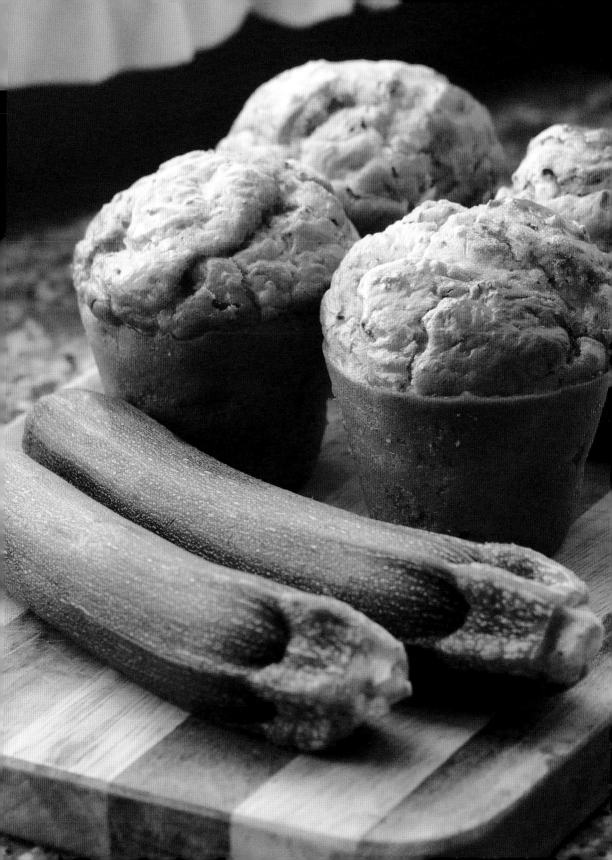

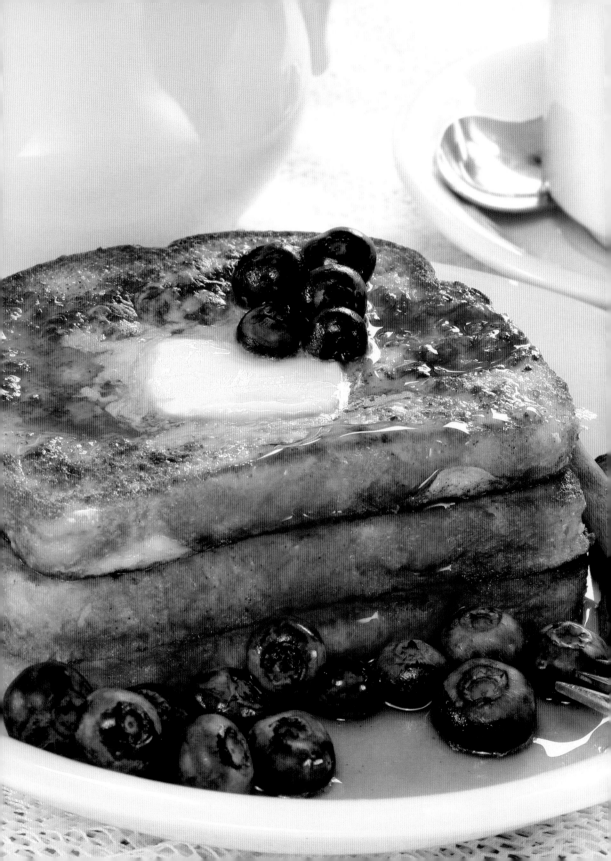

Quick and Easy Cinnamon French Toast

Pure vanilla extract and cinnamon essential oil add a memorable rich flavor to French toast. Use your favorite bread: white, whole-wheat, French or Italian. Enjoy all the health benefits of your essential oils. Remember the Citrus and Spice Blend is very potent with antimicrobial action.

Makes 4 servings

1 egg, beaten

1 tsp pure vanilla extract

Cinnamon essential oil (or Citrus and Spice Blend [page 360])

¼ cup (60 ml) milk

4 slices bread

Pure maple syrup

In small bowl, beat the egg, vanilla and essential oil together. Whisk in the milk. Next, dip the bread slice in the egg mixture, turning to coat both sides evenly.

Cook the bread slices on a lightly oiled griddle or skillet on medium heat until browned on both sides. Serve with pure maple syrup.

Lunch Recipes

For midday nutrition that's light and easy, soup is one of the most nutritious, delicious and satisfying meals for lunch. These two recipes are quick and easy to make and packed full of flavor. You can make both of these soup dishes ahead, refrigerate and warm them for your lunch the next day.

Thai Pepper Soup

If you're feeling chilled to the bone, this soup will warm you through and put a smile on your face. Plus all the health benefits and potent antimicrobial action to keep you healthy and enjoying life. Very yummy!

Makes 4 servings

2 (12-oz [355-ml]) jars roasted red peppers

1 large onion, chopped

2 tsp (6 g) garlic, minced

1 small jalapeño pepper, seeded and chopped

1 (14.5-oz [430-ml]) can tomatoes

1 (13.5-oz [400-ml]) can coconut milk

½ tbsp (7 ml) honey

1–3 drops Thai Pepper Lemongrass Blend (page 354)

½ tsp salt, optional

In a large pot (or crock pot) add the roasted red peppers (fluid and all), onion, garlic, jalapeño, tomatoes, coconut milk, honey and Thai Pepper Lemongrass Blend. Bring the soup to a low simmer on medium-low heat for 30–45 minutes, until it's completely heated and the flavors are blended.

Pour the soup through a strainer into a bowl to remove the vegetable pieces. Place the remaining liquid back into the soup pot. Add the vegetables to a food processor or blender and purée. Pour the puréed vegetables back into the soup pot and stir to blend the flavors together. Ladle the soup into bowls and serve warm. Season with salt if desired. Enjoy with warm rolls or a fresh salad.

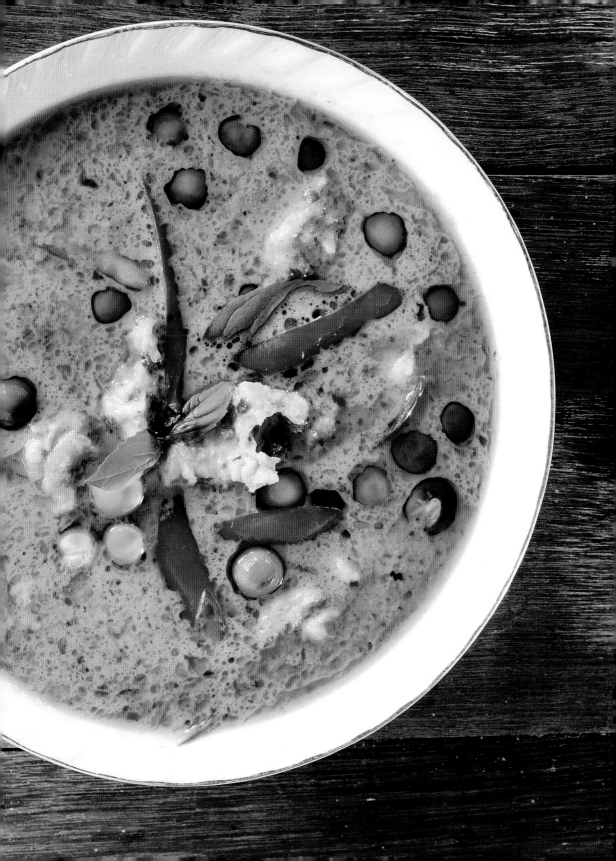

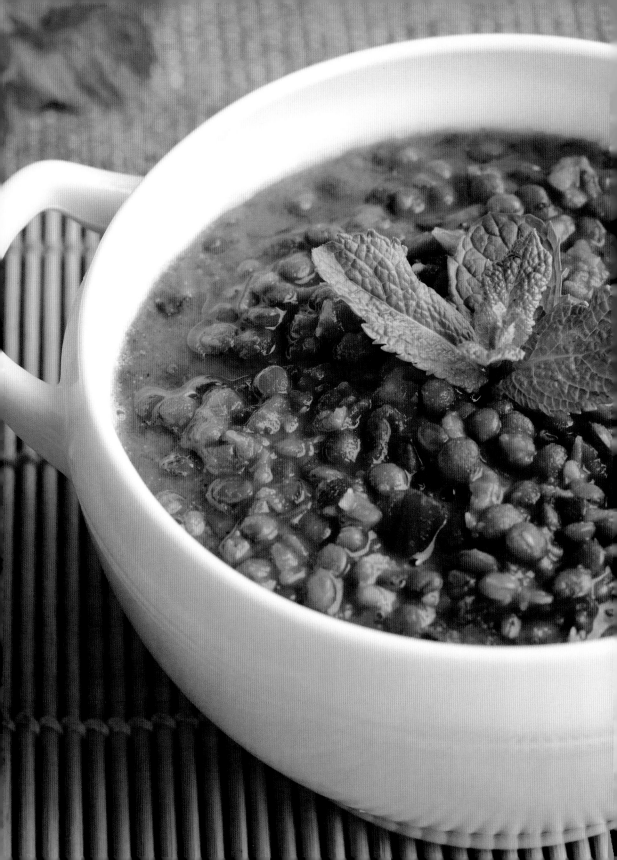

French Lentil Soup

This soup uses the small, green, Puy lentils that are claimed to have gastronomic qualities. These small, green lentils come from the region of Le Puy in France and are protected throughout the European union. Puy lentils hold their shape much better than the more familiar brown lentils that tend to fall apart during the cooking process. Puy lentils have a characteristic peppery flavor, cook quickly and are delicious. The warm, spicy and memorable medley of flavors will stimulate your appetite and satisfy your need for nourishment.

Makes 6 servings

2 cups (400 g) small French green lentils, soaked for 45 minutes

2 dozen baby carrots

1 medium onion, sliced

2 stalks celery, sliced

4 medium potatoes, chopped

3 medium broccoli buds, sliced

1–3 drops All-Purpose Herbal Blend (page 363) or Italian Blend (page 353)

1–2 tbsp (15–30 g) Celtic salt, or to taste

In a heavy soup pot (or crock pot), cook the pre-soaked French lentils in 6–8 cups (1.4–1.9 L) of water. Less water makes a thicker soup. Bring to a slow, simmering boil on medium-low heat. Then lower the heat and allow the lentils to maintain a steady simmer for 30 minutes, stirring occasionally, until the lentils are soft and the soup is beginning to thicken slightly. Add the washed and prepared veggies. Allow the soup to come to a simmering boil. Then turn off the heat and let the soup rest for 5 minutes.

At the end of the cooking process, just before serving, add the essential oil blend and season with salt. Let the soup rest for another 5 minutes before serving. Serve as a main dish with some crusty sourdough bread and a fresh green salad. This soup makes for wonderful quick and yummy leftovers for lunch the next day.

Appetizers

The importance of creating just the right appetizers for your main course cannot be overstated. These tempting recipes will stimulate your appetite and set the mood for what's to come for your entire meal.

Pita and Hummus Dip

A Mediterranean specialty that's sweet, tart and savory; and sure to please every palate. Superb as a side dish or alone as a quick and healthy snack between meals. Delight your palate with the Greek Spice Blend, with oils known for their potent antimicrobial action.

Makes 4 servings

4 pita pockets, cut into triangles

1 (12-oz [340-g]) can chickpeas

1 cup (170 g) red peppers, sautéed

¼ cup (55 g) raw tahini

1–3 drops Greek Spice Blend (page 359)

3–4 cloves fresh garlic

2 tbsp (2 g) cilantro, finely chopped

Preheat the oven to 400°F (205°C). Place the pita triangles on a large baking sheet prepared with olive oil. Bake 5–7 minutes, until light golden brown and not too crisp.

Rinse and drain the can of chickpeas. Place the drained chickpeas in a blender and add the sautéed red peppers, tahini, 1–3 drops of the Greek Spice Blend and garlic cloves. Blend until smooth. Season to taste with salt, if desired.

Transfer the hummus to a dish and top with cilantro. Serve with toasted pita triangles arranged alongside.

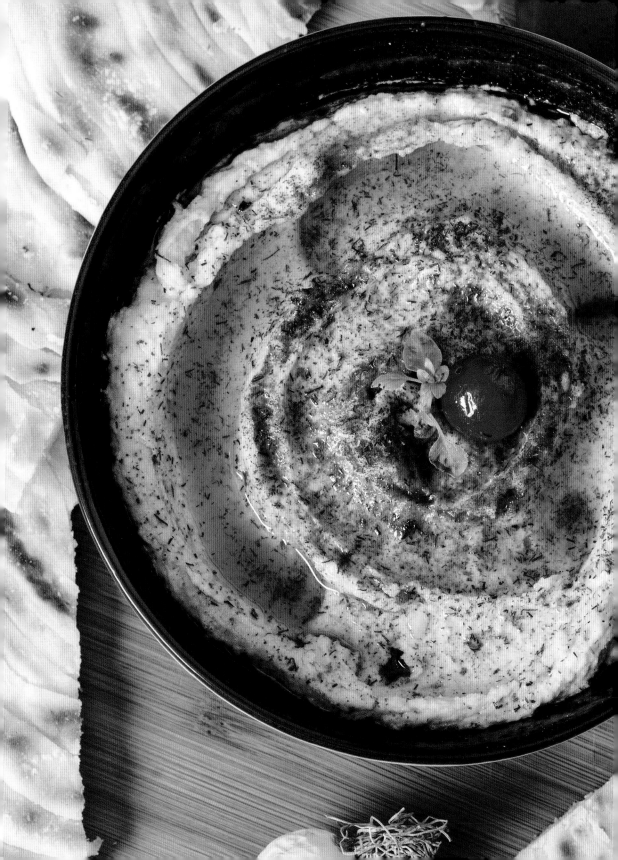

Avocado Crostini

These bright, flavorful and tasty nibbles are perfect before dinner. A creamy, crunchy treat full of spice that's sure to please. Plus the healthy goodness of your essential oils.

Makes 4–6 servings

1 French baguette, cut into ¼-inch (0.6-cm) rounds

4 avocados, medium-ripe, peeled and pitted

2 tbsp (2 g) fresh cilantro, finely chopped

2 oz (55 g) fresh goat cheese

1–3 drops Italian Blend (page 353)

1 scallion, fresh and finely chopped

½ jalapeño pepper, seeded and minced

1 clove garlic, fresh and minced

Salt, to taste

½ cup (80 g) cherry tomatoes, chopped

Preheat the oven to 400°F (205°C). Put the baguette rounds on a baking sheet prepared with oil and toast until lightly golden, 2–4 minutes. Remove from the oven.

Place the avocado in a blender, along with the cilantro, goat cheese, spice blend, scallion, jalapeño pepper and garlic. Blend together until smooth. Season to taste with salt, if desired. Optionally, you can use a fork to mash the ingredients together until blended.

Scoop the avocado mixture onto the baguette rounds and garnish with chopped cherry tomatoes.

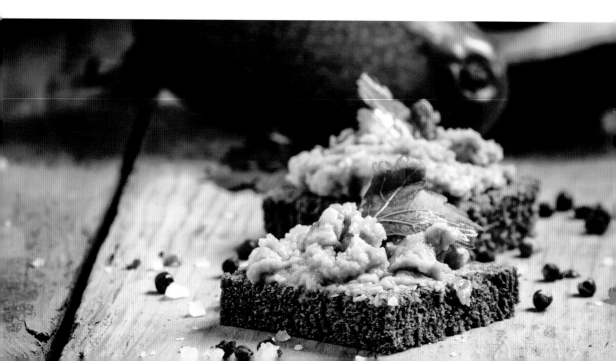

Dinner Recipes

Dinner is the guest of honor at your meal. It is the heart and soul that nourishes and sustains body and mind.

Angel Hair Pasta with Spicy Shrimp

A favorite among pasta lovers, filled with satisfying, buttery sweetness and spice that's round and smooth to the palate. Plus all the fun and healthy goodness of your essential oils, made with love and sure to satisfy.

Makes 4 servings

~~~~~~

12 oz (340 g) angel hair pasta

1 tbsp (15 ml) olive oil

2 cloves garlic, finely chopped

1 lb (455 g) medium shrimp, peeled and deveined

¾ cup (177 ml) dry white wine

Kosher salt (optional)

2 tbsp (43 g) butter

1–3 drops Indian Spice Blend (page 357)

Cook the angel hair pasta according to the directions on the package. Drain and return the pasta to the pot. Heat the olive oil in a large skillet over medium-low heat. Add the garlic to the skillet, stirring until soft, about 1 minute (do not let it brown). Add the shrimp, wine and salt, if desired, to taste. Simmer until the shrimp become opaque, 2–3 minutes. Then stir in the butter and Indian Spice Blend. Finally, toss the pasta and shrimp mixture together. Serve with a fresh green salad and warm baguette.

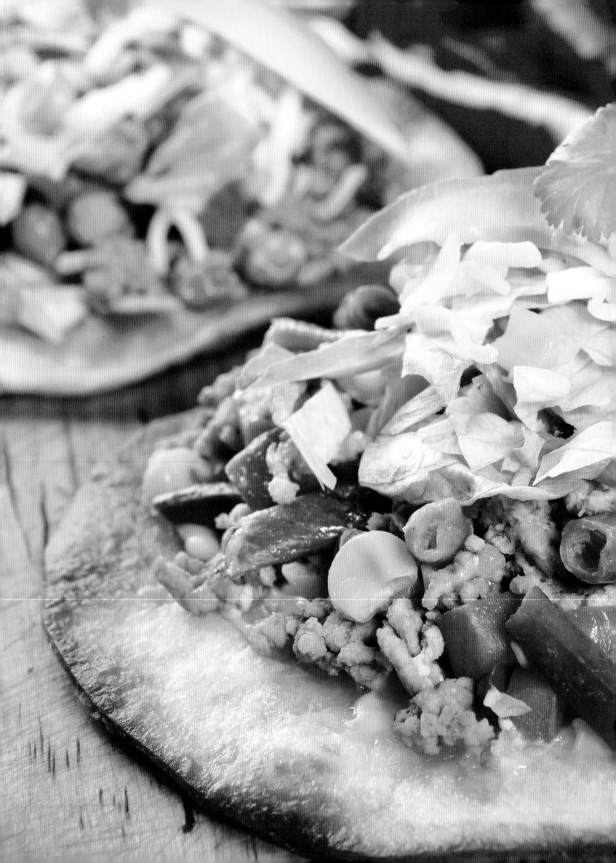

Roasted Vegetable and Refried Bean Tostadas

These vegetarian-inspired Mexican tostadas are rich with hot spicy flavor and texture that will titillate and satisfy your senses. Packed with all the wholesome benefits of essential oils to stimulate digestion and naturally strengthen your immune system.

Makes 4 servings

4 tbsp (60 ml) olive oil

10 oz (285 g) Champignon mushrooms, cleaned and quartered

2 medium zucchinis, thinly sliced

2 red bell peppers, cut into 1½-inch (3.8-cm) pieces

1–3 drops Mexican Spice Blend (page 358)

Kosher salt, optional

8 corn tortillas

1 (15-oz [425-g]) can refried beans

4 oz (115 g) cheddar cheese, grated

Sour cream

Cilantro, fresh chopped

Hot salsa, fresh or from a jar

Preheat the oven to 450°F (232°C). In a large pan, add 2 tablespoons (30 ml) of olive oil and warm over medium-low heat. When the oil is warmed, add the mushrooms, zucchini, red bell peppers and Mexican Spice Blend. Sauté the vegetables until they reach your desired tenderness (5–15 minutes). At the end of the cooking process, season to taste with salt if desired. Transfer the cooked vegetables to a medium bowl. You can substitute any vegetable in the recipe if you like.

Place the tortillas on baking sheets prepared with olive oil. Brush the tortillas lightly with the remaining olive oil, and then spread with refried beans and sprinkle with cheddar. Bake until the beans are warmed through and the cheddar is melted, about 5–10 minutes. Top with sautéed vegetables, sour cream, cilantro and salsa.

Salad Dressings

A variety of pleasing aromas and flavors sure to please and gracefully enhance your salad.

Italian Dressing

Classic Italian dressing that's rich with flavor and packed with savory sweetness. Tastes like freshly picked herbs from your garden. The oils are not only delicious, but full of antibacterial properties to nourish and build your immune system, as well as stimulate your digestion.

Makes 4-6 servings

6 tbsp (90 ml) extra virgin olive oil

2 tbsp (30 ml) red or white wine vinegar

2 medium cloves fresh garlic, chopped

2 tbsp (5 g) fresh parsley, chopped

1 tsp dried basil, crumbled

¼ tsp dried crushed red pepper

1 drop Italian Blend (page 353)

Salt, to taste (optional)

In a small bowl, combine all the ingredients and whisk together. Season to taste with salt, if desired. You can prepare this ahead of time and keep it in a sealed jar in the refrigerator.

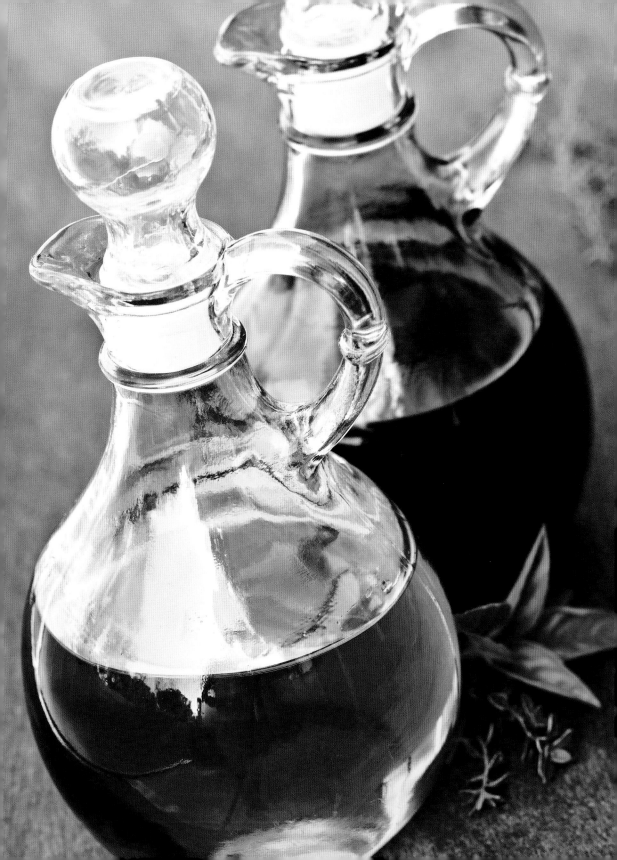

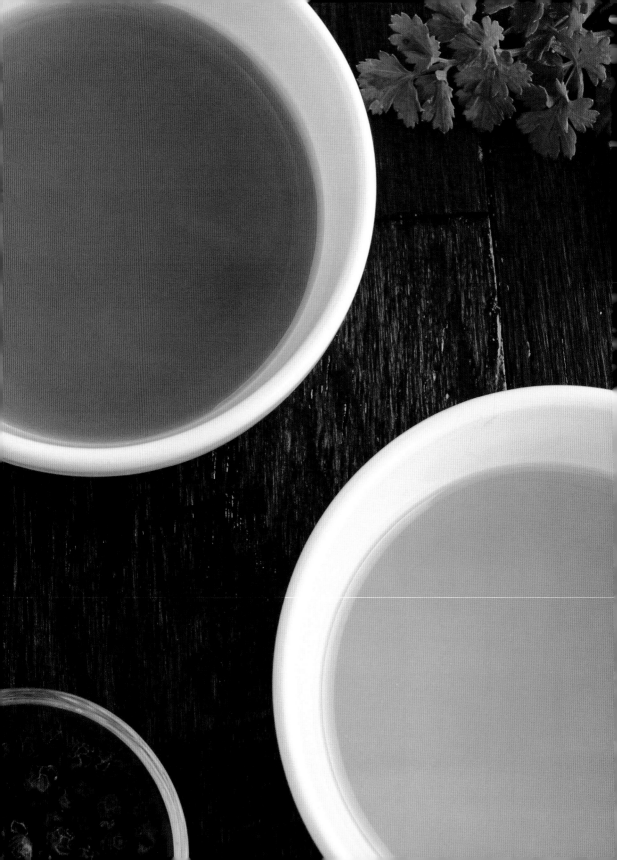

Sweet and Sour Dressing

Delicious sweet and sour flavors blend harmoniously for a delightful Asian-inspired dressing to use with your favorite dishes and salads. Plus all the numerous health benefits of essential oils, including antimicrobial action.

Makes 4–6 servings

6 tbsp (90 ml) extra virgin olive oil

2 tbsp (30 ml) red wine vinegar

¼ tsp honey

¼ tsp grated onion

⅛ tsp celery seed

⅛ tsp dry mustard

⅛ tsp paprika

1 drop Thai Pepper Lemongrass Blend (page 354)

Salt, to taste

Combine all the ingredients in a jar, shake well and chill in the refrigerator. Shake before serving. Pour on top of your favorite tossed salad greens or raw vegetables and serve.

Drinks and Beverages

The easiest way to use essential oils to flavor your drinks and beverages is simply to add a drop of a single oil or a blend of oils into some sort of carrier like a teaspoon of honey or maple syrup. Then stir into a hot or cold beverage like water, tea or milk to enjoy a refreshing break in your day.

The essential oils most often used for making a hot drink are peppermint, fresh ginger root, cinnamon leaf and lemon.

Here are a few recipes to get you started using essential oils in your beverages and drinks.

Lemongrass Black Tea

A surprisingly fresh infusion of lemongrass smooths the bitterness of black tea, adding lift that inspires, like a beautiful bouquet of flavors. Great as a morning brew before work or for an afternoon break in your day. Lemongrass oil has a regulating and tonic action on your body, mind and emotions.

Makes 100 1-cup (237-ml) servings

½ lb (227 g) black tea
10 drops lemongrass essential oil

Put your favorite black tea in a glass container that has a tight fitting lid, or you can use tea bags if you prefer. Dispense 10 drops of lemongrass oil on a paper towel and lay on top of your loose black tea or tea bags. Seal the jar with the tight-fitting lid and leave for 7 days. The scent of lemongrass will be absorbed into the tea leaves. After 7 days, remove the paper towel, prepare and serve your tea as you like it and enjoy.

Keep your lemongrass-scented black tea sealed tightly and store in a cool, dry place like a cupboard. If stored properly, scented tea will usually last up to 6 months.

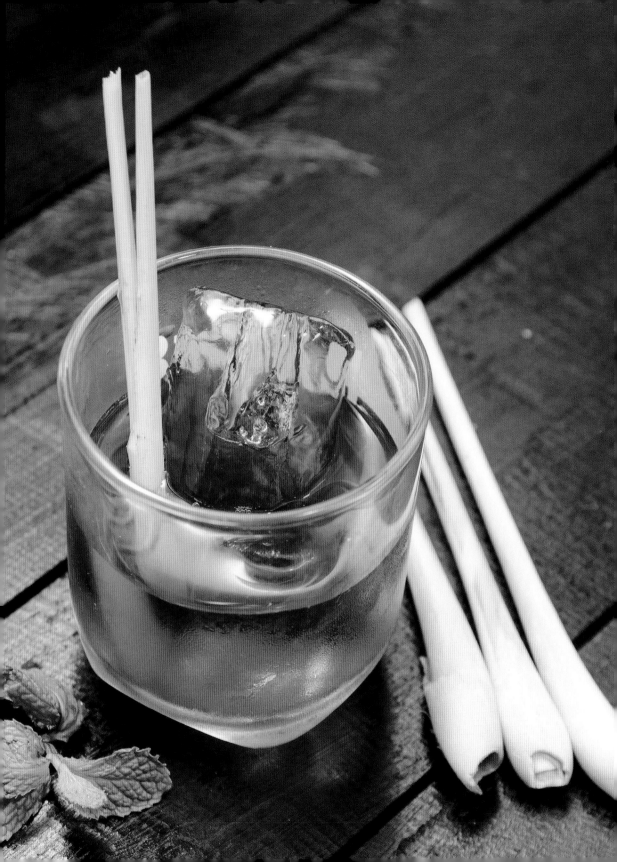

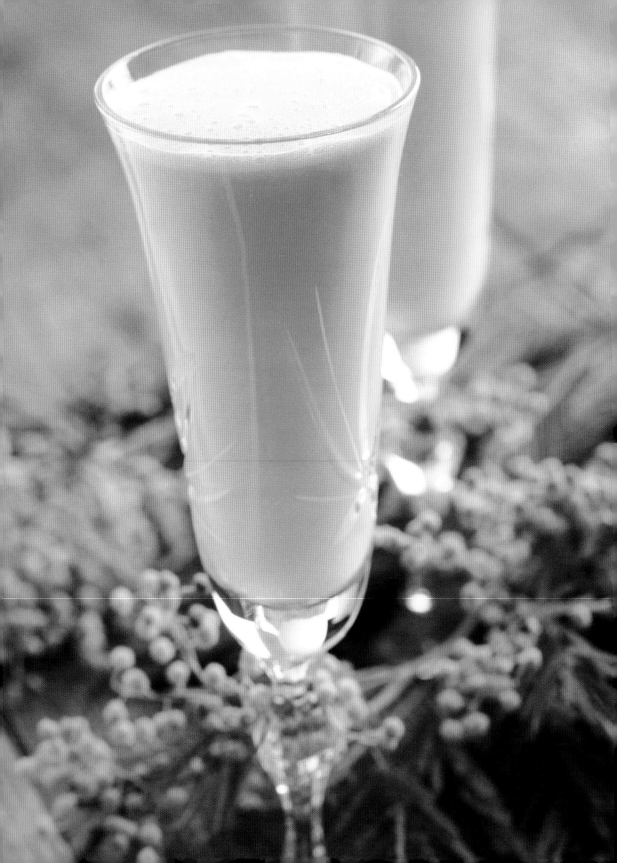

Mimosas

Mimosa cocktails made with dry, sparkling wine and fresh orange juice create a celebratory mood and are a favorite to serve at brunch. Quick and simple to make, mimosas will make your brunch a memorable and an enjoyable experience for everyone. Sweet orange essential oil is a natural antiseptic cleanser and is often referred to as the "happiness oil."

Makes 8 mimosa cocktails

1 (25-oz [750-ml]) bottle chilled dry sparkling wine

3 cups (710 ml) chilled orange juice (freshly squeezed is best!)

1–3 drops sweet orange essential oil

½ cup (118 ml) orange liqueur (Grand Marnier recommended; optional)

Fill 8 champagne flutes half full with chilled sparkling wine. Top with orange juice into which you've stirred your sweet orange essential oil. Add 1 tablespoon (15 ml) per glass of Grand Marnier, if you're using it. Serve immediately.

Venus Martini

One of the all-time honored classic cocktails, the martini dates back to the mid-1800s. If you only want to try making one cocktail, consider making the Venus Martini. A memorable, sweet and sensual delight—it will be the rave at your next gathering! Rose oil is known for freeing your emotions, and it will stimulate and delight your erotic senses.

Makes 1 martini

Ice

1 part (1½ oz) vanilla vodka (I prefer Absolut)

3 parts (4½ oz) strawberry nectar

1 drop rose essential oil

Fresh strawberries for garnish

1 part (1½ oz) half and half or cream (optional)

Half fill a shaker or blender with ice. Add the vanilla vodka, strawberry nectar (into which you've stirred your rose essential oil). Shake or blend well. Strain if shaken, or pour if blended, into an empty iced martini glass. Garnish with a fresh strawberry. If you want a creamy martini, substitute 1 part (1½ oz) half and half or cream for one part strawberry nectar.

For a stronger drink, you can increase the vodka part and decrease the strawberry nectar.

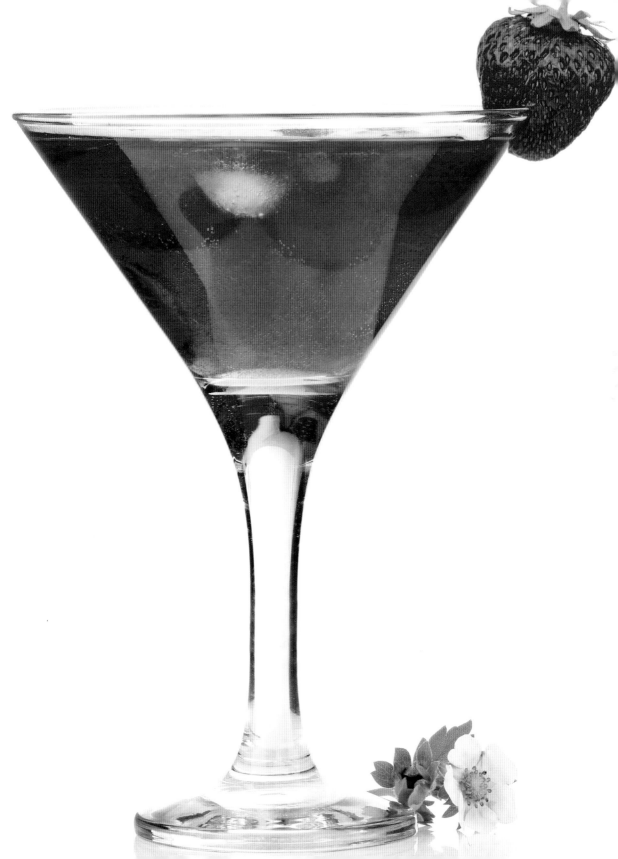

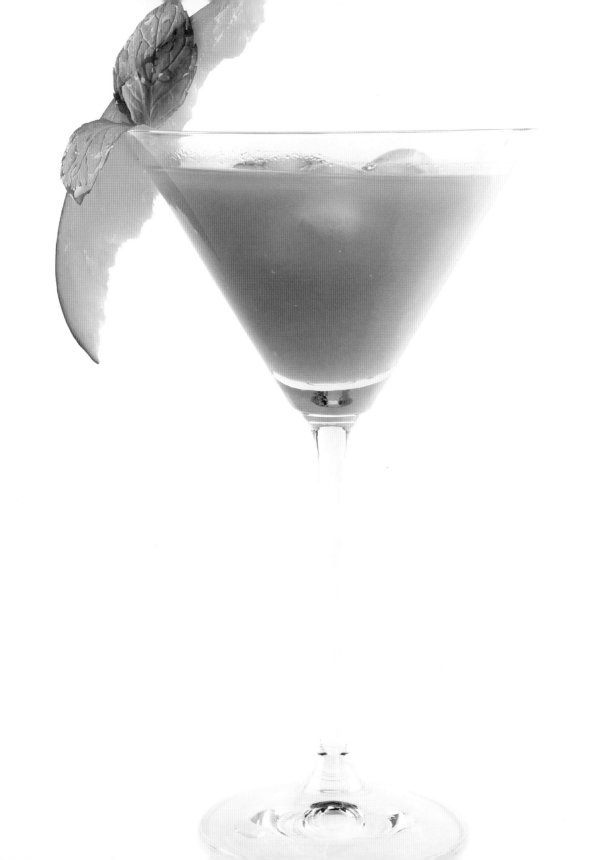

Sunshine Martini

A bright and delicious mimosa alternative that's just as yummy served with Sunday brunch. The fresh and tangy aroma of sweet orange oil is refreshing and highly favored as a remedy to shift heavy or serious moods.

Makes 1 martini

Ice

1 part (1½ oz) vanilla vodka (I prefer Absolut)

2 parts (3 oz) passion fruit liqueur (I prefer X-rated)

4 parts (6 oz) mango nectar

1 drop sweet orange essential oil

Watermelon for garnish

Half fill a shaker or blender with ice. Add the vanilla vodka, passion fruit liqueur, mango nectar and sweet orange essential oil. Shake or blend well. Strain if shaken, or pour if blended, into an empty iced martini glass. Use a watermelon scoop and add a watermelon round on top as garnish.

Chocolate Mint Martini

If you want to try only two cocktail recipes, make this your second choice. It's a splendid sweet, minty and chocolate concoction that begs for a second round. A stimulant and natural relaxant in small amounts, peppermint oil will help you stay alert, yet relaxed, as you enjoy a sociable evening with family and friends.

Makes 1 martini

Ice

1 part (1½ oz) vanilla vodka (I prefer Absolut)

2 parts (3 oz) coffee-flavored liqueur (I prefer Kahlua)

1 part (1½ oz) half and half or cream

1 drop peppermint essential oil

Chocolate-covered coffee beans for garnish

Half fill a shaker or blender with ice. Add the vanilla vodka, coffee-flavored liqueur, half and half and peppermint oil. Shake or blend well. Strain if shaken, or pour if blended, into an empty iced martini glass. Garnish with a chocolate-covered coffee bean.

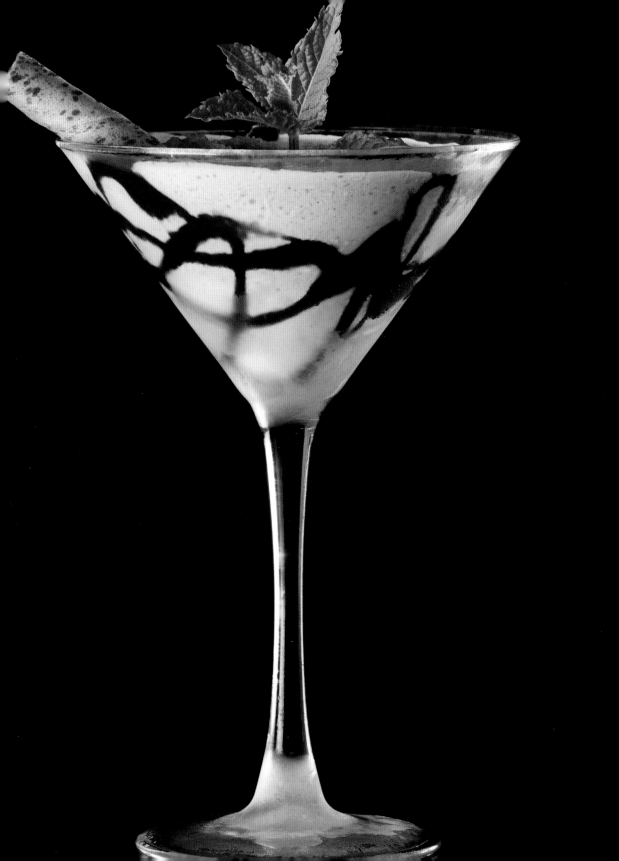

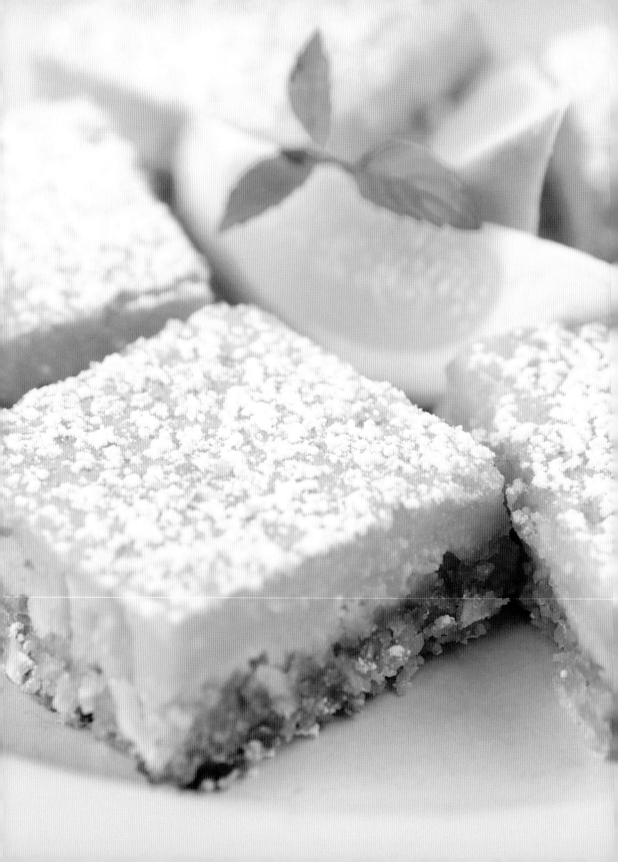

Desserts

One of the biggest industries for which essential oils are used is the food and beverage industry. Essential oils are often used to soften and add lift to food flavors in beverages and drinks and are used in many baked goods, gelatins and soft candies. For instance, small traces of rosa damascena are used to tastefully enhance strawberry, raspberry, apricot and bitter-almond food products.

The Best Lemon Bars

For a tender, flaky crust for these tart and sweet bars, the buttery dough is handmade and pre-baked so it stays light and crisp after the addition of freshly made lemon filling. Lemon essential oil will not only add an unforgettable sweet, tart tanginess to your lemon bars, it will also naturally increase your fat burning ability and boost your metabolism.

Makes about 3 dozen squares

2½ cups (315 g) all-purpose flour, sifted

¼ tsp salt (optional)

½ cup (60 g) confectioner's sugar, sifted, plus more for dusting bars

¾ cup (172 g) unsalted butter, slightly chilled and cut into small pieces

6 large eggs

3 cups (750 g) raw cane sugar

3 medium lemons, grated zest of outer lemon peel

1 cup (237 ml) freshly squeezed lemon juice (about 8 medium lemons)

1–3 drops lemon essential oil

Preheat the oven to 325°F (163°C). In a medium bowl that's been chilled, combine the flour (to which you've added salt, if desired) and confectioner's sugar. Set a little of the confectioner's sugar aside for dusting the top of the lemon bars. Use a pastry cutter or fork to cut the butter into two-thirds of the flour mixture until the butter is thoroughly covered with flour. Gently pat the buttery dough into a 9- x 13-inch (23- x 33-cm) glass baking dish.

Bake 20–25 minutes, until the crust is golden brown. Chill a medium bowl for mixing the lemon bar filling. When the crust is a golden brown, take it out of the oven and set the baking dish with the crust on a rack to cool.

Reduce the oven to 300°F (149°C). Whisk the eggs and raw cane sugar together in a chilled, medium-sized bowl. Add the lemon zest, juice and lemon essential oil and blend thoroughly together. Blend in the remaining one-third of the flour mixture.

Pour the lemon filling into the baked crust, and bake until the filling sets, about 40–45 minutes.

Cool on a rack, then refrigerate until well chilled before slicing, after 3–4 hours or more. Before serving, dust the top of the lemon bars with the extra confectioner's sugar you set aside. Slice the lemon bars into square pieces with a cold, sharp knife and serve.

Crispy Brown Sugar Chocolate Mint Chip Cookies

If you love munching on cookie dough and cookie pieces, this is the chocolate chip cookie recipe for you. During baking, the cookie dough will spread out and cover the pan, making a very flat, delicious and crispy cookie experience. These cookies are great eaten soft, gooey and warm straight out of the oven. Or you can let them cool into crispy, crunchy cookie pieces that are great for dipping in milk. As a stimulant, peppermint oil will naturally help curb your appetite and acts as an excellent digestive.

3 dozen 3-inch (8-cm) cookies

Coconut oil

½ lb (227 g) or 2 sticks unsalted butter, softened

2 cups (400 g) raw brown sugar, packed

1 cup (200 g) raw granulated cane sugar

4 eggs

2 tsp (10 ml) pure vanilla extract

2–3 drops peppermint essential oil

3 cups (375 g) all-purpose flour

¼ tsp salt (optional)

½–1 tsp baking soda

2 cups (340 g) chocolate chips

Preheat the oven to 375°F (190°C). Cover two baking sheets with coconut oil. Cream the butter in a small mixing bowl until smooth, and then blend in both sugars until smooth. Next, beat in the eggs, vanilla and peppermint oil.

In a separate large bowl, sift together the remaining dry ingredients. Then slowly stir the dry ingredients into the wet ingredients. Gently fold in the chocolate chips. Drop spoons of cookie dough onto the baking sheet. Space cookies 2 inches (5 cm) apart to allow room for them to spread.

Bake until golden brown, 8–10 minutes. Remove the cookies and break into cookie pieces or allow them to cool on a rack.

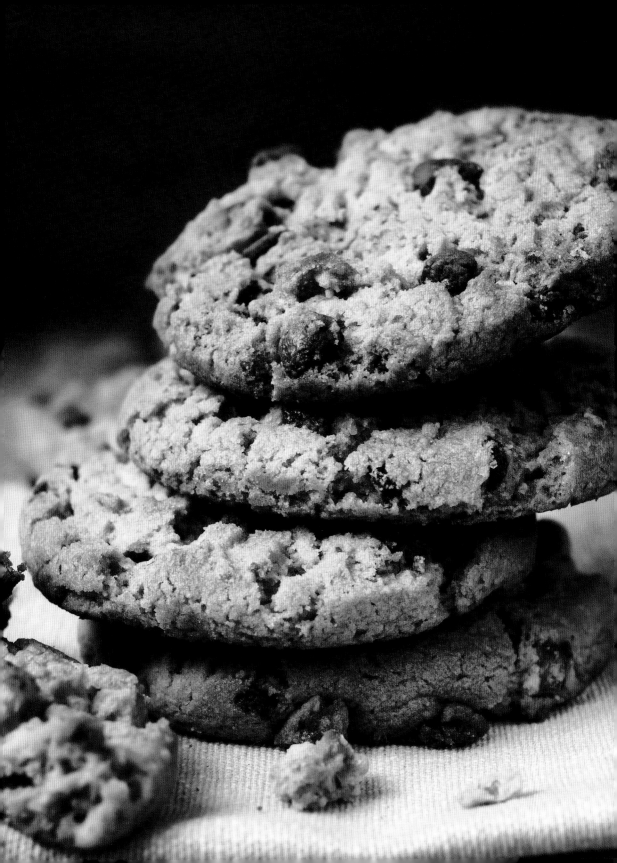

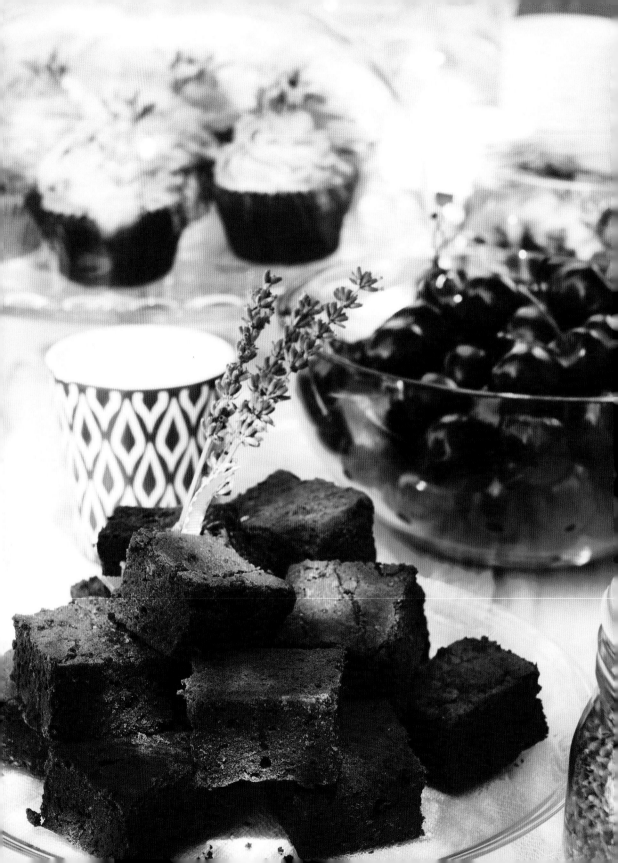

Quick-to-Make Gooey Fudgy Lavender Brownies

These brownies are indescribably delicious, rich and gooey. You'll be smacking your lips and licking your fingers to get every last morsel. Sweet, floral and slightly herbaceous, lavender essential oil will stimulate your digestion, as well as fire up your metabolism.

Makes 9 (3-inch [8-cm]) brownies

8 tbsp (115 g) unsalted butter, chilled, cut into pieces, plus more to butter pan

1 cup (125 g) all-purpose flour, sifted

¼ cup (28 g) unsweetened cocoa powder

½ tsp baking powder

½ tsp salt

8 oz (227 g) semi-sweet or bittersweet dark chocolate (bars or chips)

1–3 drops lavender essential oil

1¼ cups (315 g) raw cane sugar

3 large eggs

¼–½ cup (30–60 g) walnuts, espresso powder and chocolate chips (optional)

Preheat the oven to 350°F (177°C). Cover the bottom of a 9-inch (23-cm) square baking pan with butter. Line the bottom and two sides of the pan with a strip of parchment paper, being sure to leave 2 inches (5 cm) of the parchment paper to hang over the sides of the pan; this will make it easier to remove the brownies from the dish after baking. Butter the top of the paper, too.

Next, in a small bowl, blend together the dry ingredients including flour, cocoa, baking powder and salt. Then, place the butter and chocolate in a large bowl and put over (not in) a saucepan of gently boiling water. Melt the butter and chocolate together, stirring occasionally, until completely melted. Remove the bowl with melted butter and chocolate from the pan and blend in the lavender essential oil.

Next, add the sugar and mix together. Then, add the eggs and mix together. Next, add walnuts, espresso powder or chocolate chips, if desired. Finally, combine with the flour mixture; mix until moistened, but do not over mix. Pour the batter into the prepared pan with butter and parchment, and spread the batter evenly.

Bake brownies just until a toothpick inserted in the center comes out with a few moist crumbs (not dry), 20–30 minutes. When cooled enough, about 20–30 minutes, lift the brownies out of the pan by grasping the sides of the overhanging parchment paper. Place the brownies (and parchment paper) on a rack to cool. Place the cooled brownies on a cutting board and use a cool, damp serrated knife to cut them into 3-inch (7.6-cm) squares. Store the brownies in an airtight container in the refrigerator.

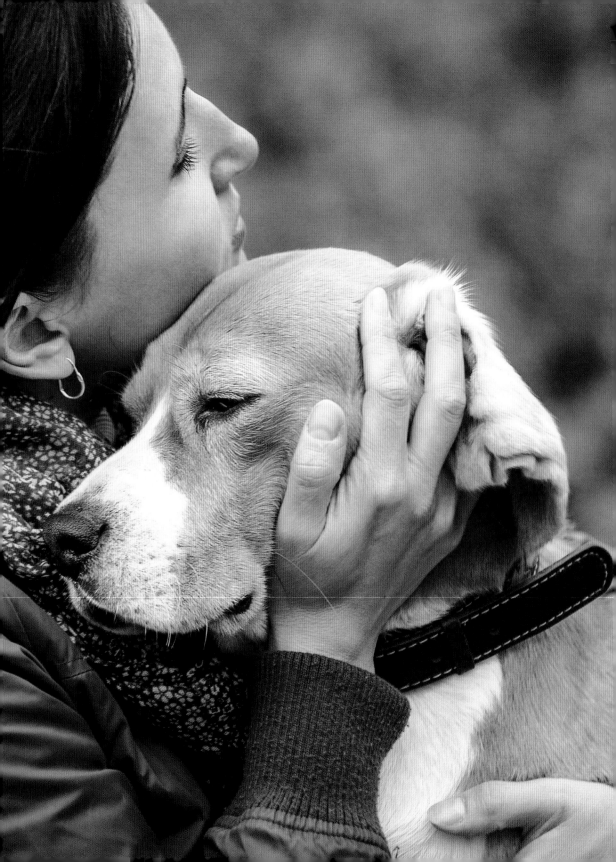

CHAPTER 20

Animals and Pets

How to Use Essential Oils with Pets and Animals

As animals have extremely sensitive olfactory senses, use these essential oils in a very weak dilution of less than 1 percent to achieve the results desired.

Essential oils can be used in pet wash, grooming spray, flea and tick prevention and treatment and muscle rub and as an antifungal. They can also be used to treat horseflies, stress and anxiety, PTSD, skin rash, burns, hair loss and more.

Suitable carriers include aloe vera, jojoba, light coconut oil or another preferred carrier for safe skin application. Compresses are also an effective method for using essential oils with animals and pets.

Use self-selection with your animal friends. Self-selection means to include them in the selection process of the essential oils to use. Pay close attention and listen to how your animal or pet responds to a tiny amount of an essential oil before using it.

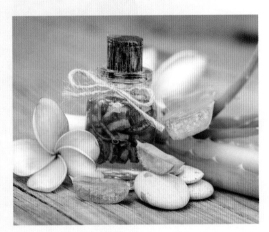

Self-selection can help determine which scents your pets enjoy and which to avoid.

CAUTION: Your animal friend's olfaction process, though similar to humans, is much more acute. Animals are super sensitive to smells. As animals have extremely sensitive olfactory senses, use essential oils in very low percentages of less than 1 percent to achieve the results desired.

CAUTION: Remember to take special care when using any essential oil on or around a cat. They simply can't metabolize essential oils the way dogs, horses and humans do. When diffusing oils for your own use, make very sure that your cat can exit the room if they choose. Hydrosols (floral waters) on the other hand, are completely safe and gentle to use with your furry friends.

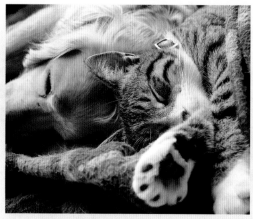

Take special care with essential oils on or around cats. (When using oils make sure your cat can exit the room.) Cats can't metabolize oils the ways dogs, horses and humans can.

List of Oils and Their Specific Uses for Your Furry Friends

- ATLAS CEDARWOOD: Grounds and stabilizes; natural insect repellent

- GERMAN CHAMOMILE: Calming and anti-inflammatory

- EUCALYPTUS RADIATA: respiratory aid; antibacterial and antiviral

- FRANKINCENSE: Comforts and relieves distress

- GERANIUM ROSEUM AND GRAVEOLENS: Insect repellent; balances

- LAVENDER: Soothes, calms and relaxes

- LEMONGRASS: Antifungal and astringent; insect repellent

- SWEET MARJORAM: Antispasmodic; pain reliever

- NEROLI: Peace and calming

- NIAOULI: Powerful antiseptic and antifungal

- PATCHOULI: Antifungal, antiseptic and insect repellent

- THYME: Powerful immune stimulant and antimicrobial

Flea and Tick Prevention and Treatment

This formula provides natural protection from pests.

To a 5-ml, colored-glass, euro-dropper bottle add:

Palmarosa: 60 drops

Lemongrass: 20 drops

Cedarwood: 20 drops

Close the cap tightly and shake the bottle vigorously to thoroughly blend the essential oils. Allow to synergize for 8 or more hours before using.

Add your essential oil blend in the proper dilution amount of 1 percent or less to a dispensing bottle filled with a carrier oil like light coconut oil. Light coconut oil is light enough to use as an aromatic, spray-on mist.

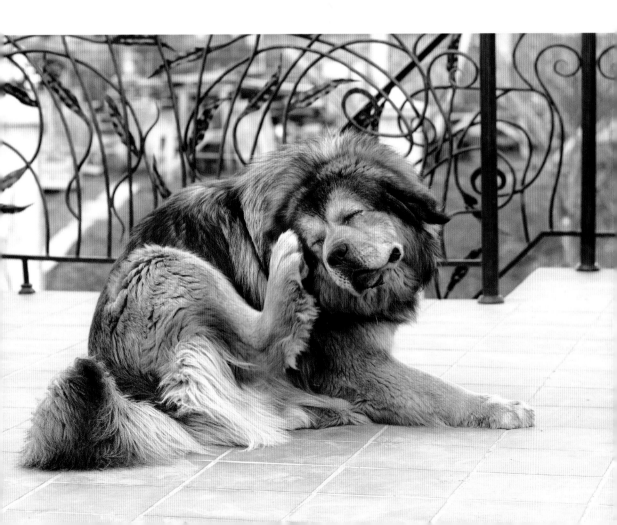

Respiratory Support

Promotes relief of breathing issues for your animal friends.

~~~~~~

To a 5-ml, colored-glass, euro-dropper bottle add:

Frankincense: 60 drops

Eucalyptus Radiata: 40 drops

Close the cap tightly and shake the bottle vigorously to thoroughly blend the essential oils. Allow to synergize for 8 or more hours before using.

Add your essential oil blend in the proper dilution amount of 1 percent or less to a dispensing bottle filled with a carrier oil like light coconut oil. Dispense 1–3 drops on a cotton ball or smell strip and allow your animal to freely sniff for 10–15 seconds to begin. Pay attention to how they respond and to notice any benefits. You may repeat up to three to four times daily.

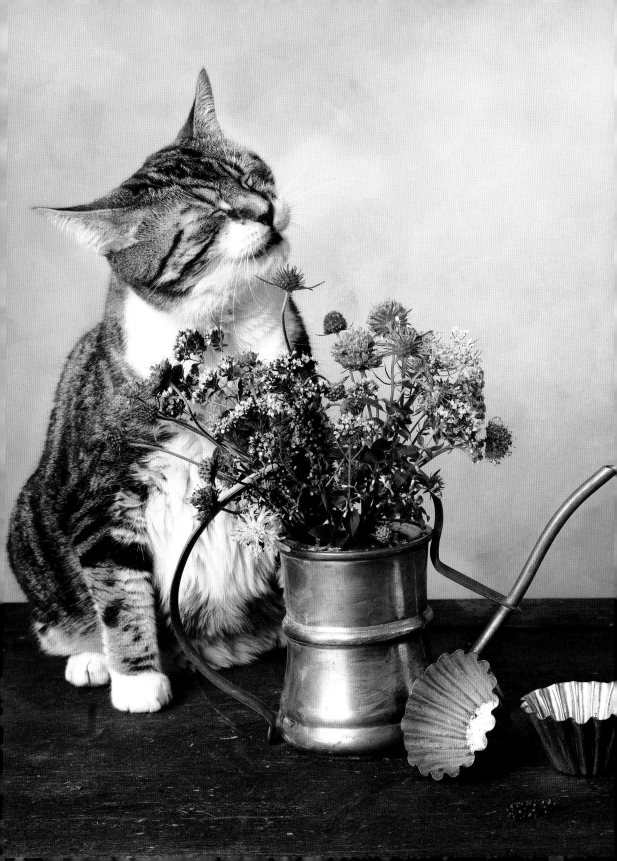

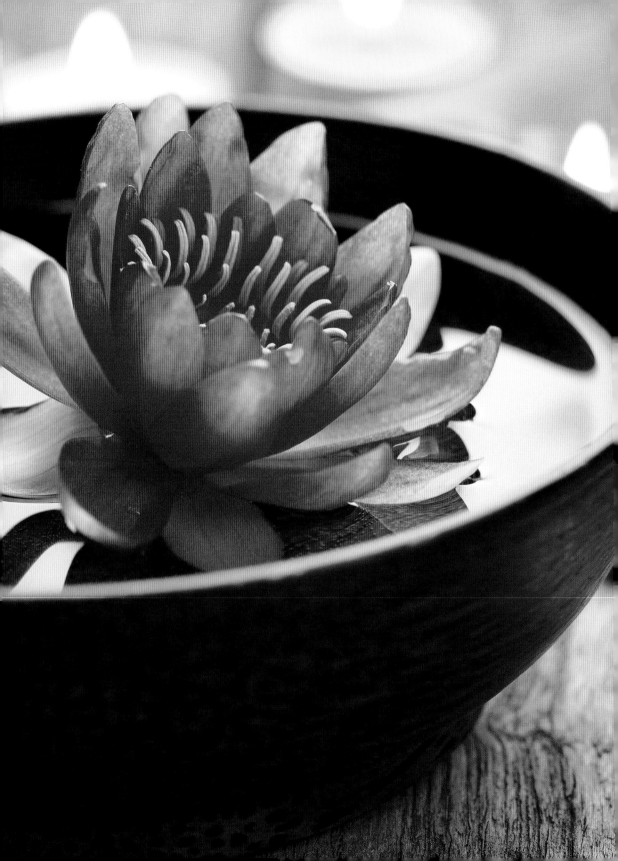

CHAPTER 21

Spiritual Blends

What are Chakras?

Chakra is a Sanskrit term meaning "disc," "spinning wheel of energy" or "wheel of light." Chakras are spiral vortices of energy that look similar in shape to our Milky Way Galaxy. Your chakras are spinning wheels of energy that connect your physical life form with your transpersonal Divine nature.

DR. CANDACE PERT'S RESEARCH

Renowned neuroscientist Dr. Candace Pert reported that, "We (humans) are quite literally hardwired for bliss." Dr. Pert's extraordinary career began in 1972 with her startling discovery of the opiate receptor. In her book, *Molecules of Emotion*, Dr. Pert, a professed Chakra buff, maps the dynamic network between emotions, the body and the mind.

Free, unimpeded circulation of prana through your chakra energy system is essential for the feeling of bliss that naturally arises with being alive.

Your regular chakra practice will assist you in clearing blockages from deep within the subconscious levels of your energy system so that you can regularly experience the state of bliss that Dr. Pert writes about.

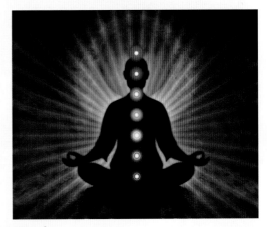

Chakras are spinning wheels of energy that connect your physical life form with your transpersonal divine nature.

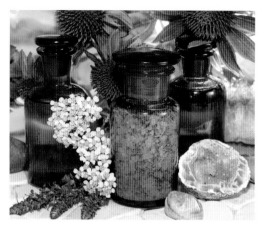

The red energy of your first chakra is vibrant and healthy when your survival needs are met.

These chakra energy centers, or chakras, connect and operate with one another within multi-dimensional planes through circuits or streams of life force energy (acupuncture meridians).

The chakras may be viewed clairvoyantly from the front, back or sides of your body and mind. I perceive chakras as balls of light like the sun. When functioning healthily, chakras appear to be vibrant and alive. For the sake of simplicity and clarity, I will speak about the nature and function for each of your chakras from a two-dimensional perspective from the front side of your body.

Essential Oils to Balance Your Chakras

THE FIRST CHAKRA (MULADHARA OR ROOT)

ELEMENT: **Earth**

COLOR: **Red**

POWER: **Stability**

Located at the end of your tailbone, this chakra is about security and survival. Its function is to support healthy skeletal and nervous systems.

Symptoms of weakness include: sciatica and reproductive issues.

Psycho-emotional signs of blockage: Chronic fear is a symptom of blockage.

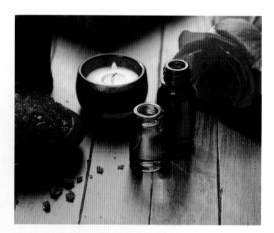

First chakra signs of blockage include chronic fear, sciatica, reproductive issues and skeletal imbalances.

First Chakra Oil Formula

Balance and strengthen your first chakra by inhaling a pure blend or anointing your chakra with a 10-percent dilution.

To a 5-ml, colored-glass, euro-dropper bottle add:

Galbanum: 1–2 drops

Helichrysum: 10 drops

Myrrh: 10 drops

Patchouli: 20 drops

Vetiver: 30 drops

Ylang Ylang III: 30 drops

Close the cap tightly and shake the bottle vigorously to thoroughly blend the essential oils. Allow to synergize for 8 or more hours before using.

Dispense 1–3 drops on a cotton ball or smell strip and inhale the aromatic vapors of your essential oil for 10–15 seconds. You may repeat as needed.

To make a ready-to-use chakra anointing oil, simply add 15–30 drops of your essential oil to a 1-ounce (30-ml) bottle of your favorite carrier oil. Shake the bottle well to disperse the oils thoroughly. Apply a few drops of your ready-to-use anointing oil at the area of your chakra.

THE SECOND CHAKRA
(SVADHISTHANA OR SEXUAL)

ELEMENT: Water

COLOR: Orange

POWER: Sexuality/sensuality

Located in the area of your lower abdomen, a healthy second chakra supports healthy relationships of all kinds, including with money.

Symptoms of weakness include: lumbar tension, chronic lower back pain, addictions and power struggles.

Psycho-emotional signs of blockage: Chronic guilt is a symptom of imbalance.

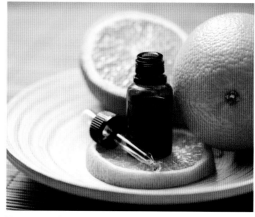

Your second chakra energy is your center of sexuality and includes relationships, including your relationship with money.

Second Chakra Oil Formula

Balance and strengthen your second chakra by inhaling a pure blend or anointing your chakra with a 10-percent dilution.

To a 5-ml, colored-glass, euro-dropper bottle add:

Rose: 10 drops

Geranium Roseum and Graveolens: 20 drops total

Sweet Orange: 20 drops

Patchouli: 10 drops

Red Mandarin: 20 drops

Ylang Ylang: 20 drops

Close the cap tightly and shake the bottle vigorously to thoroughly blend the essential oils. Allow to synergize for 8 or more hours before using.

Dispense 1–3 drops on a cotton ball or smell strip and inhale the aromatic vapors of your essential oil for 10–15 seconds. You may repeat as needed.

To make a ready-to-use chakra anointing oil, simply add 15–30 drops of your essential oil to a 1-ounce (30-ml) bottle of your favorite carrier oil. Shake the bottle well to disperse the oils thoroughly. Apply a few drops of your ready-to-use anointing oil at the area of your chakra.

THE THIRD CHAKRA (MANIPURA OR SOLAR PLEXUS)

ELEMENT: Fire

COLOR: Yellow

POWER: Desire

Located in the area of your upper abdomen, a healthy third chakra supports healthy digestion.

Symptoms of weakness include: eating disorders, digestive complaints and low self-esteem issues.

Psycho-emotional signs of blockage: Chronic shame is a symptom of imbalance.

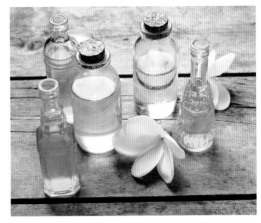

Your third chakra is your energy center for healthy digestion and self esteem.

Third Chakra Oil Formula

Balance and strengthen your third chakra by inhaling a pure blend or anointing your chakra with a 10-percent dilution.

To a 5-ml, colored-glass, euro-dropper bottle add:
Sandalwood: 20 drops
Cedarwood: 20 drops
Myrrh: 10 drops
Lemongrass: 30 drops
Lemon: 20 drops

Close the cap tightly and shake the bottle vigorously to thoroughly blend the essential oils. Allow to synergize for 8 or more hours before using.

Dispense 1–3 drops on a cotton ball or smell strip and inhale the aromatic vapors of your essential oil for 10–15 seconds. You may repeat as needed.

To make a ready-to-use chakra anointing oil, simply add 15–30 drops of your essential oil to a 1-ounce (30-ml) bottle of your favorite carrier oil. Shake the bottle well to disperse the oils thoroughly. Apply a few drops of your ready-to-use anointing oil at the area of your chakra.

THE FOURTH CHAKRA
(ANAHATA OR HEART)

ELEMENT: Air

COLOR: Green

POWER: Compassion

Located in the area of your heart, a healthy fourth chakra supports an open and compassionate heart, healthy connections with others and clairsentience.

Symptoms of weakness include: forgiveness issues and cardio-vascular and respiratory problems.

Psycho-emotional signs of blockage: Chronic depression.

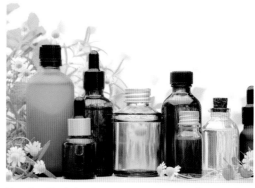

Your fourth chakra is your energy center of love and compassion toward yourself and others.

Fourth Chakra Oil Formula

Balance and strengthen your fourth chakra by inhaling a pure blend or anointing your chakra with a 10-percent dilution.

To a 5-ml, colored-glass, euro-dropper bottle add:

Bergamot: 20 drops

Rose: 10 drops

Geranium Roseum and Graveolens: 30 drops total

Ylang Ylang: 20 drops

Frankincense: 20 drops

Close the cap tightly and shake the bottle vigorously to thoroughly blend the essential oils. Allow to synergize for 8 or more hours before using.

Dispense 1–3 drops on a cotton ball or smell strip and inhale the aromatic vapors of your essential oil for 10–15 seconds. You may repeat as needed.

To make a ready-to-use chakra anointing oil, simply add 15–30 drops of your essential oil to a 1-ounce (30-ml) bottle of your favorite carrier oil. Shake the bottle well to disperse the oils thoroughly. Apply a few drops of your ready-to-use anointing oil at the area of your chakra.

THE FIFTH CHAKRA
(VISHUDDHA OR THROAT)

ELEMENT: Space/Ether

COLOR: Blue

POWER: Creativity

Located in the area of your throat, a healthy throat chakra supports open, honest communication, full self-expression and clairaudience.

Symptoms of weakness include: throat, voice, hearing and thyroid problems; headache, neck tension/pain, ringing ear or tinnitus; and rigid attitudes, fears and various phobias.

Psycho-emotional signs of imbalance: Chronic obsessive-compulsive behaviors, phobias, procrastination and indecision.

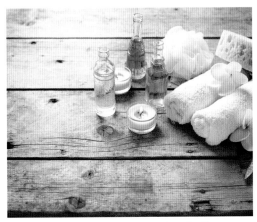

Your fifth chakra is your energy center of self expression and open, honest communications.

Fifth Chakra Oil Formula

Balance and strengthen your fifth chakra by inhaling a pure blend or anointing your chakra with a 10-percent dilution.

To a 5-ml, colored-glass, euro-dropper bottle add:
Blue Tansy: 10 drops
Lavender: 30 drops
Roman Chamomile: 20 drops
Blue Yarrow: 10 drops
Frankincense: 30 drops

Close the cap tightly and shake the bottle vigorously to thoroughly blend the essential oils. Allow to synergize for 8 or more hours before using.

Dispense 1–3 drops on a cotton ball or smell strip and inhale the aromatic vapors of your essential oil for 10–15 seconds. You may repeat as needed.

To make a ready-to-use chakra anointing oil, simply add 15–30 drops of your essential oil to a 1-ounce (30-ml) bottle of your favorite carrier oil. Shake the bottle well to disperse the oils thoroughly. Apply a few drops of your ready-to-use anointing oil at the area of your chakra.

THE SIXTH CHAKRA
(AJNA OR BROW)

ELEMENT: Light

COLOR: Indigo

POWER: Awareness

Located in the area between your eyebrows, a healthy brow chakra supports clarity, imagination and clairvoyance.

Symptoms of weakness include: Pituitary glandular disorders, headache, confusion, eye problems, learning disabilities, recurring nightmares and lack of focus and discipline.

Psycho-emotional signs of imbalance: Chronic confusion, paranoia and delusions.

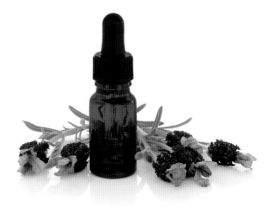

Your sixth chakra is your energy center of imagination and clear mental thinking.

Sixth Chakra Oil Formula

Balance and strengthen your sixth chakra by inhaling a pure blend or anointing your chakra with a 10-percent dilution.

To a 5-ml, colored-glass, euro-dropper bottle add:
Spikenard: 40 drops
Neroli: 40 drops
Black Pepper: 5 drops
Lemon: 5 drops
Peppermint: 10 drops

Close the cap tightly and shake the bottle vigorously to thoroughly blend the essential oils. Allow to synergize for 8 or more hours before using.

Dispense 1–3 drops on a cotton ball or smell strip and inhale the aromatic vapors of your essential oil for 10–15 seconds. You may repeat as needed.

To make a ready-to-use chakra anointing oil, simply add 15–30 drops of your essential oil to a 1-ounce (30-ml) bottle of your favorite carrier oil. Shake the bottle well to disperse the oils thoroughly. Apply a few drops of your ready-to-use anointing oil at the area of your chakra.

THE SEVENTH CHAKRA (SAHASRARA OR CROWN)

ELEMENT: Sound

COLOR: Violet

POWER: Pure Consciousness

Located in the area of the crown of your head, a healthy crown chakra supports inspiration and spirituality and gives rise to thoughts, ideas and claircognizance.

Symptoms of weakness include: Endocrine and musculoskeletal disorders, environmental hypersensitivity, manic-depressive states and psychosis.

Psycho-emotional signs of imbalance: Loss of a sense of purpose and meaning are symptoms of blockage.

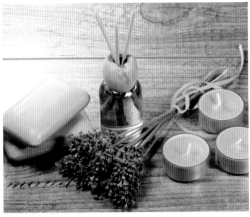

Your seventh chakra is your energy center of pure consciousness and gives rise to clear understanding.

Seventh Chakra Oil Formula

Balance and strengthen your seventh chakra by inhaling a pure blend or anointing your chakra with a 10-percent dilution.

To a 5-ml, colored-glass, euro-dropper bottle add:
Spikenard: 30 drops
Rose: 20 drops
Sandalwood: 20 drops
Neroli: 20 drops
Ylang Ylang: 10 drops

Close the cap tightly and shake the bottle vigorously to thoroughly blend the essential oils. Allow to synergize for 8 or more hours before using.

Dispense 1–3 drops on a cotton ball or smell strip and inhale the aromatic vapors of your essential oil for 10–15 seconds. You may repeat as needed.

To make a ready-to-use chakra anointing oil, simply add 15–30 drops of your essential oil to a 1-ounce (30-ml) bottle of your favorite carrier oil. Shake the bottle well to disperse the oils thoroughly. Apply a few drops of your ready-to-use anointing oil at the area of your chakra.

THE EIGHTH CHAKRA (UNIVERSAL HEART)

ELEMENT: Cosmos

COLOR: Turquoise

POWER: Cosmic Love

Located in the area above your heart, a healthy eighth chakra supports feelings of being connected and loved unconditionally by the Cosmos.

Symptoms of weakness include: Mysterious, non-responding illnesses.

Psycho-emotional signs of imbalance: Resistance to receiving love and support, disassociation and emotional numbness.

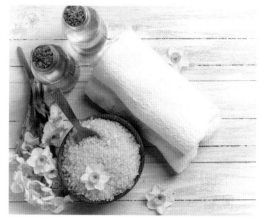

Your eighth chakra is your energy center of cosmic universal love that connects you with all life everywhere forever.

Eighth Chakra Oil Formula

Balance and strengthen your eighth chakra by inhaling a pure blend or anointing your chakra with a 10-percent dilution.

To a 5-ml, colored-glass, euro-dropper bottle add:

Melissa: 30 drops

Rose: 20 drops

Sandalwood: 20 drops

Neroli: 20 drops

Ylang Ylang: 10 drops

Close the cap tightly and shake the bottle vigorously to thoroughly blend the essential oils. Allow to synergize for 8 or more hours before using.

Dispense 1–3 drops on a cotton ball or smell strip and inhale the aromatic vapors of your essential oil for 10–15 seconds. You may repeat as needed.

To make a ready-to-use chakra anointing oil, simply add 15–30 drops of your essential oil to a 1-ounce (30-ml) bottle of your favorite carrier oil. Shake the bottle well to disperse the oils thoroughly. Apply a few drops of your ready-to-use anointing oil at the area of your chakra.

THE NINTH CHAKRA (EARTH STAR)

ELEMENT: Gaia

COLOR: Deep Green

POWER: Life Purpose

Located about 6 inches (15 cm) beneath your feet, the earth star chakra connects energetically at the pads of your feet. A balanced and healthy functioning ninth chakra supports you to feel grounded, purposeful and completely supported by life. An imbalanced ninth Chakra manifests as life purpose issues.

Symptoms of weakness include: Sore or tired feet, chronic fatigue, restless leg syndrome and leg cramps.

Psycho-emotional signs of imbalance: Feeling ungrounded, disconnected or depressed; loss of your sense of purpose, failure to thrive and poverty consciousness.

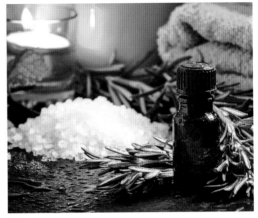

Your ninth chakra is your energy center that connects you with Gaia, Mother Earth, and ensures a strong sense of connection with your life and your purpose for being here.

Ninth Chakra Oil Formula

Balance and strengthen your ninth chakra by inhaling a pure blend or anointing your chakra with a 10-percent dilution.

To a 5-ml, colored-glass, euro-dropper bottle add:

Galbanum: 1–3 drops

Myrrh: 20 drops

Vetiver: 30 drops

Ylang Ylang III: 30 drops

Patchouli: 20 drops

Close the cap tightly and shake the bottle vigorously to thoroughly blend the essential oils. Allow to synergize for 8 or more hours before using.

Dispense 1–3 drops on a cotton ball or smell strip and inhale the aromatic vapors of your essential oil for 10–15 seconds. You may repeat as needed.

To make a ready-to-use chakra anointing oil, simply add 15–30 drops of your essential oil to a 1-ounce (30-ml) bottle of your favorite carrier oil. Shake the bottle well to disperse the oils thoroughly. Apply a few drops of your ready-to-use anointing oil at the area of your chakra.

5 ELEMENTS

Traditional Chinese medicine (TCM) is a form of medicine developed more than 2,500 years ago that is built on a foundation of Chinese medical practice that includes herbal medicine, acupuncture, exercise (qigong), massage (tui na) and diet. TCM is increasingly gaining popularity in the West and as a form of complementary alternative medicine.

One of the basic TCM principles "holds that the body's vital energy (chi or qi) circulates through channels, called meridians, that have branches connected to bodily organs and functions." The emphasis in TCM is on dynamic forces operating within the body, which, when in balance and functioning harmoniously, bring about health. Harmonious integration of the body's vital energy precedes and gives rise to the material structure.

According to TCM, there are five elements or phases characterized by five elemental qualities of nature represented by fire, earth, metal, water and wood. In classic Oriental or Chinese medicine, all disease is seen as disordered elements. Restoring the balance of the five elements and the harmonious flow of chi is at the heart of Chinese medicine.

Your meridians are the channels through which the energy of your emotions flows. The natural and free flow of life force energy (your emotion or your energy in motion) flowing through your meridians supports your health and longevity. While blocked or suppressed, emotions result in clogged meridian channels and imbalances of health.

Emotions come and go throughout your day and simply need to be experienced and allowed to move freely through your body as electro-chemical expressions of the mind's ebb and flow.

You can use essential oils to balance each of the five elements and enhance the flow of chi through the organ meridian energy channels, including the Conception Vessel (brain), Governing Vessel (nervous system) and the twelve Organ Meridians.

You do NOT have to know TCM or acupuncture to use the recommended essential oils with good results. However, to give you some reference and understanding for the dynamic force each element represents, I will give a short overview of the key functions, properties, body parts, chakras and actions associated with each of the five elements, as well as signs of balance and imbalance, keywords associated with each element and the related physical and emotional symptoms of stagnation or blockage.

In TCM, all disease is seen as disordered elements.

Fire Element Meridians

The power of fire is transformation.

ORGAN MERIDIAN CHANNELS
Small intestines (yang) and heart (yin), also includes triple warmer (yang) and pericardium (yin)

PROPERTIES OF FIRE ELEMENT
SEASON: Summer

TASTE: Bitter

EMOTION: Joy/sadness

BODY PARTS: Heart, pericardium, circulation, hormones, blood vessels, tongue, small intestine

COLOR: Red

CHAKRA: Third (Manipura) Solar Plexus

BITTER ACTION
Cooling, astringent, drying, anti-inflammatory, antibiotic, often anti-parasitic and antiviral; promotes detoxification, stimulates appetite and secretion of digestive juices throughout the gastro-intestinal system, enhances digestion and flow of bile.

A balanced fire element empowers you to trust yourself and take full responsibility for your life. There is a strong sense of self-worth and positive self-regard, as well as personal freedom and autonomy. You are a creator of your reality, and you manifest easily all that you desire in the physical world.

An imbalanced fire element may manifest as an inability to take responsibility for yourself and your life experiences. You may lack discipline and self-control, and you may blame or criticize others for your problems.

KEYWORDS:
Decisiveness, self-motivation, self-esteem, commitment, personal power, self-control, honor, integrity, self-respect, self-approval, willingness to change and take responsibility.

RELATED PHYSICAL SYMPTOMS OF IMBALANCE INCLUDE:
Light headedness, heart palpitations, poor circulation, frozen shoulder, chest pain, dark circles under eyes, hardening of the arteries, hearing difficulties, herpes, high or low blood sugar, cold sores, confusion, constipation, diarrhea, dry hair and skin, indigestion, mouth ulcers, pimples, poor circulation, fatigue, depression, anxiety, restricted diaphragm, poor muscle tone, heart attack, dislike of heat and insomnia.

RELATED EMOTIONAL STAGNATION OR BLOCKAGE INCLUDE:
Feelings of shame, victimization, need for approval, stress, anger, frustration, fear of responsibility, guilt, worry, doubt, self-esteem and commitment issues.

Essential Oils to Balance Fire Element

Promotes balance for the fire element and organ meridians.

To a 5-ml, colored-glass, euro-dropper bottle add:

Cedarwood: 20 drops

Lemon: 20 drops

Lemongrass: 20 drops

Myrrh: 20 drops

Palmarosa: 20 drops

Rosemary: 1–5 drops

Close the cap tightly and shake the bottle vigorously to thoroughly blend the essential oils. Allow to synergize for 8 or more hours before using.

When using aromatherapy to restore energetic balance and flow of chi, your results can be enhanced when accompanied by diaphragmatic breathing.

Dispense 1–3 drops on a cotton ball or smell strip and inhale the aromatic vapors of your essential oil for 10–15 seconds. You may repeat as needed. This formula may also be effective as a compress over the area being treated.

To make a ready-to-use anointing oil that you can apply directly to the area being treated, simply add 15–30 drops of your essential oil to a 1-ounce (30-ml) bottle of your favorite carrier oil. Shake the bottle well to disperse the oils thoroughly. Apply a few drops of your ready-to-use anointing oil on the area being treated.

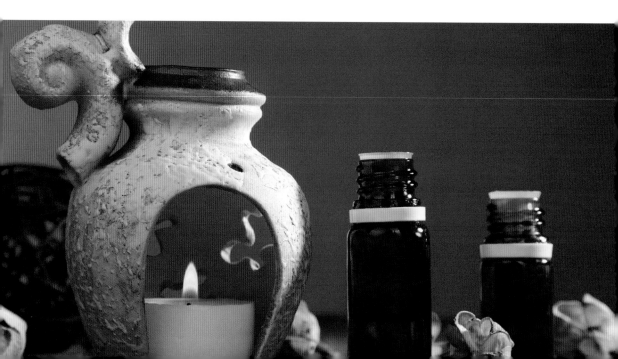

Earth Element Meridians

The power of earth is to be awakened.

ORGAN MERIDIAN CHANNELS
Stomach (yang), spleen (yin)

PROPERTIES OF EARTH ELEMENT
SEASON: Indian summer

TASTE: Sweet

EMOTION: Desire/worry

BODY PARTS: Stomach, spleen, muscles, mouth

COLOR: Yellow

CHAKRA: First (Muladhara) Root

SWEET ACTION
Warming, soothing, nourishing, body-building and tonic.

Most foods are classified as sweet. There are complex sweet flavors like grains, beans, dairy products and meat. Simple sweets are less satisfying. Examples are honey, sweet fruits and juices. Simple sweets intensify your craving for sweet rather than satisfy it.

A balanced earth element supports healthy survival instincts and being grounded.

The earth element ensures your connection to nature, universal laws and your own physical body. When the earth element is balanced, you engage with the maturation process of your life journey and walk steadily toward the fulfillment of your destiny. Earth energy awakens you to your deepest and most profound potential in which all aspects of your body, mind and spirit are integrated and expressed.

An imbalanced earth element may manifest itself as instability and an inability to create lasting and supportive structures in your life. Issues such as not belonging or feeling accepted by one's tribe can be prevalent.

KEYWORDS:
Stability, security, survival, cohesion, self-reliance, personal boundaries, synthesis, tribe and family.

RELATED PHYSICAL SYMPTOMS OF IMBALANCE INCLUDE:
Arthritis, heartburn, indigestion, shoulder and neck tension, stomach ulcer, sinusitis, eczema, rashes, fatigue, food allergies, diabetes, sweet cravings, poor lymph circulation, frequent urination, low blood sugar, insomnia, bed wetting, sciatica, constipation, obesity and ovarian, uterine, prostate and hemorrhoid conditions.

RELATED EMOTIONAL STAGNATION OR BLOCKAGE INCLUDE:
Feelings of fear that come from disconnection from one's tribe, community or family, or even from one's self.

The sense of abandonment or not belonging gives rise to feelings of frustration, rage, blocked passion, emotional instability, self-indulgence, self-centeredness, insecurity, grief, loss, depression and conflict between attachment and letting go.

Essential Oils to Balance Earth

Promotes balance for the earth element and organ meridians.

To a 5-ml, colored-glass, euro-dropper bottle add:

Galbanum: 1–5 drops

Helichrysum: 20 drops

Myrrh: 10 drops

Patchouli: 10 drops

Vetiver: 30 drops

Ylang Ylang III: 30 drops

Close the cap tightly and shake the bottle vigorously to thoroughly blend the essential oils. Allow to synergize for 8 or more hours before using.

When using aromatherapy to restore energetic balance and flow of chi, your results can be enhanced when accompanied by diaphragmatic breathing.

Dispense 1–3 drops on a cotton ball or smell strip and inhale the aromatic vapors of your essential oil for 10–15 seconds. You may repeat as needed. This formula may also be effective as a compress over the area being treated.

To make a ready-to-use anointing oil that you can apply directly to the area being treated, simply add 15–30 drops of your essential oil to a 1-ounce (30-ml) bottle of your favorite carrier oil. Shake the bottle well to disperse the oils thoroughly. Apply a few drops of your ready-to-use anointing oil on the area being treated.

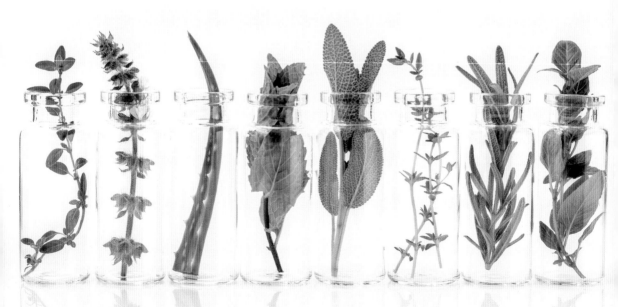

Metal Element Meridians

The power of metal is movement and integration.

ORGAN MERIDIAN CHANNELS
Large intestine (yang) and lung (yin)

PROPERTIES OF METAL ELEMENT
SEASON: Autumn

TASTE: Pungent

EMOTION: Grief

BODY PARTS: Lungs, large intestine, skin, nose

COLOR: White

CHAKRA: Fourth (Anahata) Heart

PUNGENT ACTION
Warming, dispersing and drying. Moves energy from the interior to the surface of the body, improving circulation and digestion, dispelling cold and stimulating energy flow.

A balanced metal element empowers you to experience enduring compassion and generosity for yourself and others. The nature and primary function of your heart chakra is to connect you with the kinetic experience of touching and being touched. An open, balanced and healthy metal element resonates with the feeling of a state of joy to attract experiences of abundance, prosperity and sharing. You easily feel self-love and acceptance.

Balancing the metal element promotes the healing of emotional wounds and the letting go of old issues of grief and loss, emotional heaviness, sadness, despair, depression (anger turned inward) and feelings of being unloved or unlovable.

KEYWORDS:
Compassion, empathy, trust, optimism, acceptance, forgiveness, joy, love of self and others, gratitude, integration, fulfillment, movement, sensitivity and clairsentience.

RELATED PHYSICAL SYMPTOMS OF IMBALANCE INCLUDE:
Cardiovascular and respiratory problems, allergies, heart disease, asthma, lung cancer, breast cancer, thoracic spine, pneumonia, hypertension, stroke, angina, arthritis, heart disease, shoulder girdle pain and discomfort, rotator cuff injuries, tendinitis, carpal tunnel, arm and hand pain and chronic restrictions in the upper back and thoracic area.

RELATED EMOTIONAL STAGNATION OR BLOCKAGE INCLUDE:
Unresolved grief, disappointment and loss that manifests as insensitivity, passivity, sadness, depression (anger turned inward), lack of forgiveness, anxiety and being emotionally closed.

Essential Oils to Balance Metal Element

Promotes balance for the metal element and organ meridians.

To a 5-ml, colored-glass, euro-dropper bottle add:

Bergamot: 20 drops

Frankincense: 20 drops

Helichrysum: 10 drops

Geranium Roseum and Graveolens: 10 drops each

Spikenard: 10 drops

Ylang Ylang: 20 drops

Close the cap tightly and shake the bottle vigorously to thoroughly blend the essential oils. Allow to synergize for 8 or more hours before using.

When using aromatherapy to restore energetic balance and flow of chi, your results can be enhanced when accompanied by diaphragmatic breathing.

Dispense 1–3 drops on a cotton ball or smell strip and inhale the aromatic vapors of your essential oil for 10–15 seconds. You may repeat as needed. This formula may also be effective as a compress over the area being treated.

To make a ready-to-use anointing oil that you can apply directly to the area being treated, simply add 15–30 drops of your essential oil to a 1-ounce (30-ml) bottle of your favorite carrier oil. Shake the bottle well to disperse the oils thoroughly. Apply a few drops of your ready-to-use anointing oil on the area being treated.

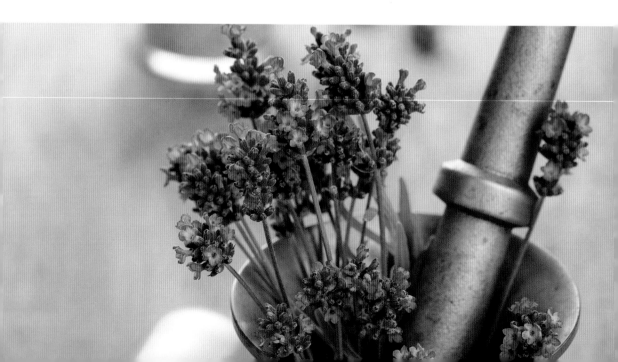

Water Element Meridians

The power of water is to overcome obstacles and act with integrity.

ORGAN MERIDIAN CHANNELS
Bladder (yang) and kidney (yin)

PROPERTIES OF WATER ELEMENT
SEASON: Winter

TASTE: Salty

EMOTION: Fear

BODY PARTS: Kidneys, bladder, ears, bones, nails, spleen

COLOR: Black

CHAKRA: Second (Svadhisthana) Sexual

SALTY ACTION
Cooling and moistening; nourishes kidneys and bladder; helps maintain fluid balance.

A balanced water element empowers you to trust the natural flow of life, giving and receiving in equal measure without difficulty. You are relaxed, calm and at ease with your life. You feel robust energy, physical power, stamina and aliveness; you shine like a star. You surrender to the process of sharing and your relationships are harmonious and deeply connected. Openness of your heart, mind and body ensure enjoyment of your life experience. You express sensuality and sexuality in a fluid and unified way. A balanced water element ensures a strong immune system and an inherent sense of physical power, health and well-being, including financial health.

An imbalanced water element may manifest as an inability to give or receive in equal measure, and you may find it difficult to surrender to "what is" and struggle with authority figures. You may be locked into the purely physical expression of your sensuality and sexuality. You may try to control situations and emotions in relationships, which may lead to repression of your needs and healthy self-expression of your truth. This is where your gun holster sits; you will either decide to react, take aim and fire or put your guns away for peaceful co-existence.

KEYWORDS:
Fluidity, giving and receiving love, communion, co-creation, procreation, endurance, self-confidence and patience.

RELATED PHYSICAL SYMPTOMS OF IMBALANCE INCLUDE:
Hot feet, leg pain, lumbar tension, lower back pain, chronic fatigue, claustrophobia, underarm and foot odor, hammer and pigeon toes, low or high blood sugar, bed wetting, kidney and bladder infection, immune disorders, skin conditions, swelling and edema, sweaty palms and feet, low energy, chronic stress, impatience, dark circles under eyes, salt craving, sensitivity to cold, impotence, frigidity, irritable bowel, painful urination, cystitis, urinary tract infection, sciatica, tight hamstrings, prostate conditions and addictions of all kinds.

RELATED EMOTIONAL STAGNATION OR BLOCKAGE INCLUDE:
Feelings of guilt or rejection. One attracts toxic environmental conditions (both internal and external) that trigger states of anxiety, fear and worry. You may be locked into power struggles with yourself or others and experience issues of rejection and victimization, jealousy and mistrust. The need for protection is often prevalent.

Essential Oils to Balance Water Element

Promotes balance for the water element and organ meridians.

To a 5-ml, colored-glass, euro-dropper bottle add:

Bergamot: 30 drops

Clary Sage: 10 drops

Geranium: 20 drops

Helichrysum: 10 drops

Lavender: 10 drops

Ylang Ylang: 20 drops

Close the cap tightly and shake the bottle vigorously to thoroughly blend the essential oils. Allow to synergize for 8 or more hours before using.

When using aromatherapy to restore energetic balance and flow of chi, your results can be enhanced when accompanied by diaphragmatic breathing.

Dispense 1–3 drops on a cotton ball or smell strip and inhale the aromatic vapors of your essential oil for 10–15 seconds. You may repeat as needed. This formula may also be effective as a compress over the area being treated.

To make a ready-to-use anointing oil that you can apply directly to the area being treated, simply add 15–30 drops of your essential oil to a 1-ounce (30-ml) bottle of your favorite carrier oil. Shake the bottle well to disperse the oils thoroughly. Apply a few drops of your ready-to-use anointing oil on the area being treated.

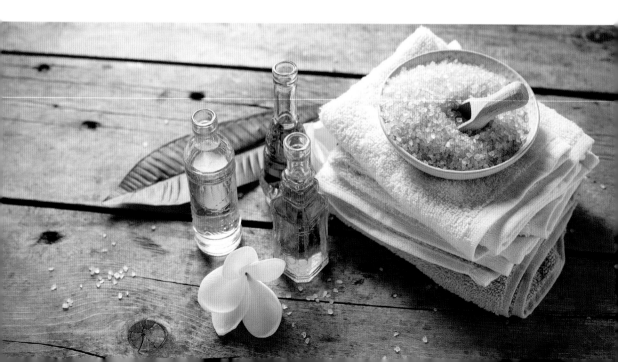

Wood Element Meridians

The power of wood is to regulate and restore.

ORGAN MERIDIAN CHANNELS

Gallbladder (yang) and liver (yin)

PROPERTIES OF WOOD ELEMENT

SEASON: Spring

TASTE: Sour

EMOTION: Anger

BODY PARTS: Liver, gallbladder, eyes, tendons

COLOR: Green

CHAKRA: Third (Manipura) Solar Plexus

SOUR ACTION

Cooling; promotes digestion, enzyme secretion and liver function.

A balanced wood element supports trust in the life process and taking full responsibility for one's life. You feel strong, stable, motivated and disciplined; you are able to easily fuel yourself with inspiration. You have a strong sense of purpose and the necessary autonomy to set and accomplish your goals. You are the creator of your life experience and easily sustain all that you desire in the physical world. You feel robust energy, physical power, stamina and aliveness. A balanced wood element supports a strong immune system.

An imbalanced wood element may manifest as a need to manipulate and control situations that may lead to repression of your needs and healthy self-expression.

KEYWORDS:

Endurance, stability, patience, decisive, motivated, disciplined, responsible and organized.

RELATED PHYSICAL SYMPTOMS OF IMBALANCE INCLUDE:

Abdominal bloating, digestive upsets, breast tenderness, cellulite, coated tongue, constipation, excessive bleeding, gout, irregular and painful menses, fatigue, flatulence, gallstones, halitosis, headaches, hemorrhoids, hepatitis, leg edema, nausea, soft nails, stiff neck and shoulders, skin conditions, varicose veins and uterine fibroids.

RELATED EMOTIONAL STAGNATION OR BLOCKAGE INCLUDE:

Feelings of guilt or shame, abandonment, rejection, anxiety, fear and worry, extreme self-criticism and unrealistic expectations of yourself and others.

Essential Oils to Balance Wood Element

Promotes balance to the wood element and organ meridians.

To a 5-ml, colored-glass, euro-dropper bottle add:

Cedarwood: 20 drops

Helichrysum: 20 drops

Myrrh: 20 drops

Rosemary: 1–5 drops

Sandalwood: 20 drops

Spikenard: 20 drops

Close the cap tightly and shake the bottle vigorously to thoroughly blend the essential oils. Allow to synergize for 8 or more hours before using.

When using aromatherapy to restore energetic balance and flow of chi, your results can be enhanced when accompanied by diaphragmatic breathing.

Dispense 1–3 drops on a cotton ball or smell strip and inhale the aromatic vapors of your essential oil for 10–15 seconds. You may repeat as needed. This formula may also be effective as a compress over the area being treated.

To make a ready-to-use anointing oil that you can apply directly to the area being treated, simply add 15–30 drops of your essential oil to a 1-ounce (30-ml) bottle of your favorite carrier oil. Shake the bottle well to disperse the oils thoroughly. Apply a few drops of your ready-to-use anointing oil on the area being treated.

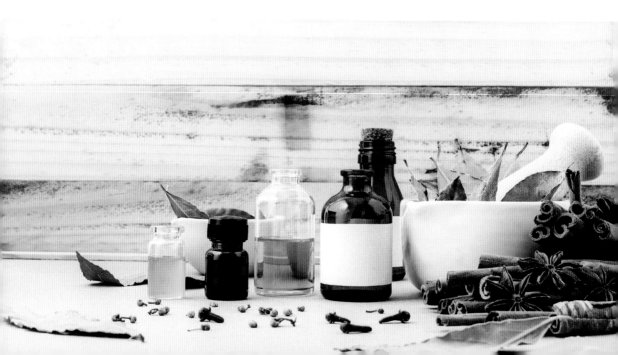

PLANETARY ELIXIRS

Pure essential oils can be used to enhance the planetary rulers for each of your zodiac signs and help ameliorate harsh influences in your natal chart or by transit. Popular sun sign astrology gives a very narrow view of the astrological influences affecting us at any given time. As a metaphysician and practicing astrologer for more than thirty years, I've learned how to make a very complex subject, your personal astrology, very simple to navigate.

With this simple guide, essentially all you need to do is tune into how you're feeling. Then select the planet that governs that key feeling or issue that you're wanting to experience more of or less of and use the essential oil or planetary elixir to experience results.

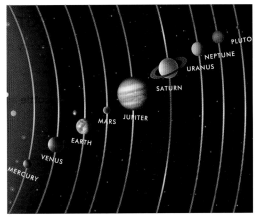

Essential oils can be used to balance your relationship with the stars.

Sun Planetary Elixir

SUN (LEO): Personal will, life force essence, the hero, the star.

To a 5-ml, colored-glass, euro-dropper bottle add:

Helichrysum: 40 drops

Ginger: 10 drops

Lemon: 20 drops

Sweet Orange: 20 drops

Cinnamon Leaf: 10 drops

Rosemary: 1–5 drops

Close the cap tightly and shake the bottle vigorously to thoroughly blend the essential oils. Allow to synergize for 8 or more hours before using.

Dispense 1–3 drops on a cotton ball or smell strip and inhale the aromatic vapors of your planetary elixir for 10–15 seconds. You may repeat as needed. This elixir is also effective when diffused into the air or used as an aromatic mist.

To make a ready-to-use Sun Planetary Elixir, simply add 15–30 drops of your synergy blend to a 1-ounce (30-ml) bottle of your favorite carrier oil. Shake the bottle well to disperse the oils thoroughly. Apply a few drops of your ready-to-use blend to your heart area, as well as on the back of your neck and behind both ears.

Moon Planetary Elixir

MOON (CANCER): Emotional needs, security issues, home, family.

To a 5-ml, colored-glass, euro-dropper bottle add:

Roman Chamomile: 20 drops

Clary Sage: 10 drops

Geranium: 20 drops

Ylang Ylang: 20 drops

Red Mandarin: 20 drops

Spikenard: 10 drops

Close the cap tightly and shake the bottle vigorously to thoroughly blend the essential oils. Allow to synergize for 8 or more hours before using.

Dispense 1–3 drops on a cotton ball or smell strip and inhale the aromatic vapors of your planetary elixir for 10–15 seconds. You may repeat as needed. This elixir is also effective when diffused into the air or used as an aromatic mist.

To make a ready-to-use Moon Planetary Elixir, simply add 15–30 drops of your synergy blend to a 1-ounce (30-ml) bottle of your favorite carrier oil. Shake the bottle well to disperse the oils thoroughly. Apply a few drops of your ready-to-use blend to your heart area, as well as on the back of your neck and behind both ears.

Mercury Planetary Elixir

MERCURY (VIRGO AND GEMINI): Communications and ways of connecting.

To a 5-ml, colored-glass, euro-dropper bottle add:

Cedarwood: 20 drops

Myrrh: 10 drops

Lemongrass: 30 drops

Ylang Ylang: 30 drops

Frankincense: 10 drops

Close the cap tightly and shake the bottle vigorously to thoroughly blend the essential oils. Allow to synergize for 8 or more hours before using.

Dispense 1–3 drops on a cotton ball or smell strip and inhale the aromatic vapors of your planetary elixir for 10–15 seconds. You may repeat as needed. This elixir is also effective when diffused into the air or used as an aromatic mist.

To make a ready-to-use Mercury Planetary Elixir, simply add 15–30 drops of your synergy blend to a 1-ounce (30-ml) bottle of your favorite carrier oil. Shake the bottle well to disperse the oils thoroughly. Apply a few drops of your ready-to-use blend to your heart area, as well as on the back of your neck and behind both ears.

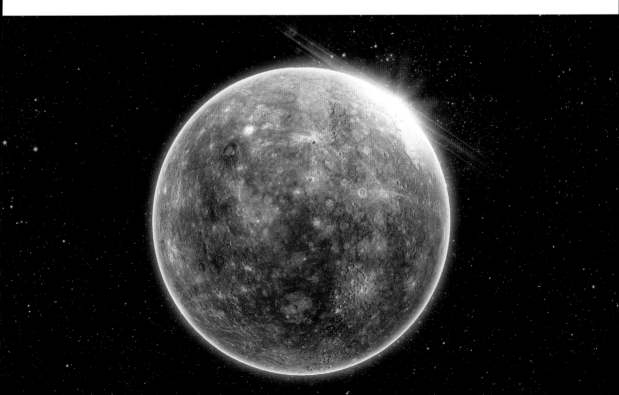

Venus Planetary Elixir

VENUS (TAURUS AND LIBRA): Personal love; what attracts you and gives you pleasure.

To a 5-ml, colored-glass, euro-dropper bottle add:

Rose: 10 drops

Geranium Roseum and Graveolens: 10 drops each

Ylang Ylang: 20 drops

Neroli: 20 drops

Sandalwood: 20 drops

Patchouli: 10 drops

Close the cap tightly and shake the bottle vigorously to thoroughly blend the essential oils. Allow to synergize for 8 or more hours before using.

Dispense 1–3 drops on a cotton ball or smell strip and inhale the aromatic vapors of your planetary elixir for 10–15 seconds. You may repeat as needed. This elixir is also effective when diffused into the air or used as an aromatic mist.

To make a ready-to-use Venus Planetary Elixir, simply add 15–30 drops of your synergy blend to a 1-ounce (30-ml) bottle of your favorite carrier oil. Shake the bottle well to disperse the oils thoroughly. Apply a few drops of your ready-to-use blend to your heart area, as well as on the back of your neck and behind both ears.

Mars Planetary Elixir

MARS (ARIES): Desire, drive, ambition, ego, taking action.

To a 5-ml, colored-glass, euro-dropper bottle add:

Cedarwood: 20 drops

Myrrh: 20 drops

Lemon: 10 drops

Sandalwood: 20 drops

Patchouli: 10 drops

Helichrysum: 10 drops

Palmarosa: 10 drops

Close the cap tightly and shake the bottle vigorously to thoroughly blend the essential oils. Allow to synergize for 8 or more hours before using.

Dispense 1–3 drops on a cotton ball or smell strip and inhale the aromatic vapors of your planetary elixir for 10–15 seconds. You may repeat as needed. This elixir is also effective when diffused into the air or used as an aromatic mist.

To make a ready-to-use Mars Planetary Elixir, simply add 15–30 drops of your synergy blend to a 1-ounce (30-ml) bottle of your favorite carrier oil. Shake the bottle well to disperse the oils thoroughly. Apply a few drops of your ready-to-use blend to your heart area, as well as on the back of your neck and behind both ears.

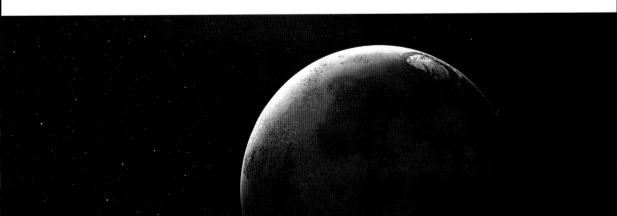

Jupiter Planetary Elixir

JUPITER (SAGITTARIUS): Expands whatever it touches and brings good fortune, enthusiasm and optimism.

To a 5-ml, colored-glass, euro-dropper bottle add:

Sweet Orange: 30 drops

Cinnamon Leaf: 10 drops

Ginger: 10 drops

Helichrysum: 20 drops

Sandalwood: 20 drops

Frankincense: 10 drops

Close the cap tightly and shake the bottle vigorously to thoroughly blend the essential oils. Allow to synergize for 8 or more hours before using.

Dispense 1–3 drops on a cotton ball or smell strip and inhale the aromatic vapors of your planetary elixir for 10–15 seconds. You may repeat as needed. This elixir is also effective when diffused into the air or used as an aromatic mist.

To make a ready-to-use Jupiter Planetary Elixir, simply add 15–30 drops of your synergy blend to a 1-ounce (30-ml) bottle of your favorite carrier oil. Shake the bottle well to disperse the oils thoroughly. Apply a few drops of your ready-to-use blend to your heart area, as well as on the back of your neck and behind both ears.

Saturn Planetary Elixir

SATURN (CAPRICORN): Brings structure and gives form, rules, authority and limitations.

To a 5-ml, colored-glass, euro-dropper bottle add:

Cedarwood: 30 drops

Myrrh: 20 drops

Sandalwood: 30 drops

Galbanum: 1–5 drops

Vetiver: 10 drops

Ylang Ylang III: 10 drops

Close the cap tightly and shake the bottle vigorously to thoroughly blend the essential oils. Allow to synergize for 8 or more hours before using.

Dispense 1–3 drops on a cotton ball or smell strip and inhale the aromatic vapors of your planetary elixir for 10–15 seconds. You may repeat as needed. This elixir is also effective when diffused into the air or used as an aromatic mist.

To make a ready-to-use Saturn Planetary Elixir, simply add 15–30 drops of your synergy blend to a 1-ounce (30-ml) bottle of your favorite carrier oil. Shake the bottle well to disperse the oils thoroughly. Apply a few drops of your ready-to-use blend to your heart area, as well as on the back of your neck and behind both ears.

Uranus Planetary Elixir

URANUS (AQUARIUS): Radical breakthrough, visionary, pioneer and freedom urge.

To a 5-ml, colored-glass, euro-dropper bottle add:

Cedarwood: 20 drops

Myrrh: 20 drops

Ylang Ylang: 20 drops

Frankincense: 20 drops

Bergamot: 20 drops

Black Spruce: 1–5 drops

Close the cap tightly and shake the bottle vigorously to thoroughly blend the essential oils. Allow to synergize for 8 or more hours before using.

Dispense 1–3 drops on a cotton ball or smell strip and inhale the aromatic vapors of your planetary elixir for 10–15 seconds. You may repeat as needed. This elixir is also effective when diffused into the air or used as an aromatic mist.

To make a ready-to-use Uranus Planetary Elixir, simply add 15–30 drops of your synergy blend to a 1-ounce (30-ml) bottle of your favorite carrier oil. Shake the bottle well to disperse the oils thoroughly. Apply a few drops of your ready-to-use blend to your heart area, as well as on the back of your neck and behind both ears.

Neptune Planetary Elixir

NEPTUNE (PISCES): Perfect ideal, dreams, illusions and unconscious patterns, self-sabotage, addiction.

To a 5-ml, colored-glass, euro-dropper bottle add:

Sandalwood: 20 drops

Myrrh: 20 drops

Black Spruce: 1–5 drops

Thyme: 10 drops

Sweet Marjoram: 20 drops

Bergamot: 20 drops

Helichrysum: 10 drops

Close the cap tightly and shake the bottle vigorously to thoroughly blend the essential oils. Allow to synergize for 8 or more hours before using.

Dispense 1–3 drops on a cotton ball or smell strip and inhale the aromatic vapors of your planetary elixir for 10–15 seconds. You may repeat as needed. This elixir is also effective when diffused into the air or used as an aromatic mist.

To make a ready-to-use Neptune Planetary Elixir, simply add 15–30 drops of your synergy blend to a 1-ounce (30-ml) bottle of your favorite carrier oil. Shake the bottle well to disperse the oils thoroughly. Apply a few drops of your ready-to-use blend to your heart area, as well as on the back of your neck and behind both ears.

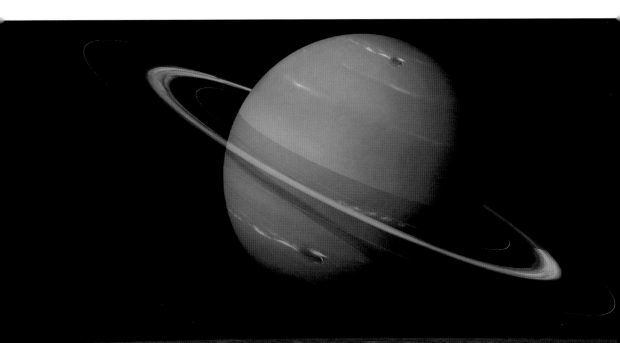

Pluto Planetary Elixir

PLUTO (SCORPIO): Death, destruction, rebirth, regeneration, healing and power, bad habits, quiet shame, hidden motives.

To a 5-ml, colored-glass, euro-dropper bottle add:

Helichrysum: 30 drops

Spikenard: 30 drops

Cypress: 10 drops

Sweet Marjoram: 10 drops

Black Pepper: 5 drops

Lemon: 15 drops

Close the cap tightly and shake the bottle vigorously to thoroughly blend the essential oils. Allow to synergize for 8 or more hours before using.

Dispense 1–3 drops on a cotton ball or smell strip and inhale the aromatic vapors of your planetary elixir for 10–15 seconds. You may repeat as needed. This elixir is also effective when diffused into the air or used as an aromatic mist.

To make a ready-to-use Pluto Planetary Elixir, simply add 15–30 drops of your synergy blend to a 1-ounce (30-ml) bottle of your favorite carrier oil. Shake the bottle well to disperse the oils thoroughly. Apply a few drops of your ready-to-use blend to your heart area, as well as on the back of your neck and behind both ears.

ANGEL THERAPY

Angels have been around since the dawn of time as God's messengers. The word angel itself is found in many languages that all share the Latin root word *angelus*, which means "messenger." It also comes from the Greek word *ángelos*. The easiest way I've come to understand angels is that they represent the perfect idea that life has when creating anything in the manifest world.

The founder of modern day angel therapy is Dr. Doreen Virtue, who has published more than fifty books and oracle card decks on the subject. The basis for angel therapy is that by connecting and communicating with angels, healing may occur.

The legend of the spiritual heavens has it that there are four primary angels, or archangels, that act as guardians of the world. They are Gabriel, Michael, Raphael and Uriel.

Each of these archangels has a particular task to fulfill as God's messenger. Each aromatherapy blend of select essential oils was formulated to match the angel's signature purpose and carries the scent of its perfume.

Gabriel

TO SUPPORT YOUR WORK AS A MESSENGER

Protector of the element of water, the word Gabriel is derived from Hebrew and means "God is my strength." Gabriel is the angel that oversees conception, birth and the adoption of a child and helps those whose purpose in life involves art and communication.

An angel of mercy and compassion, Gabriel helps to purify the body, mind and emotions of those called to be writers, counselors, therapists and teachers. Gabriel is considered the patron of postal workers, clergy and those in the communications field.

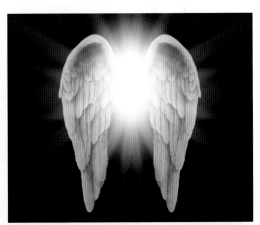

The four primary angels that act as guardians of the world are Michael, Raphael, Uriel and Gabriel.

Gabriel Angel Therapy Oil

To support healthy connections and communications.

To a 5-ml, colored-glass, euro-dropper bottle add:
Neroli: 40 drops
Rose: 20 drops
Ylang Ylang: 20 drops
German Chamomile: 10 drops
Helichrysum: 10 drops

Close the cap tightly and shake the bottle vigorously to thoroughly blend the essential oils. Allow to synergize for 8 or more hours before using.

Dispense 1–3 drops on a cotton ball or smell strip and inhale the aromatic vapors of your Gabriel Angel Therapy Oil for 10–15 seconds. You may repeat as needed. This formula is also effective when diffused into the air or used as an aromatic mist.

To make a ready-to-use angel therapy oil, simply add 15–30 drops of your synergy blend to a 1-ounce (30-ml) bottle of your favorite carrier oil. Shake the bottle well to disperse the oils thoroughly. Apply a few drops of your ready-to-use blend to your heart area, as well as on the back of your neck and behind both ears.

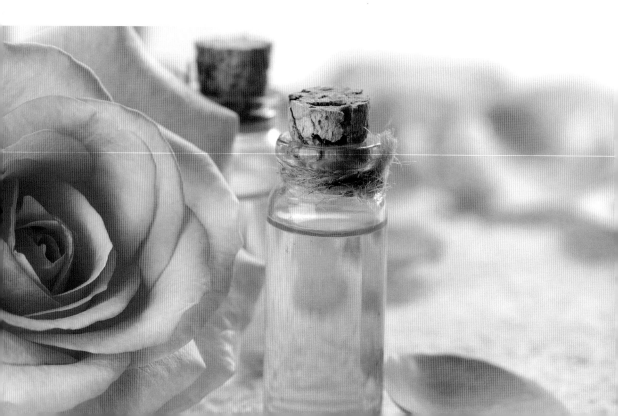

Michael

TO SUPPORT YOUR INNER SPIRITUAL WARRIOR

In Hebrew the name Michael means "Who is like God." Archangel Michael is the warrior and protector angel who rids you of fear and cuts your cords of attachment. Leader of all the archangels, Michael is the protector of the fire element. Michael upholds fair and balanced life outcomes and helps you to clarify and make changes to fulfill your life purpose. Michael is the angel of strength and courage and the patron of those in the legal and military professions.

Michael Angel Therapy Oil

For protection, strength and courage in order to overcome fear and procrastination.

To a 5-ml, colored-glass, euro-dropper bottle add:

Cedarwood: 40 drops

Myrrh: 30 drops

Black Spruce: 1–5 drops

Thyme: 10 drops

Black Pepper: 10 drops

Lemon: 10 drops

Close the cap tightly and shake the bottle vigorously to thoroughly blend the essential oils. Allow to synergize for 8 or more hours before using.

Dispense 1–3 drops on a cotton ball or smell strip and inhale the aromatic vapors of your Michael Angel Therapy Oil for 10–15 seconds. You may repeat as needed. This formula is also effective when diffused into the air or used as an aromatic mist.

To make a ready-to-use angel therapy oil, simply add 15–30 drops of your synergy blend to a 1-ounce (30-ml) bottle of your favorite carrier oil. Shake the bottle well to disperse the oils thoroughly. Apply a few drops of your ready-to-use blend to your heart area, as well as on the back of your neck and behind both ears.

Raphael

TO SUPPORT YOUR INNER HEALER

Raphael's name in Hebrew means "God heals." Archangel Raphael is the protector of the air element and the angel of joy, love and laughter. His primary role is to oversee all physical healing for both animals and humans. Raphael helps you to heal your mind and soul and to overcome all forms of human suffering, including addictions. Raphael is the patron of those in the healing and medical professions.

Raphael Angel Therapy Oil

To support healing and work as a healer.

To a 5-ml, colored-glass, euro-dropper bottle add:

Helichrysum: 20 drops

Frankincense: 20 drops

Palmarosa: 20 drops

Sweet Marjoram: 20 drops

Cypress: 10 drops

Myrrh: 5 drops

Rosemary: 5 drops

Close the cap tightly and shake the bottle vigorously to thoroughly blend the essential oils. Allow to synergize for 8 or more hours before using.

Dispense 1–3 drops on a cotton ball or smell strip and inhale the aromatic vapors of your Raphael Angel Therapy Oil for 10–15 seconds. You may repeat as needed. This formula is also effective when diffused into the air or used as an aromatic mist.

To make a ready-to-use angel therapy oil, simply add 15–30 drops of your synergy blend to a 1-ounce (30-ml) bottle of your favorite carrier oil. Shake the bottle well to disperse the oils thoroughly. Apply a few drops of your ready-to-use blend to your heart area, as well as on the back of your neck and behind both ears.

Uriel

TO SUPPORT YOUR INNER LIGHT AND ILLUMINATION

Uriel's name in Hebrew means "God's light" because he illuminates and brings clarity into the darkest situations, as well as encourages prophetic visions. Protector of the earth element, Uriel helps with healing and recovery in the aftermath of natural disasters or difficult transitions in life. Uriel helps you to find the perfect solutions to your problems and pass all of your tests. The angel of wisdom and brilliant ideas, Uriel is the patron of music and literature.

Uriel Angel Therapy Oil

To support your spiritual understanding.

To a 5-ml, colored-glass, euro-dropper bottle add:

Frankincense: 20 drops

Cinnamon Leaf: 20 drops

Ginger: 10 drops

Helichrysum: 10 drops

Peppermint: 10 drops

Black Pepper: 10 drops

Lemongrass: 10 drops

Lemon: 10 drops

Close the cap tightly and shake the bottle vigorously to thoroughly blend the essential oils. Allow to synergize for 8 or more hours before using.

Dispense 1–3 drops on a cotton ball or smell strip and inhale the aromatic vapors of your Uriel Angel Therapy Oil for 10–15 seconds. You may repeat as needed. This formula is also effective when diffused into the air or used as an aromatic mist.

To make a ready-to-use angel therapy oil, simply add 15–30 drops of your synergy blend to a 1-ounce (30-ml) bottle of your favorite carrier oil. Shake the bottle well to disperse the oils thoroughly. Apply a few drops of your ready-to-use blend to your heart area, as well as on the back of your neck and behind both ears.

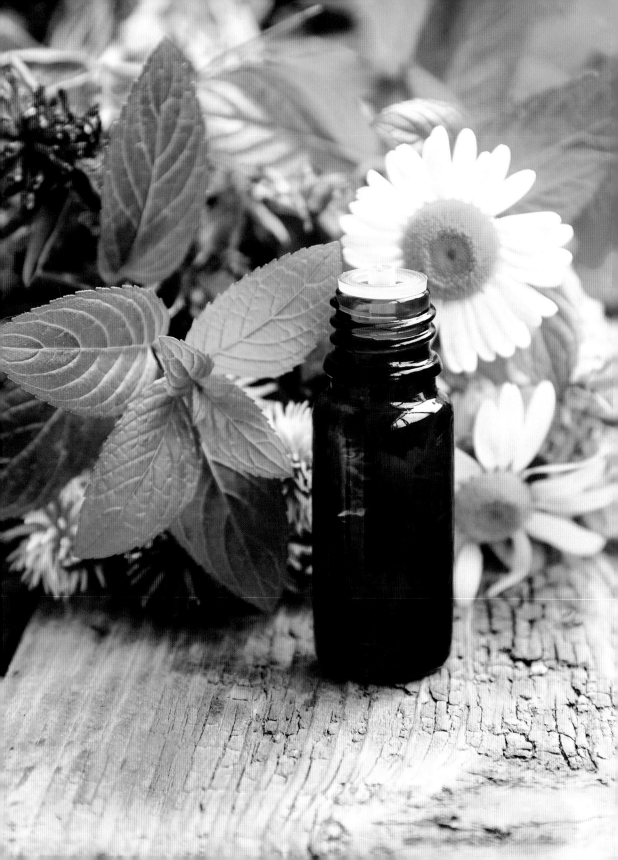

Essential Oils Quick Reference Guides

Safety and Dilution Guide

Below are sample dilution guidelines I use for my aromatherapy products.

GUIDE FOR STANDARD DILUTION OF ESSENTIAL OILS IN CARRIER OIL

ADULTS (25+ YEARS): 15 drops EO in 1 ounce (30 ml) of carrier oil

CHILDREN AGE EIGHTEEN AND OLDER: 10 drops EO in 1 ounce (30 ml) of carrier oil

CHILDREN AGE TEN TO EIGHTEEN: 6-9 drops EO in 1 ounce (30 ml) of carrier oil

CHILDREN AGE FIVE TO TEN: 5 drops EO in 1 ounce (30 ml) of carrier oil

CHILDREN AGE FOUR AND THE ELDERLY AND INFIRM: 4 drops EO in 1 ounce (30 ml) of carrier oil

CHILDREN AGE THREE: 3 drops EO in 1 ounce (30 ml) of carrier oil

CHILDREN AGE TWO: 2 drops EO in 1 ounce (30 ml) of carrier oil

NEWBORN TO CHILDREN AGE TWO: 1 drop in 1 ounce (30 ml) of carrier oil

GENERAL FLUID CONVERSION GUIDE

1 ml = 20 drops EO
3.75 ml = 1 dram = ⅛ oz = 75 drops EO
5 ml = 1 tsp = 100 drops EO
15 ml = 3 tsp (1 tbsp) = ½ oz = 300 drops EO
30 ml = 2 tbsp = 8 drams = 1 oz = 600 drops EO

DILUTION GUIDE FOR SAFE SKIN APPLICATION

How much essential oil should you put into your carriers for safe skin application? Generally, effective blends for adults are made using a dilution ratio of 1, 2 or 3 percent of essential oil to the carrier. Perfume oils are higher dilutions of 5–10 percent.

1% Dilution (5–6 drops per ounce [30 ml] carrier): Use for children under twelve, seniors over sixty-five, pregnant women and people with long-term illnesses or immune system disorders. A 1-percent dilution is a good place to start with individuals who are generally sensitive to aromas, chemicals or other environmental pollutants.

2% Dilution (10–12 drops per ounce [30 ml] carrier): Use for general health and skincare, natural perfumes, bath products and your everyday blends.

3% Dilution (15–18 drops per ounce [30 ml] carrier): Use for specific application blends and acute health conditions (i.e. treating a cold or flu, pain relief and sports blends).

5% Dilution (28–30 drops per ounce [30 ml] carrier): Use for sports massage blends, natural perfumes and short-term treatment for specific, acute health conditions.

10% Dilution (58–60 drops per ounce [30 ml] carrier): Very expensive essential oils like rose, helichrysum and neroli are often made available in a 10-percent dilution of carrier oil. Essential oil blends for natural perfumes and specific applications may sometimes also be found in 10-percent dilutions.

Medical Terms: Primary Actions and Effects

ADAPTOGENS/REGULATORS: substances that promote beneficial adaptation to change; refers to the pharmacological concept whereby administration results in stabilization of physiological processes and promotion of homeostasis or balance

ANALGESIC: pain reliever

ANTIDEPRESSANT: alleviates or prevents depression, lifts mood, counters melancholia

ANTI-INFLAMMATORY: reduces inflammation resulting from injury or infection

ANTI-INFECTIOUS/ANTIMICROBIAL: kills microorganisms or inhibits their growth

ANTI-PARASITIC: inhibits and destroys growth of parasites

ANTISPASMODIC: calms nervous and muscular spasms; for pain and indigestion

CARMINATIVE/STOMACHIC: settles digestive system, relieves intestinal gas

CICATRIZANT: wound healing; promotes formation of scar tissue

DIGESTIVE/STOMACHIC: aids and promotes appetite and assists digestion of food

EXPECTORANT/MUCOLYTIC: promotes removal of mucus from respiratory system

FUNGICIDAL: prevents and destroys fungal infection

INSECT REPELLANT/INSECTICIDE: repels and destroys insects

RUBEFACIENT: increases local blood circulation causing analgesic effect

SEDATIVE: promotes calming and tranquilizing effect and induces sleep

STIMULANT: raises levels of physiological or nervous activity in the body; good for convalescence and physical fatigue

URINARY TRACT ANTISEPTIC: inhibits growth of microorganisms in the urinary tract

Psycho-emotional Aromatherapy Chart (Super Oils)

Action	Problem	EO Solution
REGULATOR OR ADAPTOGEN (EITHER STIMULANT OR SEDATIVE)	Manic/depressive, extreme mood swings, depressive anxiety, hormone imbalance	bergamot, geranium, rose, ylang ylang III, sandalwood, cedarwood, blue yarrow, helichrysum, frankincense, palmarosa
MOTIVATING	Lethargy, boredom, issues of low self-worth, immune depression	grapefruit, rosemary, peppermint, lemongrass, eucalyptus, thyme
SEDATIVE	Fear, stress, worry, insomnia, irritability, anxiety, anger issues	chamomile, sandalwood, ylang ylang III, red mandarin, melissa, neroli, spikenard, vetiver
STIMULANT	Mental fatigue, poor memory, poor concentration, inability to focus	lemon, peppermint, cinnamon, rosemary
UPLIFTING (MOOD ENHANCER)	Loss of inspiration, lack of direction, aimless, purposeless	grapefruit, ylang ylang, tangerine, black spruce, peppermint, lemon
RELAXANT	Stressed, uptight, control issues	clary sage, geranium, sandalwood, ylang ylang, sweet marjoram, palmarosa, lavender, frankincense
EUPHORIC	Depression, lack of self-confidence, moody	neroli, ylang ylang, grapefruit, clary sage, spikenard
APHRODISIAC	Shyness, isolation, loneliness, frigidity, emotional coldness, withdrawal, impotence, loneliness	sandalwood, cinnamon, ginger, clary sage, rose, patchouli

APPENDIX 2

Symptoms Guide: Super Oils to Use

ADAPTOGEN/REGULATOR: bergamot, geranium, ylang ylang III, rose, frankincense, sandalwood

ALLERGIES: blue tansy, hyssop, ammi visnaga, chamomile, lemongrass, spikenard

ANXIETY/FEAR/WORRY: bergamot, vetiver, ylang ylang, rose, neroli, melissa, geranium, clary sage, chamomile, red mandarin, black spruce, black pepper

CIRCULATION: rosemary, cinnamon, ginger, peppermint, cypress, black pepper, black spruce

DEPRESSION: bergamot, sandalwood, geranium, rose, neroli, melissa, frankincense, ylang ylang, grapefruit, black spruce, sweet orange

CONGESTION/COUGH: eucalyptus, lemon, cinnamon, ginger, rosemary, hyssop

CRAMPS/SPASMS: peppermint, black pepper, sweet marjoram

DETOXIFICATION: juniper berry, lemon, rosemary

DIGESTIVE: ginger, peppermint

FUNGAL INFECTION: palmarosa, thyme, oregano, tea tree, grapefruit

HORMONE BALANCE: geranium, rose, bergamot, clary sage

INFECTION: palmarosa, eucalyptus, clove, cinnamon, thyme, oregano, ravensara, tea tree, ledum

INFLAMMATION/BURNS: chamomile, helichrysum, lavender, blue tansy, blue yarrow

INJURY/WOUND HEALING: helichrysum, rose, chamomile, sweet marjoram, rosemary

INSECT REPELLANT: palmarosa, rose, geranium, patchouli, peppermint, cedarwood, lemongrass

PAIN RELIEF: chamomile, peppermint, sweet marjoram, black pepper, ginger, black spruce

PARASITES: cinnamon, clove bud

RESPIRATORY: eucalyptus, hyssop, ledum, ammi visnaga, frankincense, blue tansy

SEDATIVE: spikenard, vetiver, ylang ylang III, chamomile, red mandarin, lavender, clary sage

SKINCARE/BURNS: geranium, carrot seed, lavender, chamomile, rose, ylang ylang, galbanum, frankincense, myrrh, sandalwood, patchouli, cypress

STIMULANT: rosemary, ginger, lemon, peppermint, black pepper

URINARY TRACT INFECTION: juniper berry, lemon, rosemary

WEIGHT CONTROL: grapefruit, lemon

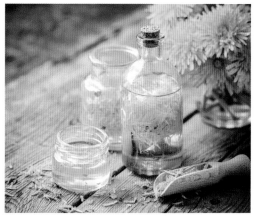

Key oils to relieve pain, inflammation and speed healing are helichrysum, chamomile, lavender, blue tansy and blue yarrow.

Further Reading, Resources and References

The Practice of Aromatherapy: A Classic Compendium of Plant Medicines and Their Healing Properties, by Jean Valnet MD and Robert B. Tisserand

Aromatherapy Workbook, by Marcel Lavabre

The Secret Teachings of Plants: The Intelligence of the Heart in the Direct Perception of Nature, by Stephen Harrod Buhner

Clinical Aromatherapy: Essential Oils in Practice, by Jane Buckle

The Art of Aromatherapy: The Healing and Beautifying Properties of the Essential Oils of Flowers and Herbs, by Robert Tisserand

The Aromatherapy Practitioner Reference Manual (2 Volumes), by Sylla Sheppard-Hanger

The Blossoming Heart: Aromatherapy for Healing and Transformation, by Robbi Zeck ND

The Complete Book of Essential Oils & Aromatherapy, by Valerie Ann Worwood

Aromatherapy for Healing the Spirit: Restoring Emotional and Mental Balance with Essential Oils, by Gabriel Mojay

Animal Aromatherapy Certification Course® by Kelly Holland Azzaro

The Magic of Ayurveda Aromatherapy: Discover the Magic & Rare & Unique Ayurveda Aromatherapy Oils in Harmony with Universal Healing Success, by Farida S. Irani

The Chemistry of Essential Oils, by David G. Williams

Aromatherapy: The Complete Guide to Plant and Flower Essences for Health and Beauty, by Daniele Ryman

Complete Aromatherapy Handbook: Essential Oils for Radiant Health, by Susanne Fischer-Rizzi

Aromatherapy for Health Professionals, 2nd edition, by Len and Shirley Price

Aromatherapy Workbook: A Complete Guide to Understanding and Using Essential Oils, by Shirley Price

Medical Aromatherapy: Healing with Essential Oils, by Kurt Schnaubelt

International Fragrance Association, http://www.ifra.org/

Essential Oils Safety: A Guide for Health Care Professionals, 2nd Edition by Robert B. Tisserand

Acknowledgments

For my son, Ezra, my inspiration, who never gave up on me!

To my agent, Marilyn Allen, who, like an angel, found me and guided me through the publishing process.

Big thank you to my editor, Liz Seise, my publisher, Will Kiester and the Page Street team for their invaluable assistance in birthing a truly great book!

About the Author

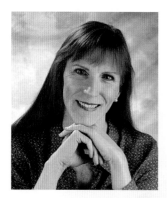

KG is an earth-loving aromatherapist, metaphysical coach and holistic health educator of more than 35 years. She is passionate about helping others become the person they most want to be, by living a full life.

Born and raised in Wilmington, North Carolina, KG knew from a very young age she wanted to help people feel better. She realized early on it was the way people were thinking that caused most, if not all, of their problems. KG became passionate about changing the way people think about their life situations. After college, and with nothing more than a desire to help people overcome their challenges, she began pursuing her dream.

After discovering the work of Carl Jung and Rudolph Steiner, KG traveled to the Findhorn community in Scotland and became even more immersed in transformational healing. After being introduced to essential oils, she realized that she had found what she had been looking for her whole life. One sniff of pure plant essences can instantly shift a person's thinking and mental attitude.

KG is proud to have created a socially conscious online presence that positively touches hundreds of thousands of lives around the world. Her online aromatherapy training and metaphysical coaching programs help people, like you, live true to themselves, free to take meaningful action and create a life they love. She lives in Ashland, Oregon.

Index

A

Abies sibirica, 54. *See also* Siberian balsam; silver fir

absolute oil extraction, 19

Achillea millefolium, *65*, 148–50, *148*, *150*. *See also* blue yarrow

acupuncture, 416

adaptogens, 446

adulterant, 23

air freshener, 48, 334

Air Freshener Formula, 334

alcohol, 66

allergic reactions, 53

Allergic Skin Reaction Relief Formula, 199, 202

allergies, 446

All-Purpose Herbal Blend, 363, 371

All-Purpose Household Surface Cleaner Formula, 338

aloe vera gel, 67

alopecia, 281–82, 282

alpha-tocopherol, 40

Ammi visnaga, *60*, 97–98, *97*, *98*, 446, 447. *See also* khella plant seeds

amygdala, 27

Angel Hair Pasta with Spicy Shrimp, 375

angel therapy, 437–41

   Gabriel Angel Therapy Oil, 438

   Michael Angel Therapy Oil, 439

   Raphael Angel Therapy Oil, 440

   Uriel Angel Therapy Oil, 441

animals, 399–403

   Flea and Tick Prevention and Treatment, 400

   Respiratory Support, 402

Anthemis nobilis, 87. *See also* chamomile

anxiety, 446

anxiety relief, 256

Anxiety Relief Formula, 256

Aphrodite Perfume Oil Formula, 315

appetizers, 372

   Pita and Hummus Dip, 372

aromatherapy, 20

   aromatherapy blending guide, 157–60

   aromatherapy blends, 67

   aromatherapy delivery pathways, *30*

   aromatherapy formulas, 163–71, 164, 167, 168, 170, 171

   aromatherapy journals, 65

   aromatherapy massage, 23

   aromatherapy sprays, 47–48, 66, *66*

   aromatherapy terms, 23–25

   brief history of, 22–23

   Calming Formula, 168

   how it works, 26–27

   Muscle Pain Relief Formula, 171

   Relaxation Formula, 164

   Restorative Formula, 170

   Sports Injury Formula, 167

aromatherapy formulas, 163–71

   Calming Formula, 168

   Muscle Pain Relief Formula, 171

   Relaxation Formula, 164

   Restorative Formula, 170

   Sports Injury Formula, 167

aromatherapy journals, 65

Arthritis Pain Relief Formula, 186

astringent, 270

Athlete's Foot Formula, 203, 205

atlas cedarwood, *60*, 99–100, *99*, *100*, 198, 252, 260, 319, 344, 400

atomizers, 66, *66*

attention, 348

Audacity Men's Cologne Formula, 319

autonomic nervous system (ANS), 324

Avocado Crostini, 374, *374*

avocados, 66

Ayurvedic medicine, 22

B

babies, 321–27

   baby massage, 323–26, *325*

   teething solutions, 326–27

background information, 19

baking soda, 66, 291

basil, 54, 151, 174, 190, 344, 348, 352, 353, 354, 357, 359, 363

basins, 67

baths, 40–41, *40–41*

bath salts, 66, 291–92

beauty treatments. *See* spa and beauty treatments

beeswax, 45–46, *46*, 67, 274, 311

bentonite green clay, 233

bergamot, *57*, 69–70, *69*, 164, 209, 228, 240, 251, 252, 256, 259, 260, 261, 315, 322, 410, 424, 434, 435, 446

The Best Lemon Bars, *392*, 393

Betula lenta, 151

beverages, 19, 382

    Chocolate Mint Martini, 390

    Lemongrass Black Tea, 382

    Mimosas, 385

    Sunshine Martini, 389

    Venus Martini, 386

birch, 151, 213, 285

black pepper, 54, *60*, 101, *101*, 183, 184, 186, 187, 190, 228, 319, 330, 338, 347, 352, 354, 357, 359, 363, 412, 435, 439, 441, 446, 447

black spruce, *60*, 102, *102*, 170, 315, 319, 333, 334, 344, 434, 435, 439, 446

blending supplies, 159–60

blood vascular system, 27

blue tansy, *60*, 103, *103*, 194, 197, 200, 211, 231, 411, 446, 447

blue yarrow, *65*, 199, 200, 231, 282, 302, 411, 447

body butters, 44, *45*, 67, 274

    beeswax, 45–46, *46*

    cocoa butter, 45

    Healing and Regenerative Body Butter Formula, 311–13

    shea butter, 45

body freshener, 48

body masks, 66

    French Clay Body Mask Formula, 308–10

body massage carrier oils, 39

    sesame oil, 39

    sweet almond oil, 39

    vitamin E oil, 40, *40*

    wheat germ oil, 40

body scrubs, 44–45, *45*, 293

body skin toners. *See* skin toners

body wraps, 43, *43*

Boswelia carterii, 74–75. *See also* frankincense

Boswelia frereana, *58*, 74–75. *See also* frankincense

botanical species, 57

bottles

    glass dropper, 65

    glass euro-dropper, 67

    glass misting/atomizer, *66*

breakfast recipes, 364–67

    Quick and Easy Cinnamon French Toast, 367

    Zucchini Citrus and Spice Muffins, 364

breast health, 243

Breast Health Massage Formula, 246

breast massage, 243

brown sugar, 293

brunch recipes, 364–67

    Quick and Easy Cinnamon French Toast, 367

    Zucchini Citrus and Spice Muffins, 364

brushes, 65

Burn Care Formula, 193

burns, 447

butters, 67, 274, 311–13. *See also* body butters

C

Calming Formula, 168

Cananga odorata, 54, *59*, 93–95. *See also* ylang ylang

cardamom, 352, 357

carrier oils, 23, 55, *55*, 60, 65, 293, 307, 326

    face carrier oils, 36, 36–38, *36*, *37*, 38, 38–39, *38*, *39*

    vegetable carrier oils, *55*, 65

carrot seed, *61*, 104, *104*, 204, 266, 267, 268, 273, 280, 297, 298, 305, 308, 323, 447

cassia, 352, 360

cats, 400

cedarwood, 282, 319, 344, 348, 400, 409, 418, 426, 429, 433, 439, 447

Cedrus atlantica, *60*, 99–100. *See also* atlas cedarwood

Celtic salt, 44, *44*, 66, *66*, 233, 291

chakras, 405–6, *405*, *406*, 413

    Eighth Chakra Oil Formula, 414

essential oils to balance, 406

Fifth Chakra Oil Formula, 411

First Chakra Oil Formula, 407

first chakras, 406, *406*

Fourth Chakra Oil Formula, 410

Ninth Chakra Oil Formula, 415

second chakra, 408

Second Chakra Oil Formula, 408

Seventh Chakra Oil Formula, 413

Sixth Chakra Oil Formula, 412

Third Chakra Oil Formula, 409

Chamaemelum nobile, 59, 87. *See also* Roman chamomile

chamomile, *62*, 87, *87*, 168, 179, 255, 411, 428, 446, 447

    blue Moroccan chamomile, *60*, 103, *103*

    German chamomile, 114–15, *114–15*, 179, 183, 184, 187, 193, 194, 197, 199, 200, 204, 211, 214, 217, 256, 267, 270, 301, 322, 323, 326, 400, 438

    Roman chamomile, *59*, 87, *87*, 168, 256, 322, 411, 428

childbirth, 321–22

children, 53, 321–27. *See also* babies

Chocolate Mint Martini, 390, *391*

Chronic Skin Conditions Formula, 301

Cinnamomun zeylanicum, 54, *61*, 105. *See also* cinnamon leaf

cinnamon, 54, 105–6, *105*, 315, 352, 357, 359, 367, 446, 447

cinnamon leaf, *61*, 208, 233, 235, 330, 333, 334, 344, 347, 360, 427, 432, 441, 446

circulation, 446

Citrus and Spice Blend, 360, 364, 367

Citrus aurantium, 63, 128–29. *See also* neroli

Citrus bergamia, 57, 69–70. *See also* bergamot

Citrus deliciosa, 64, 134. *See also* red mandarin

Citrus limonum, 58, 82–84

Citrus paradisi, 62, 118–19. *See also* grapefruit

Citrus sinensis, 64. *See also* sweet orange

clary sage, *61*, 107–8, *107*, 164, 214, 239, 240, 242, 246, 251, 255, 282, 291, 322, 424, 428, 446, 447

clay, 66

    bentonite green clay, 233

    French Clay Body Mask Formula, 308, 308–10, *309–10*

    French Clay Facial Mask, 273

    French green clay, 273, 308

    French pink clay, 273, 308

    green clay, 233, 273, 291, 308

    pink clay, 273, 291, 308

cleaning products

    Air Freshener Formula, 334

    All-Purpose Household Surface Cleaner Formula, 338

    Deodorizer Formula, 333

    Dish Wash Formula, 341

    Dryer Formula, 337

    eco-friendly Cleaning Supplies, 338

    to eliminate odors, 333, 334

    Washer Formula, 337

Cleansing and Detoxification Formula, 219

clove, 54, 109, *109*, 235, 352, 357, 360

clove bud, *61*, 205, 207, 208, 233, 446, 447

cocoa butter, 45, 274, 311

coconut oil, 36, 36–38, *36*, *37*, 67, 233, 273, 274, 294, 311

Cocos nucifera, 36. *See also* coconut oil

cold air diffiusion, 31, *31*

cold press expression, 23

cold press extraction, 23

cold pressing, 19

Cold Sore Formula, 289

colognes. *See* Love and Romance Blends

Commiphora myrrha, 63, 126–27. *See also* myrrh

Complete Skincare Beauty Treatment Program, 263

compresses, 41–42, *41*

congestion, 446

Constipation Relief Formula, 190

cooking, 48–49, *48*, *49*, 351–97

coriander, 22, 352, 357, 363

cosmetics, 19

cotton balls, 65

cough, 446

cramps, 446

cream, 66

creams, 67

creativity, stimulating, 347

Crispy Brown Sugar Chocolate Mint Chip Cookies, 394, *395*

culinary wellness oils and blends, 351–63

    All-Purpose Herbal Blend, 363

    Citrus and Spice Blend, 360

    Greek Spice Blend, 359

    Indian Spice Blend, 357

    Italian Blend, 353

    Mexican Spice Blend, 358

    Thai Pepper Lemongrass Blend, 354

cumin, 352, 354, 357, 358, 363

Cupressus sempervirens, *61*, 110–11. *See also* cypress

curiosity, stimulating, 347

Cymbopogon citratus, *62*, 122–23. *See also* lemongrass

Cymbopogon flexuosus, 122–23. *See also* lemongrass

Cymbopogon martinii, *63*, 131–32. *See also* palmarosa

cypress, *61*, 110–11, *110–11*, 164, 167, 177, 180, 183, 184, 185, 186, 188, 190, 200, 209, 213, 219, 235, 239, 242, 266, 270, 285, 306, 330, 333, 334, 338, 341, 435, 440, 446, 447

D

daily life

    Focus Support and Pay Attention Formula, 348

    Improve Productivity Formula, 344

    Stimulate Curiosity and Creativity Formula, 347

Daucus carota, *61*, 104. *See also* carrot seed

delivery (childbirth), 321–22

delivery pathways, *30*

dentistry, preventative, 232

Deodorizer Formula, 333

depression, 259–60, 446

    depression relief, 259–60

    Depression Relief Formula, 259

    Depression Relief Formula 2, 260

desserts

    The Best Lemon Bars, 393

    Crispy Brown Sugar Chocolate Mint Chip Cookies, 394

    Quick-to-Make Gooey Fudgy Lavender Brownies, 397

detoxification, 446

Devic kingdom, 16

diet-induced weight gain, 220

diffuser, 23

digestive, 446

dilusion guide, 34

dilution, 23, *34*, 65

    dilution guide, 34, 34–35, 443–44

    safe skin application, 35, *35*

dinner recipes, 375–77

    Angel Hair Pasta with Spicy Shripm, 375

    Roasted Vegetable and Refried Bean Tostadas, 377

direct inhalation method, 29, *29*, 31

Dish Wash Formula, 341

distillation, 22, 23

drinks. *See* beverages

Dry, Chapped Lips Formula, 286

Dry and Mature Skin Formula, 307

Dryer Formula, 337

E

earth element meridians, 419–20

eating intuitively, 220

eco-friendly Cleaning Supplies, 338

    All-Purpose Household Surface Cleaner Formula, 338

    Dish Wash Formula, 341

eggs, 66

eighth chakra, 414

Eighth Chakra Oil Formula, 414, *414*

electro-chemical effects, *32*

endocrine system, 27

Energy Clearing Formula, 330

enthusiasm, 249–50

environmental fragrance, 31

Epsom salts, 66, 203, 208, 247, 291

Eros Aphrodisiac Formula, 316

essences, 19

essential oils, 23, 293. *See also specific oils*

    culinary, 352

    in daily life, 343–49

    how to use, 29–49

    inhalation of, 26–27, *26*, *27*

    most commonly used, 69–97

    pure, 69–97

    in the workplace, 343–49

Essential Oils to Balance Earth Element, 420

Essential Oils to Balance Fire Element, 418

Essential Oils to Balance Metal Element, 422

Essential Oils to Balance Water Element, 424

Essential Oils to Balance Wood Element, 426

eucalyptus, *58*, 71–73, *71*, *73*, 163, 174, 176, 337, 446, 447

   Eucalyptus globulus, 71–73, 163, 235

   Eucalyptus radiata, 402

   Eucalyptus radiata, 71–73, 231, 235, 400

Eugenia caryophyllata, 54, *61*, 109. *See also* clove bud

Exfoliating Sugar Scrub Oils Formula, 293

exfoliating sugar scrubs, 292, 293

   Exfoliating Sugar Scrub Oils Formula, 293

   pH Balancing Honey Lemon Sugar Facial Scrub Formula, 294

expression, 19, 23

extraction, 19, 23, 57

eyes, accidental application in, 55

F

face butters, 274

face carrier oils, 36–38

   coconut oil, 36, 36–38, *36*, *37*

   jojoba oil, 38, *38*

   rosehip seed oil, 38–39, *39*

Facial and Body Toner Formula (Normal to Dry Skin), 270

facial masks, 42, *43*, 66

facial scrubs, 44, 66

facial skincare, 36, *36*

facial skin toners, 48. *See also* skin toners

facial steams, 33–34, *34*, 67, *67*

FDA, 48

fear, 446

Female Toner, 239

fennel, 225

Ferula galbaniflua, *61*, 112–13. *See also* galbanum

Fibroids Formula, 245, 247

Fibromyalgia Pain Relief Formula, 185

fifth chakra, 411

Fifth Chakra Oil Formula, 411, *411*

Findhorn, 16

fire element meridian, 417–18, *418*

First Chakra Oil Formula, 407

five elements, 416–17, 416–27, *416*

   Essential Oils to Balance Earth Element, 420

   Essential Oils to Balance Fire Element, 418

   Essential Oils to Balance Metal Element, 422

   Essential Oils to Balance Water Element, 424

   Essential Oils to Balance Wood Element, 426

fixative, 24

flavoring, 19, 48–49, *48*, *49*

Flea and Tick Prevention and Treatment, 400

focusing, 348

Focus Support and Pay Attention Formula, 348

food, 19, 24, 48–49, *48*, *49*, 351–97

Foot Bath for Athlete's Foot or Toenail Fungus, 203

footbaths, 67, 203, 208

fourth chakra, 410

Fourth Chakra Oil Formula, 410

fractionated coconut oil, 36–38

fragrance, 22, 24. *See also* Love and Romance Blends; perfumes

frankincense, *58*, 74–75, *75*, 170, 177, 231, 235, 239, 252, 261, 268, 270, 291, 315, 322, 330, 347, 400, 402, 410, 411, 429, 432, 434, 440, 441, 446, 447

French Clay Body Mask Formula, 308, 308–10, *309–10*

French Clay Facial Mask, 273

French green clay, 273, 308

French Lentil Soup, *370*, 371

French pink clay, 273, 308

fungal infection, 446

G

Gabriel, 437–38

Gabriel Angel Therapy Oil, 438

galbanum, *61*, 112–13, *112–13*, 170, 209, 267, 407, 415, 420, 433, 447

Gattefossé, René-Maurcie, 20

Gaultheria procumbens, 54. *See also* wintergreen

GC/MS (Gas Chromatograph/Mass Spectrometer), 24

generally regarded as safe (GRAS), 48, 55

generic names, 57

geranium, 76–77, *77*, 239, 259, 266, 311, 424, 428, 446, 447

   Pelargonium graveolens, *58*, 76–77, 193, 197, 199, 204, 235, 240, 242, 250, 251, 255, 260, 261, 264, 268, 270, 273, 276, 280, 297, 302, 306, 307, 322, 400, 408, 410, 430

Pelargonium roseum, 58, 76–77, 193, 197, 199, 204, 235, 240, 242, 246, 250, 251, 255, 260, 261, 264, 268, 270, 273, 276, 280, 297, 302, 306, 307, 322, 400, 408, 410, 430

Geranium Bourbon, 298

German chamomile, 114–15, *114–15*, 179, 183, 184, 187, 193, 194, 197, 199, 200, 204, 211, 214, 217, 256, 267, 270, 301, 322, 323, 326, 400, 438

ginger, 22, 54, *62*, 116–17, *116–17*, 171, 186, 187, 191, 246, 315, 319, 352, 427, 432, 441, 446, 447

    Citrus and Spice Blend, 360

    Indian Spice Blend, 357

    Thai Pepper Lemongrass Blend, 354

glycerin, 270

grapefruit, *62*, 118–19, *118–19*, 222, 250, 347, 446, 447

Greek Spice Blend, 359, 372

green tea, 341

grief, 261

Grief and Loss Formula, 261

H

Hair and Scalp Treatment Program, 281

hair and scalp treatments, 279–85

    Hair and Scalp Treatment Program, 281

    Scalp Massage Oil, 285

    Scalp Reconditioning Formula, 280

    Stop Hair Loss (Alopecia) Formula, 282

hair loss, stopping, 281–82

Headache Relief Blend, 163

Headache Relief Formula, 174

Headache Relief Formula 2, 176

Healing and Regenerative Body Butter Formula, 311–13

Healing Bath Salts Formula, 291, 291–92

healing blends, 173–217

    Allergic Skin Reaction Relief Formula, 199, 202

    Arthritis Pain Relief Formula, 186

    Athlete's Foot Formula, 203, 205

    Burn Care Formula, 193

    Constipation Relief Formula, 190

    Fibromyalgia Pain Relief Formula, 185

    Foot Bath for Athlete's Foot or Toenail Fungus, 203

    Headache Relief Formula, 174

    Headache Relief Formula 2, 176

    Healing Bath Salts Formula, 291

    Herpes Formula, 209–10

    Leg Cramp Relief Formula, 188

    Migraine Relief Formula, 177

    Mosquito and Insect Protective Repellent Formula, 198

    Muscle Pain Relief Formula, 180

    Nausea Relief Formula, 191

    Nerve Pain Relief Formula, 184

    Pain Relief Formula, 179

    Poison Ivy and Oak Irritation Relief Formula, 200

    Ringing Ear Relief Formula, 213

    Ringworm Formula, 211–12

Scar Formula, 203

Sciatica Pain Relief Formula, 183

Sleep Formulas, 214, 217

Sunburn Relief Formula, 194

Tendinitis Relief Formula, 187

Toenail Fungus Formula, 207

UV Radiation Burn Relief Formula, 197

Warm Bath Treatment, 202

Warts Formula (non-genital), 208

healing salves, 67

healthy lifestyle, 219–47

    Breast Health Massage Formula, 246

    Cleansing and Detoxificaction Formula, 219

    eating intuitively, 220

    Female Toner, 239

    Fibroids Formula, 245

    Hormone Balance Formula, 240

    Hot Flash Relief Formula, 242

    Natural Re-Mineralizing Toothpaste Formula, 233

    Oral Health Program, 232

    Recovery after Illness Formula, 235

    Rejuvenating and Healing Forumla, 235

    Sitz Bath, 247

    Steam Inhalation to Support Respiratory System Formula, 231

    Stop Smoking Formula and Treatment, 228

    Stop Smoking Program, 226–27

Weight Loss Formula 2, 225

Weight Loss Formula and Treatment, 222

weight loss program, 220

women's health formulas, 239, 240, 242, 245, 246, 247

helichrysum Italian everlasting, *58*, 78–79, *79*, 167, 179, 180, 187, 188, 193, 194, 197, 199, 200, 204, 209, 211, 213, 245, 261, 267, 268, 277, 285, 288, 297, 301, 302, 306, 307, 311, 407, 420, 424, 426, 427, 431, 432, 435, 438, 440, 441, 447

Helichrysum italicum, *58*, 78–79. *See also* helichrysum Italian everlasting

herbal infused oils, 24, *24*

herbalism, 24

herbal medicine, 24

Herpes Formula, 209–10

hippocampus, 27

holy basil, 352

    Indian Spice Blend, 357

    Thai Pepper Lemongrass Blend, 354

honey, 66, 294

hormonal system, 27

hormone balance, 446

Hormone Balance Formula, 240

Hot Flash Relief Formula, 242

hot oils, 54–55

household cleaning products, 19

household products, 329–41

    Air Freshener Formula, 334

    All-Purpose Household Surface Cleaner Formula, 338

    Deodorizer Formula, 333

Dish Wash Formula, 341

Dryer Formula, 337

eco-friendly Cleaning Supplies, 338

to eliminate odors, 333, 334

Energy Clearing Formula, 330

Washer Formula, 337

humidifier, 67

hydrosol, 24

hypothalamus gland, 27

hyssop, *62*, 120, *120*, 231, 446, 447

Hyssopus officinalis, *62*, 120. *See also* hyssop

I

Immune Stimulant Blend, 163

Improve Productivity Formula, 344

incense, 19

Indian Spice Blend, 357

    Angel Hair Pasta with Spicy Shrimp, 375

Indian tantric practices, 22

Indus Valley, 22

infection, 446

inflammation, 447

infused oil, 24, *24*, *25*

injury, 447

insect repellant, 447

insoluble, 24

integrative health care, 20

internal use, 55

Italian Blend, 353

    Avocado Crostini, 374

    Italian Dressing, 378

Italian Dressing, 378

J

jars, 67

jojoba oil, organic, 38, *38*

juniper berry, 151, 174, 213, 219, 245, 285, 330, 338, 446, 447

Juniperus communis, 151. *See also* juniper berry

Jupiter Planetary Elixir, 432

K

khella plant seeds, 97–98

L

labor, 321–22

laundry care, 337

Lavandula angustifolia, *58*, 80–81, 163. *See also* lavender

lavender, *58*, 80–81, *81*, 163, 164, 168, 174, 176, 177, 180, 184, 188, 193, 194, 197, 204, 207, 209, 211, 214, 235, 239, 245, 264, 270, 286, 291, 298, 305, 308, 311, 322, 337, 341, 352, 397, 400, 411, 424, 447

ledum, *62*, 121, *121*, 235, 446, 447

Ledum groenlandicum, *62*, 121. *See also* ledum

Leg Cramp Relief Formula, 188

lemon, *58*, 82–84, *82*, *84*, 174, 191, 205, 207, 208, 209, 213, 219, 222, 225, 231, 233, 235, 242, 245, 246, 250, 259, 285, 294, 306, 330, 333, 334, 337, 338, 341, 344, 348, 352, 409, 412, 418, 427, 431, 435, 439, 441, 446, 447. *See also Citrus limonum*

    The Best Lemon Bars, 393

    Citrus and Spice Blend, 360

Thai Pepper Lemongrass Blend, 354

lemongrass, *62*, 122–23, *122–23*, 170, 180, 198, 242, 334, 347, 352, 400, 409, 418, 429, 441, 446, 447. *See also Cymbopogon citratus*

Flea and Tick Prevention and Treatment, 400

Lemongrass Black Tea, 382

Thai Pepper Lemongrass Blend, 354

Lemongrass Black Tea, 382, *383*

lemons, 294

lemon tea tree, 198

Leptospermum scoparium, 151, 163. *See also* manuka

Lift the Mood Formula, 251

Lift the Spirits Formula, 250

limbic system, 27

lime, 352

Citrus and Spice Blend, 360

Mexican Spice Blend, 358

Thai Pepper Lemongrass Blend, 354

liniment, 24

lip balms, 67, 286

Cold Sore Formula, 289

Dry, Chapped Lips Formula, 286

Severely Dry, Cracked, Chapped Lips, 288

location, 57

loss, 261

Love and Romance Blends, 315–19

Aphrodite Perfume Oil Formula, 315

Audacity Men's Cologne Formula, 319

Eros Aphrodisiac Formula, 316

lunch recipes, 368–71

French Lentil Soup, 371

Thai Pepper Soup, 368

M

manuka, 151, 163

marjoram, 88, *88*, 163, 167, 168, 171, 174, 176, 179, 180, 183, 184, 185, 186, 187, 188, 190, 352, 400, 435, 440, 447

All-Purpose Herbal Blend, 363

Greek Spice Blend, 359

Italian Blend, 353

Mars Planetary Elixir, 431

masks, 42, 66

body masks, 66, 308–10

facial masks, 42, *43*, 66

French Clay Body Mask Formula, 308, 308–10, *309–10*

French Clay Facial Mask, 273

massage, 23, 27

baby massage, 323–26, *325*

Calming Formula, 168

massage oil blends, 164, 167, 168, 170, 171, 285

Muscle Pain Relief Formula, 171

Relaxation Formula, 164

Restorative Formula, 170

Scalp Massage Oil, 285

Sports Injury Formula, 167

Matricaria chamomila, *62*, 114–15. *See also* chamomile

Matricaria recutita, 114–15

Mature Skincare Formula, 268

Maury, Madame, 23

medical terms, 444

medicinals, 19–21, 22

meditation, 252

Meditation Formula, 252

Melaleuca alternifolia, 54, *59*, 89. *See also* tea tree

melissa, *63*, 124–25, *124–25*, 414, 446

Melissa officinalis, *63*, 124–25. *See also* melissa

Mentha x piperita, 54, *59*, 85–86, 163. *See also* peppermint

Mercury Planetary Elixir, 429

metal element meridians, 421–22

metaphysical healing, 16

Mexican Spice Blend, 358

Roasted Vegetable and Refried Bean Tostadas, 377

Michael, 439

Michael Angel Therapy Oil, 439

micro diffusion, *33*

Migraine Relief Formula, 177

Mimosas, *384*, 385

Moisture Balancing and Healing for All Skin Types Formula, 305

mood, 251

Moon Planetary Elixir, 428

Moroccan blue chamomile, *60*, 103, *103*

Mosquito and Insect Protective Repellent Formula, 198

motherhood, 321–27

sleep remedies, 322–23

Muscle Pain Relief Formula, 171, 180

myrrh, 22, *63*, 126–27, *126–27*, 170, 204, 207, 208, 209, 219, 235, 252, 266, 270, 277, 288, 315, 330, 407, 409, 415, 418, 420, 426, 429, 431, 433, 434, 435, 439, 440, 447

N

names, 57

Nardostachys jatamansi, 151. *See also* spikenard

Natural Re-Mineralizing Toothpaste Formula, 233

Nausea Relief Formula, 191

neat, 24

Neolithic era, 22

Neptune Planetary Elixr, 435

neroli, *63*, 128–29, *128–29*, 316, 322, 400, 412, 413, 414, 430, 438, 446

Nerve Pain Relief Formula, 184

nerves, 27

niaouli, 400

ninth chakra, 415

Ninth Chakra Oil Formula, 415, *415*

Normal to Dry Skincare Formula, 264

notes, 24

nutmeg, 352

    Citrus and Spice Blend, 360

    Greek Spice Blend, 359

O

oats, 202

Ocimum basilicum, 54, 151. *See also* basil

odors, eliminating, 333, 334

oil pulling, 234, *234*

Oily Skincare Formula, 266

Oily Skin Formula, 306

ointments, 67

old brain, 27

olfactory, 24

olfactory nerves, 27

Oral Health Program, 232

    Natural Re-Mineralizing Toothpaste Formula, 233

oregano, 54, *63*, 130, *130*, 209, 233, 235, 337, 352, 446

    Greek Spice Blend, 359

orifice reducer, 24

Origanum marjorana, *59*, 88, 163. *See also* marjoram

Origanum vulgare, 54, *63*, 130, *130*. *See also* oregano

P

pain relief, 447

Pain Relief Formula, 179

palmarosa, *63*, 131–32, *131–32*, 198, 199, 200, 204, 209, 211, 239, 240, 242, 245, 264, 267, 270, 282, 289, 301, 302, 306, 307, 347, 400, 418, 431, 440, 446, 447

parasites, 447

patchouli, *63*, 133, *133*, 198, 222, 270, 288, 315, 319, 400, 407, 408, 415, 420, 430, 431, 447

patch test, 25

Pelargonium graveolens, *58*, 76–77. *See also* geranium

Pelargonium roseum, *58*, 76–77. *See also* geranium

peppermint, 54, *59*, 85–86, *85*, 163, 167, 171, 174, 176, 177, 179, 180, 185, 186, 188, 190, 191, 198, 225, 233, 242, 246, 250, 330, 333, 334, 337, 338, 344, 348, 352, 412, 441, 446, 447

    Chocolate Mint Martini, 390

    Crispy Brown Sugar Chocolate Mint Chip Cookies, 394

    Thai Pepper Lemongrass Blend, 354

perfumes/perfume oil, 19, 47–48, *47*, *48*. *See also* Love and Romance Blends

Pert, Candace, 405

pets, 399–403

    essential oils to use for, 400

    Flea and Tick Prevention and Treatment, 400

    Respiratory Support, 402

pharmaceuticals, 19

pH Balancing Honey Lemon Sugar Facial Scrub Formula, 294, *295*

photosensitizing, 53

phytochemicals, 25

phytomedicinals, 25

Picea mariana, 60, 102. *See also* black spruce

pink clay, 291

pink grapefruit, 225

Pinus sylvestris, 54. *See also* Scotch pine

Piper nigrum, 54, *60*, 101. *See also* black pepper

Pita and Hummus Dip, 372, *373*

pituitary gland, 27

planetary elixirs, 427–36

Jupiter Planetary Elixir, 432

Mars Planetary Elixir, 431

Mercury Planetary Elixir, 429

Moon Planetary Elixir, 428

Neptune Planetary Elixir, 435

Pluto Planetary Elixir, 435

Saturn Planetary Elixir, 433

Sun Planetary Elixir, 427

Uranus Planetary Elixir, 434

Venus Planetary Elixir, 430

plants, parts of, 57

Pluto Planetary Elixir, 435

Pogostemon cablin, *63*, 133. *See also* patchouli

Poison Ivy and Oak Irritation Relief Formula, 200

poultices, 25, 42, *42*

pregnancy, 53, 321–22

Premature Aging Skincare Formula, 276

primary actions and effects, 444

productivity, improving, 344

Prunus amygdalus var. dulcis, 39. *See also* sweet almond oil

psycho-emotional aromatherapy chart, *445*

purified water, 66

Q

Quick and Easy Cinnamon French Toast, 367

Quick-to-Make Gooey Fudgy Lavender Brownies, *396*, 397

R

Raphael, 440

Raphael Angel Therapy Oil, 440

ravensara, 289, 446

Recovery after Illness Formula, 235

red mandarin, *64*, 134, *134*, 168, 214, 217, 256, 261, 291, 322, 408, 428, 446, 447

reference guides, 443

    dilution guide, 443–44

    medical terms, 444

    primary actions and effects, 444

    psycho-emotional aromatherapy chart, *445*

    safety guide, 443–44

Regulating All Skin Types Formula, 298

Regulating and Balancing, Wound Healing, Problem Skin Formula, 302

regulators, 446

Rejuvenating and Healing Forumla, 235

relaxation and emotional support formulas, 249–62

    Anxiety Relief Formula, 256

    Depression Relief Formula, 259

    Depression Relief Formula 2, 260

    Grief and Loss Formula, 261

    Lift the Mood Formula, 251

    Lift the Spirits Formula, 250

    Meditation Formula, 252

    Stress Relief Formula, 255

Relaxation Formula, 164

Repair Butter Essential Oil Formula, 274

repair butters for body and face, 274

reptilian brain, 27

resin tapping, 19

resources, 448

respiratory, 447

respiratory steam, 34

respiratory steams, 67

Respiratory Support, 402

Restorative Formula, 170

Rig Veda, 22

Ringing Ear Relief Formula, 213

Ringworm Formula, 211–12

Roasted Vegetable and Refried Bean Tostadas, *376*, 377

robes, 65

Roman chamomile, *59*, 87, *87*, 168, 256, 322, 411, 428

room deodorizer, 48

Rosa damascena, *64*

Rosa damascena, *64*, 139–41. *See also* rose otto

Rosa rubignosa, 38–39. *See also* rosehip seed oil

rose, 194, 204, 209, 239, 261, 267, 268, 270, 276, 311, 315, 316, 408, 410, 413, 414, 430, 438, 446, 447

    Venus Martini, 386

rosehip seed oil, 38–39, *39*

rosemary, *64*, 135–38, *135–36*, 219, 235, 280, 348, 353, 359, 363, 418, 426, 427, 440, 446, 447 rosemary verbenone, 228, 266, 282, 307, 308, 344, 352

rose otto, *64*, 139–41, *139–40*

rose petals, *19*

Rosmarinus officinalis ct verbenone and cineole, *64*, 135–38. *See also* rosemary

S

safe use, 51–55

    reducing risk of sensitization, 52–53

    safe skin application, 35, *35*

    safety guide, 443–44

sage, 352

    All-Purpose Herbal Blend, 363

salad dressings, 378

    Italian Dressing, 378

    Sweet and Sour Dressing, 381

salt glow treatments, 297, 307

    Regulating All Skin Types Formula, 298

    Skin Healing and Regeneration Formula, 297

salts, 44, *44*, 208

    bath salts, 66, 291–92

    Celtic salt, 44, *44*, 66, *66*, 233, 291

    detoxifying and purifying, *66*

    Epsom salts, 66, 203, 208, 247, 291

    Healing Bath Salts Formula, 291, 291–92

    sea salt, 44, *44*, 66, 203, 208, 247, 307

    smelling salts, 66

salves, 67

Salvia sclarea, 61, 107. *See also* clary sage

sandalwood, 22, *64*, 142–44, *142–44*, 286, 311, 315, 316, 319, 322, 409, 413, 414, 426, 430, 431, 432, 433, 435, 446, 447

San Diego, California, 16

Santalum album, *64*, 142–44. *See also* sandalwood

Saturn Planetary Elixir, 433

Scalp Massage Oil, 285

Scalp Reconditioning Formula, 280

scalp treatments. *See* hair and scalp treatments

Scar Formula, 203

scents, 19

Sciatica Pain Relief Formula, 183

Scotch pine, 54

scrubs, 44, 66

    body scrubs, 44–45

    Celtic sea salt, 44–45, *44*, *45*

    facial scrubs, 44

    salt, 44–45, *44*, *45*

    sea salt, 44–45, *44*, *45*

sea salt, 44, *44*, 66, 203, 208, 247, 307

sebum, 25

second chakra, 408, *408*

Second Chakra Oil Formula, 408

sedative, 447

self-selection, 53, 399

Sensitive Skincare Formula, 267

sensitization, reducing risk of, 52–53

sesame oil, 39, *39*

Sesamum indicum, 39. *See also* sesame oil

seventh chakra, 413

Seventh Chakra Oil Formula, 413

Severely Dry, Cracked, Chapped Lips, 288

Severely Dry and Cracked Skin Formula, 277

shea butter, 45, 67, 274, 311

shelf life, 154–55

Siberian balsam, 54

silver fir, 54

Simmondsia californica, 38. *See also* jojoba oil, organic

single note, 25

Sitz Bath, 247

sixth chakra, 412

Sixth Chakra Oil Formula, 412, *412*

skin brush, 65

skin brushing, *46*

skincare, 447

skincare formulas, 264–77

    Chronic Skin Conditions Formula, 301

    Dry and Mature Skin Formula, 307

    Facial and Body Toner Formula (Normal to Dry Skin), 270

    Healing and Regenerative Body Butter Formula, 311–13

    Mature Skincare Formula, 268

    Moisture Balancing and Healing for All Skin Types Formula, 305

    Normal to Dry Skincare Formula, 264

Oily Skincare Formula, 266

Oily Skin Formula, 306

Premature Aging Skincare
Formula, 276

Regulating and Balancing,
Wound Healing, Problem Skin
Formula, 302

Repair Butter Essential Oil
Formula, 274

repair butters for body and
face, 274

Sensitive Skincare Formula, 267

Severely Dry and Cracked Skin
Formula, 277

Skin Healing and Regeneration
Formula, 297

skin irritation, 52–54, 55, *55*

skin test, 54

skin toners, 269

Facial and Body Toner Formula
(Normal to Dry Skin), 270

skin types, 264

sleep remedies, 214, 217, 322–23,
323

smelling salts, 66

soaps, 19

soluble, 25

solvent extraction, 19

Sore Muscle Blend, 163

spa and beauty treatments,
263–313

bath salts, 291–92

Chronic Skin Conditions
Formula, 301

Cold Sore Formula, 289

Complete Skincare Beauty
Treatment Program, 263

Dry, Chapped Lips Formula,
279–85

Dry and Mature Skin Formula,
307

Exfoliating Sugar Scrub Oils
Formula, 293

exfoliating sugar scrubs, 292–94

Facial and Body Toner Formula
(Normal to Dry Skin), 270

hair and scalp treatments,
279–85

Healing and Regenerative Body
Butter Formula, 311–13

Healing Bath Salts Formula,
291–92

lip balms, 286–89

Mature Skincare Formula, 268

Moisture Balancing and Healing
for All Skin Types Formula,
305

Normal to Dry Skincare
Formula, 264

Oily Skincare Formula, 266

Oily Skin Formula, 306

pH Balancing Honey Lemon
Sugar Facial Scrub Formula,
294

Premature Aging Skincare
Formula, 276

Regulating All Skin Types
Formula, 298

Regulating and Balancing,
Wound Healing, Problem Skin
Formula, 302

Repair Butter Essential Oil
Formula, 274

repair butters for body and
face, 274

salt glow treatments, 297

Scalp Massage Oil, 285

Scalp Reconditioning Formula,
280

Sensitive Skincare Formula, 267

Severely Dry, Cracked, Chapped
Lips, 288

Severely Dry and Cracked Skin
Formula, 277

skincare formulas, 264, 264–77,
266, 267, 268, 270, 273, 274,
276, 277, 301, 302, 305, 306,
307, 308–10, 311–13

skin toners, 270

spasms, 446

species, 57

spikenard, 22, 151, 211, 214, 217, 252,
255, 256, 277, 301, 305, 322, 347,
412, 413, 426, 428, 435, 446, 447

Spiritual Blends, 405–41

Eighth Chakra Oil Formula, 414

Fifth Chakra Oil Formula, 411

First Chakra Oil Formula, 407

Fourth Chakra Oil Formula, 410

Ninth Chakra Oil Formula, 415

Second Chakra Oil Formula, 408

Seventh Chakra Oil Formula, 413

Sixth Chakra Oil Formula, 412

Third Chakra Oil Formula, 409

Sports Injury Formula, 167

stagnant energy, clearing, 329–41

steam distillation, 19

Steam Inhalation to Support
Respiratory System Formula, 231

stevia leaf, 233

stimulant, 447

Stimulate Curiosity and Creativity Formula, 347

Stop Hair Loss (Alopecia) Formula, 282

Stop Smoking Formula and Treatment, 228

Stop Smoking Program, 226–27, 228

storage, 153–55

stress relief, 255

Stress Relief Formula, 255

sugar, *45*, 66, 293, 294

Sunburn Relief Formula, 194

Sun Planetary Elixir, 427

Sunshine Martini, *388*, 389

supplemental oils, 60–65, 97–151

supplies, 57–67

    additional, 65–66–67

    optional, 67

    supplemental oils, 60–65

    what to have on hand, 57

sweet almond oil, 39, *39*

Sweet and Sour Dressing, 381

sweet basil, 352, 353, 359, 363

sweet marjoram, *59*, 88, *88*, 167, 168, 171, 176, 179, 180, 183, 184, 185, 186, 187, 188, 190, 352, 353, 359, 363, 400, 435, 440, 447

sweet orange, *64*, 190, 222, 225, 259, 260, 315, 352, 360, 385, 389, 408, 427, 432, 446

symptoms guide, 446–47

synergistic (term), 25

synergy blends, 65, 274

synthetic (term), 25

synthetic fragrance oils, 22

T

Tanacetum annuum, *60*, 103. *See also* Moroccan blue chamomile

tangerine, 259

tea, Lemongrass Black Tea, 382

tea tree, 54, *59*, 89–90, *89*, *90*, 198, 205, 208, 235, 289, 446

teething solutions, 326–27

Tendinitis Relief Formula, 187

Thai Pepper Lemongrass Blend, 354, 368, 381

Thai Pepper Soup, 368, *368*

therapeutic uses, 29

    cold air diffusion, 31, *31*

    direct inhalation method, 29, *29*, 31

    environmental fragrance, 31

    facial steam, 33–34, *34*

    micro diffusion, *33*

    respiratory steam, 34

    ultrasonic micro diffusion, 33, *33*

third chakra, 409, *409*

Third Chakra Oil Formula, 409

thyme, 54, *64*, 146–47, *146–47*, 205, 207, 208, 209, 233, 235, 282, 352, 400, 435, 439, 446

    All-Purpose Herbal Blend, 363

    Greek Spice Blend, 359

    Italian Blend, 353

    Mexican Spice Blend, 358

Thymus vulgaris, 54, *64*, 146–47. *See also* thyme

Tisserand, Robert, 20, 23

Toenail Fungus Formula, 203, 207

toothpaste, 233

towels, 65

Traditional Chinese Medicine, 416

transformational healing arts, 16

Tritcum vugare, 40. *See also* wheat germ oil

turmeric, 352

    All-Purpose Herbal Blend, 363

    Indian Spice Blend, 357

    Mexican Spice Blend, 358

U

ultrasonic micro diffusion, 33, *33*

Uranus Planetary Elixir, 434

Uriel, 441

Uriel Angel Therapy Oil, 441

urinary tract infection, 447

UV Radiation Burn Relief Formula, 197

V

Valnet, Jean, 22, 23

vascular system, 27

vegetable carrier oil, *55*, 65

vegetable glycerin, 67, 311

vegetable oil, 273

Venus Martini, 386, *387*

Venus Planetary Elixir, 430

vetiver, *59*, 91–92, *91*, 164, 217, 255, 256, 280, 322, 407, 415, 420, 433, 446, 447

Vetiveria zizaniodes, *59*, 91–92. *See also* vetiver

viscosity, 25

vitamin E oil, 40, *40*, 274, 311

volatile, 25

volatilization, 25

W

Warm Bath Treatment, 202

Warts (non-genital) Formula, 208

washcloth, 65

Washer Formula, 337

water

    fresh spring, 270

    purified, 66, 233, 270, 273, 308

    spring, 273

water element meridians, 423–24

weight control, 447

    Weight Loss Formula 2, 225

    Weight Loss Formula and Treatment, 222

    weight loss program, 220-21

wheat germ oil, 40

wintergreen, 54

witch hazel, 66

women's health

    breast health, 243

    breast massage, 243

women's health formulas, 239

    Breast Health Massage Formula, 246

    Female Toner, 239

    Fibroids Formula, 245, 247

    Hormone Balance Formula, 240

    Hot Flash Relief Formula, 242

    Sitz Bath, 247

wood element meridians, 425–26

workplace environment

    Focus Support and Pay Attention Formula, 348

    Improve Productivity Formula, 344

    Stimulate Curiosity and Creativity Formula, 347

worry, 446

wound healing, 447

wraps, 42

    body wraps, 43, *43*

Y

yarrow, *65*, 148–50, 199, 200, 282, 302, 411, 447

ylang ylang, 54, *59*, 93–95, *93*, *94*, *95*, 168, 179, 180, 183, 184, 185, 186, 199, 204, 214, 217, 251, 252, 256, 259, 260, 261, 264, 268, 270, 273, 276, 280, 282, 286, 291, 298, 305, 308, 311, 315, 316, 319, 407, 408, 410, 413, 414, 415, 420, 424, 428, 429, 430, 433, 434, 438, 446, 447

Z

Zingiber officinale, 54, *62*, 116–17. *See also* ginger

Zucchini Citrus and Spice Muffins, 364